The Languages of the Brain

The Languages of the Brain

Edited by
Albert M. Galaburda
Stephen M. Kosslyn
Yves Christen

Harvard University Press
Cambridge, Massachusetts
London, England / 2002

Printed in the United States of America

Library of Congress Cataloging-in-Publication Data

The languages of the brain / edited by Albert M. Galaburda, Stephen M. Kosslyn, Yves Christen.
p. ; cm.
Includes bibliographical references and index.
ISBN 0-674-00772-7 (alk. paper)
1. Language acquisition. 2. Cognition. 3. Neurolinguistics. 4. Nonverbal communication. I. Galaburda, Albert M., 1948– II. Kosslyn, Stephen Michael, 1948– III. Christen, Yves.
[DNLM: 1. Cognition—physiology—Congresses. 2. Language—Congresses. 3. Brain—physiology—Congresses. 4. Concept Formation—Congresses. 5. Nonverbal Communication—psychology—Congresses. BF 455 L2877 2002]
QP399 .L375 2002
153.6—dc21 2002069094

Contents

Preface

Every generation feels that it is living through the worst violence that has ever visited the planet. True or not, our time is no different from any other in that violence is at least partly the result of poor understanding and inadequate communication. How we think, learn, and communicate depends to a large extent on language, broadly conceived. Certainly, we communicate with certain signs and symbols that signal concepts. But behind these signs and symbols are other "languages," languages of thought. These languages constrain and convey the fabric of our minds, and we must understand the entire panoply of "languages" of the brain if we are to understand how humans think, learn, and communicate. The more we know about these forms of language, the closer we shall be to solving the myriad problems besieging human societies, including violence.

In this book, we have brought together an unusual combination of contributions. We hope that the connections among the various strands illustrated here—both those made explicit and those apparent only in the breach—will inspire others to continue to study the languages of the brain.

The essays in this volume began their lives at a conference, "The Languages of the Brain," sponsored by the Harvard University Interfaculty Initiative in Mind/Brain/Behavior and the IPSEN Foundation. We are grateful to the Mind/Brain/Behavior Initiative, especially Anne

Harrington and Jerome Kagan; to the IPSEN Foundation of France, especially Jacqueline Mervaillie, for the opportunity to join together several flavors of biological and social scientists to talk about the languages of the brain; and to the Dana Foundation, for its steadfast support of the Mind/Brain/Behavior Initiative. The congenial Parisian atmosphere and the individual energies bulldozed through the barriers of jetlag, leading to the remarkable interchange of ideas presented here. We also thank Elizabeth Knoll and the rest of the Harvard University Press staff, especially Elizabeth Gilbert and Kirsten Giebutowski, as well as Gjergj Lazri, Debbie Bell, Jennifer Shephard, and Bill Thompson for their help in turning good intentions into written contributions.

The Languages of the Brain

Introduction

Albert M. Galaburda, Stephen M. Kosslyn,
and Yves Christen

The only way we can convey our thoughts in detail to another person is through verbal language. Although paintings, theater, and other nonverbal means of expression convey information, they lack the precision of language and its range of content. Does this imply that our thoughts themselves ultimately rely on language? Can it be that the "language of thought" is not simply a metaphor, but is to be taken literally—that thoughts are actually verbal? Is there only a single way in which thoughts can occur? In this book, we argue to the contrary, that there are multiple possible "languages of thought" and that different languages play different roles in life of the mind.

As we use the term here, a "language" is conceived very broadly, as a system with three major components: representations of information, representations of relations, and a set of rules for how the relations can be used to combine and manipulate representations. Each of these categories can be broken down into more fine-grained ones, such as representations of objects, actions, and qualities, and relations that specify conjunction, inclusion, and possession. In this sense, language is not just about communication. It is used to represent the world and one's interpretation of it; it is used to organize information, to help store information in memory, and to reason about the world and one's place in it. This conception of language opens the door to the idea that there is more than one "language of thought," more than one way to think.

We can delineate two major classes of languages of thought: verbal and nonverbal. Each of these classes can in turn be further divided. For example, verbal language includes one's mother tongue, second languages (learned either as an adult or as a child), recovered language ("learned" after brain damage), degenerate forms in dementing illnesses, anomalous forms in learning disabilities, the special tongues of twins and other groups, and sign language. Verbal language (at least some features of it) is not modality specific; it can be represented auditorily (speech), visually (writing), and in the tactile modality (Braille). Similarly, we can further divide nonverbal language. It includes the language of emotions, expressed through facial expression, body language, and affective speech prosody; the visual languages, expressed through mental imagery and art; the motor languages, expressed by pantomime, sports, and dance; and the language of quantities and size expressed through numbers, which also has a verbal component, a separate symbolic representation, and a nonsymbolic representation (see Chapter 11).

The notion that humans rely on multiple languages of thought flies in the face of much of the common wisdom in various fields (for example, see Fodor, 1975). The idea that human thought relies on something akin to verbal language has been taken seriously at least since the battle between Bishop Berkeley and John Locke. Berkeley argued that mental images could not be vehicles of thought, primarily because they are ambiguous (for example, an image of an apple could represent an apple, fruit, motherhood, worm food, and so on) and because they cannot directly represent categories (an image is an image of a particular thing). As Berkeley pointed out, in spite of these limitations of images we clearly can think unambiguous thoughts—when thinking about a port, we are not confused about whether we are thinking about wine or a safe harbor. And we can think about categories, such as triangles in general without reference to any particular set of angles. Thus, he argued, images cannot be the basis of thinking—in present terms, they cannot be a language of thought.

However, words per se suffer some of the same problems as images, namely that they are ambiguous. If words were the language of thought, one could be confused about which "port" one had in mind when thinking the word. But this is not the case. Such considerations led Gottlob Frege to conceive the notion of a proposition, which is the sense underlying a statement. A given statement in a natural language (like English or French) may be ambiguous, but each of the possible interpretations corresponds to a single underlying proposition. On this view, what distinguishes the two interpretations of "The sailor liked the port" is the fact that there are two distinct propositions it could express (the sailor liked the safe harbor or the sailor liked the wine). Depending on which meaning one has in mind, different propositions are present. This idea led to the claim that thought relies on *propositional representations.* Such representations are language-like, but unambiguous; they capture the gist of a statement (for example, see Pylyshyn, 1973).

Even if we concede that propositional representations are—if only by virtue of their lack of ambiguity—central to thinking, this does not rule out crucial roles for other forms of representations. Images and words, for example, may be akin to scribblings on a notepad. Such representations may allow us not only to store information but also to operate on it in various ways. In fact, researchers have discovered working memory structures that are specialized for verbal versus spatial information (for example, Smith and Jonides, 1999). Many of the chapters in this volume explore specific situations in which words and images play key roles in our thought processes.

The first evidence that thought does in fact involve more than verbal language may have come from the study of brain-damaged patients. In 1861 Paul Broca presented the case of Leborgne and called the left third frontal convolution of the left frontal lobe "le siège de la parole" (the seat of the word); this area soon became identified with language production. Shortly thereafter, Carl Wernicke presented cases in which he showed a crucial role for the left posterior temporal lobe in comprehending language. As patients with brain lesions were studied with growing frequency, it became clear that thought does not depend on language. Some of the crucial observations focused on what was impaired and what was spared in aphasia (language disruptions following brain damage). The patients of interest had problems with language even though their input/output mechanisms were intact (they could hear well and could move their vocal apparatus well). Rather, they had difficulty with the central aspects of language processing—the very aspects that presumably are used in cognition. Nevertheless, careful observers noted that patients who could not comprehend or produce verbal language well were not particularly impaired in other ways. For example, they managed their daily affairs, they recognized familiar faces, some could remember songs, they gave evidence that they knew what was happening around them. If verbal language were all that we used in thinking, then these patients should have had more pervasive deficits. Such observations suggested that these patients still had the use of some "languages of thought." But what are these "languages"? And how do they interact with verbal language? These are the central topics of this book.

Human beings have sometimes been characterized as the animal that uses language. Recently, however, evidence has been produced that bees have a kind of language, and that chimpanzees can be taught to use rudimentary forms of language. Does this mean that the use of languages does not distinguish humans? Not exactly. First, it is not clear that these other "languages" really qualify as language, even in the broad way that we characterize the term. Do these other animals really use rules to combine representations? Second, even if other animals do have some capacity to use a kind of language, their languages do not have the richness or power of human languages. Even if they can combine representations in novel ways, it is not clear how many options are in their repertoire. For instance, chimpanzees can learn "words" for book, pencil, and touch, but there is no evidence that they can distinguish between the two commands "touch the book with the pencil" and "touch the book and the pencil," which a small child can do (Bowerman, 1973; Slobin, 1985). Similarly, although the brains of apes share many similarities to the human brain, there are differences that are visible with the naked eye. The human brain is larger and more finely folded than the chimpanzee brain. Neuroanatomy must speak to the functional differences between the species.

The present volume is intended to broaden our conception of the languages of thought and how they can be brought to bear in a wide range of activities. Three broad themes are evident. First, the languages of thought are really "languages of the brain." The brain is obviously the organ of thought, and it is its representational systems that we hope to understand. Second, languages are embedded in processing systems. We conceive of languages not simply in the abstract, but in terms of mechanisms that represent and process information; each language of the brain is only a part of a broader system. Third, history, context, and culture interact with the languages of the brain. Not only are the contents of our thoughts dictated in large part by our personal histories, but these contents direct our interactions with the world—and thereby lead us to produce certain kinds of cultural creations that in turn influence the contents of other people's thoughts. We consider each general theme in turn.

The Languages of Thought Are Really "Languages of the Brain"

A central assumption of many of the chapters below is that it is most profitable to consider the nature of thought not solely in the abstract, but rather as embodied processing. Much (although, as you will see here, not all) of the insights about the distinctions among different languages of thought have hinged on studying the brain. Thus in this volume we speak of "languages of the brain," not languages of thought.

The distinction between the different types of languages of the brain has been documented by many sources of data. First, there have been studies of countless patients with brain injury, which have demonstrated dissociations between verbal language, visual imagery, and motor control (for example, see Jeannerod, 1998; Farah, 1990).

Second, different forms of language have different developmental schedules, and break down separately in developmental disorders. For instance, developmental dyslexics have trouble with some aspects of verbal language, whereas patients with Williams syndrome are dreadful at visuo-spatial tasks while being relatively good at linguistic tasks and very good at face recognition tasks (Bellugi and Morris, 1995).

Third, diseases that cause degeneration of the brain, such as Alzheimer's disease and Parkinson's disease, also reveal dissociations between different representational systems—which is evidence for the distinctions among them. Alzheimer's disease is usually a mixed disorder affecting visuo-spatial abilities, some aspects of verbal language, and memory, but on occasion one sees relatively isolated loss in one cognitive function for some time before the others begin to fail (Petersen, 1998). Visuo-motor abilities are strikingly affected in Parkinson's disease.

Fourth, neuroimaging has allowed us to observe the workings of the brain not only when a person produces observable behavior, for example by speaking, but also when a person merely thinks. Working with a living, nonlesioned subject has many advantages; for example, one need not worry about possible compensations and other complications that may muddy the path of inference from damaged to normal brains (but may not: Caramazza and Badecker, 1991; Caramazza, 1992; Kosslyn and Intrilligator, 1992). Studies of the activation of the brain while people perform a particular mental task have clearly indicated that the different representational systems rely on the operation of different sets of brain areas (for example, Posner and Raichle, 1994).

These classes of converging evidence have convincingly led to a kind of topology of thought, which inscribes the substrate of mental processes onto the geography of the brain. Mental objects may now be thought of as having a material reality, and it is clear that different types of thinking arise from the joint action of different areas of the brain working in concert. Philosophers will undoubtedly find of interest an idea expressed by Jean-Pierre Changeux (1983), namely that we now have at our disposal physical traces of access to meaning. The fact that neuroimaging can highlight brain areas involved in perception, memory, motor control, and so on thus leads to a true semantic geography. Subjectivity becomes, in a certain sense, accessible to objectivity.

We must temper our enthusiasm for the new neuroimaging techniques, however, because of their limited resolution, both spatially and temporally. Such limitations imply that a family of distinct languages of the brain might, with our present coarse techniques, appear to be one and the same. When more finely honed tools become available, we may distinguish a larger number of types of representations than is currently evident. Moreover, our knowledge is limited by the kinds of questions we have chosen to put to the machines. At present, we are just beginning to learn where and how the psychological activity responsible for mental processes and behaviors are seated in the brain. As we begin to think about the nature of such processing in more sophisticated ways, we will design more subtle and penetrating experiments. The recognition of these limitations, however, should not undermine the utility of attempting to pinpoint the physical traces of access to different "languages of the brain." Technological and conceptual progress will refine our knowledge of the nature of understanding and thought.

Languages Are Embedded in Processing Systems

The reflections in this introduction underscore the contributions of functional neuroanatomy. They teach us that the world of the mind can be explored like a continent, that is to say, with the help of geographers' methods. The reader who is knowledgeable about metaphysics may think that this is a new way of searching for the location of the soul or, in keeping with modern assumptions, the location of the many, perhaps modular souls, in such a way that little progress would have been made since Descartes if not for the appearance of progress due to new techniques. Of course, this is not the case: none of the projects summarized in this volume have the aim of showing how all knowledge of a certain sort converges onto a single center (the soul, as it were). The common goal, rather, is to delineate processing systems. No single area working alone accomplishes very much; it is only through the joint activity of many areas that the brain gives rise to cognition. Many empirical results indicate that different systems of brain areas (which sometimes are partially overlapping) underlie different sorts of processing. In this volume, most researchers focus on one piece, one facet, of a particular system and show how it relates to other perceptual and cognitive processes, interconnected and heterarchical.

How do we characterize the different "languages"? We begin with the assumption that different languages of the brain correspond to different processing systems. In thinking about how to characterize these systems, it is useful to draw a distinction between the format of a language and its content. The *format* is the type of code used, such as the difference between Morse code, French, and written Arabic. These are different systems of notation, with different rules for interpreting the marks. For example, the same symbol, "A," can mean different things depending on the format of the language. If this is taken as a letter in written English, it is an indefinite article; if we take it as a picture, it could stand for a flock of geese heading south for the winter. In order for a representation to be a repository of information, it must be embedded in a broader processing system in which it is interpreted in a particular way. One advantage of turning to the brain is that it gives us a handle on how to think about the relation between representations and the processes that interpret them (for example, see Chapters 12–14, 16).

In contrast to the format, the *content* is the information that is conveyed by such codes. It is possible to represent the same content using different formats; the information in this sentence, for example, could be conveyed using Morse code, French, and so on. The flock of geese could be described or depicted in a painting, or even mimicked by a talented mime. However, and this is an essential point, the differences in format among different languages of the brain leads them to represent particular content more or less easily. For example, imagine the uppercase letter "N," and rotate it 90 degrees clockwise? Can you "see" that it is another letter? To do this using a description of the shape would be awkward, but to use an image (which depicts, rather than describes) is relatively straightforward. Some aspects of knowledge cannot be easily represented or processed in one particular language, but instead lend themselves to a different type of language. All languages of the brain are not equally adequate for representing all types of thoughts, as implied by sayings such as "A picture is worth a thousand words."

We have suggested that mental images are one "language of thought," and this topic is addressed in several chapters. But what about the previously noted objections of the good Bishop Berkeley? The key is that the different languages are interconnected. Not only is each language a processing system—with its distinctive representations and processes—but the languages as a whole are themselves part of an even larger, more inclusive processing system. If one forms a mental image, it is "under a description": you know what it stands for—you are not confused about whether that image of an apple stands for apple or worm food. The notion of being "under a description" implies that the representations in one language have a relation to those in another language. Thus the same image would have different relations to different verbal descriptions, for example (see Chapter 12).

By the same token, words such as "courage," "violence," and "sex" often elicit strong visceral sensations. One could say that such words are abstract because they do not have perceptual links to vision and hearing, but to the extent that they have perceptual links to specific visceral sensations, they are concrete. Similarly, try thinking about how to explain the color pink to someone who has been blind from birth. The different languages necessarily must be interrelated: it is possible to describe what you see, draw what you hear described, and so on. Somehow we translate from one system to another.

It may be tempting (as it was to Pylyshyn, 1973) to argue that all languages of the brain ultimately must be translated into a common underlying language—propositional representations. According to this view, propositional representations are actually doing all of the work in cognition. However, this argument does not wash. To translate between languages (as any speaker of two natural languages knows), all that is necessary are translation rules between the different languages; there is no need to pass through a common code to make the interconnections (think of how dictionaries work). Indeed, if the only way that the system could translate from one type of representation to another, say from L-1 to L-2, was via a third, intermediate representation, L-3 (that is, converting L-1 to L-3, and then L-3 to L-2), what would allow the translation to that intermediate representation (that is, how would one get from L-1 to L-3)? Anderson (1978) long ago pointed out that the notion that an intermediate representation is necessary to connect different types of representations leads one into the trap of an infinite regress: Each pair would require an intermediate representation (for example, to get from L-1 to L-3, we need L-4), but to get to that, yet another intermediate representation between it and the first one (that is, L-5, between L-1 and L-4) would be required, and then yet another would need to be sandwiched in between the first and this new one, and so on and so on.

Indeed, part of the progress evident in this volume is a rejection of the idea that there is a single "seat" or "center" for any specific ability, or that there is a single code that all information ultimately must be translated into. The distributed nature of the "languages of the brain" rejects the notion that there is a homunculus, a little man inside who watches what's going on and pulls the strings. As is true for the idea of a universal intermediate representation, this notion of a center for an ability simply pushes the problem back a step: What is going on in the homunculus that allows it to know how to respond? Is there another homunculus in it, and so on, in infinite regress? Similarly, merely having activation in a given area does not constitute comprehension; comprehension only arises through a set of interrelations among different representations, which may imply possible behaviors.

In this volume we explore some of the distinct characteristics of different languages of the brain. For example, verbal language has unique syntactic combinatorial properties that are not the same as the combinatorial properties of other languages of the brain. Although all languages share the requirement that there be rules that dictate how representations can be combined, the rules differ considerably. Verbal language may be the only type in which the representations of things are in "form classes" (parts of speech), and the form classes dictate the appropriate application of combinatorial rules. That is, the syntax of verbal language hinges on whether words are nouns, verbs, and so on—not on their specific meanings. There is no obvious parallel in other modalities. In addition, verbal language is superior at representing abstract concepts. Try to get a picture in your mind of the concept of "courage" per se (without resorting to a visual memory of a movie or a cartoon depicting someone in a courageous act). Hard to do, if not impossible.

However, it may be overly simplistic to think of "verbal language" as a single language of the brain. There exist variants in verbal languages, linguistic diversity even within a culture, for instance in the language of teenagers and of specialized professionals. It would be interesting to know exactly what is invariant in this linguistic variance, and whether such variance implies a distinct "language" (or dialect) of the brain. Take, for instance, the anecdotal reports of aphasic bilingual patients who lose abilities in one but not in the other language. Such reports imply that different verbal languages are represented differently in the brain. Does this imply that the different languages can play different roles in thinking? Might it be that romantic thoughts would be better couched in mental French than in mental English?

In contrast, the depictive features of visual languages emphasize shapes and visual properties (texture, color, and so on) rather than time. And the dynamic qualities of motoric representations emphasize changes in location and position over time. Such properties are likely to be just as unique to those languages as are the unique features of verbal languages. Depending on what content is being conveyed, different languages of the brain are more or less useful.

Despite these differences, the different brain languages probably also share properties. These common properties may arise from the fact that all languages draw on representations of concepts and categories. These representations specify not only individual cases, in specific circumstances, but also relations among more than one concept or category in more general circumstances. An important motivation for putting diverse discussions of different languages of the brain in a single volume is to explore the question of what properties the languages of the brain may share, and in what manner and to what extent they interact in the representation and manipulation of knowledge. All representations, be they the most concrete perceptual or the most abstract conceptual, can be used to specify the ways in which characteristics or properties are associated with objects or events.

Thus in thinking about the relations among languages, we must consider the ways in which various types of representations work together, which may not always be obvious. In fact, Bernard Mazoyer, Emmanuel Mellet, and Nathalie Tzourio argue in Chapter 12 that in some situations systems of representations may even be inhibitory. This may result from the fact that two languages may share end organs—try whistling a tune while laughing. Or the competition may be more central—try imagining a tune while reading silently. Yet in other cases there is clear cooperation, such as in the visual imagery that occurs when reading.

Another thread that runs through many of the chapters is that meaning is to be found in the interactions among languages of the brain. The meaning of a work of art, for example, is to be understood in terms of the associations it brings to mind, and their influence on one's subsequent cognition and behavior.

In addition, some of the chapters emphasize the possibility that motor processes play a key role in thought. This notion has not received its due in mainstream psychology, particularly in North America. Here we explore the notion that motor processes may even be involved in "intentionality." In particular, the anticipation of making a movement and of perceiving the consequences of making a movement may correspond to "intentionality."

History, Context, and Culture

All of the languages of the brain serve to represent content. But where does that content come from? Another theme explored in the volume is that the content of mental processes can only be understood from the point of view of the history of the individual and the species. That is, history is registered in part via the experiences of the individual (firsthand experience via perception and secondhand experience via verbal language) and in part via the evolution of the species. Our brains are not blank slates, general purpose machines. As Elizabeth Spelke points out in Chapter 15, brain function is structured even at a very early age, perhaps too early to be accounted for solely by appeal to experience. In all cases, history initially affects representations, which then affect other representations (for example, the visual can be described verbally, which in turn gives rise to propositional representations).

As discussed in Section 2, meaning may depend largely on history, on one's experience with a particular kind of stimulus or event. Clearly, the meanings of words are to be understood only in terms of their history, what one has been taught to associate with that sound.

The importance of history emphasizes another crucial fact about the languages of the brain: they function in a context, which is both social and cultural. That is, not only do events in the world result in representations in the different languages, but such representations in turn lead us to affect the world. Section 6 considers the applied uses of different languages, such as graphic arts and even advertising. The different languages lead to different externalizations, different physical manifestations in the world—which then feed back to serve as stimuli for other people, evoking internal representations. Our products are bridges between representations in the languages of our brains and the corresponding languages in the brains of others. In addition, the fact that the brain is situated in the world implies that the study of the anatomic substrate of thought is not enough to develop even a neurological theory of mind, let alone a fuller theory that takes into account the interactions between the person and the world.

These observations imply that we should not think narrowly about the importance of understanding the languages of the brain. The study of languages of the brain is obviously of interest to neurologists and psychologists, but it is also rich in its potential for those in other fields of knowledge.

This book is organized along two broad poles in the classification of the brain's languages: verbal and nonverbal. Within each broad category we have three subcategories, each of which addresses some particular aspect of the languages of the brain. Our goal was to cast light on as many facets as possible, but to include enough material on each to expose the depth of the different topics. We also sought subject matter that would illustrate the similarities and differences among the different languages. In addition, we selected topics on which there has been demonstrable progress.

The research summarized in this volume is only a small taste of what is to come. "Can the brain understand the brain?" David Hubel was asking this question twenty years ago, and other researchers, clinicians, philosophers, and even theologians have asked it again and again since then. Even if the complexity of the task makes us doubt ever being able to understand everything, we cannot help but notice the great progress made since Hubel posed his question, and hope for even more in the next decade and beyond.

References

Anderson, J. R. 1978. Arguments concerning representations for mental imagery. *Psychological Review, 85,* 249–277.

Bellugi, U., and C. A. Morris, eds. 1995. Williams Syndrome: From cognition to gene. *Genetic Counseling, 6,* 131–192.

Bowerman, M. 1973. *Early syntactic development: A cross-linguistic study with special reference to Finnish.* Cambridge: Cambridge University Press.

Caramazza, A. 1992. Is cognitive neuropsychology possible? *Journal of Cognitive Neuroscience, 4,* 80–95.

Caramazza, A., and W. Badecker. 1991. Clinical syndromes are not God's gift to cognitive neuropsychology: A reply to a rebuttal to an answer to a response to the case against syndrome-based research. *Brain and Cognition, 16,* 211–227.

Changeux, J.-P. 1983. *L'homme neuronal.* Paris: Fayard.

Farah, M. 1990. *Visual agnosia: Disorders of object recognition and what they tell us about normal vision.* Cambridge: MIT Press.

Fodor, J. A. 1975. *The language of thought.* New York: Crowell.

Jeannerod, M. 1997. *The cognitive neuroscience of action.* Oxford: Blackwell Publishers.

——— 1998. *The neural and behavioural organization of goal-directed movements.* Oxford: Clarendon Press/Oxford University Press.

Kosslyn, S. M., and J. M. Intrilligator. 1992. Is cognitive neuropsychology plausible? The perils of sitting on a one-legged stool. *Journal of Cognitive Neuroscience, 4,* 96–106.

Petersen, R. C. 1998. Clinical subtypes of Alzheimer's disease. *Dementia and Geriatric Cognitive Disorders 9,* Suppl. 3, 16–24.

Posner, M. I., and M. E. Raichle. 1994. *Images of mind.* New York: Scientific American Library/Scientific American Books.

Pylyshyn, Z. W. 1973. What the mind's eye tells the mind's brain: A critique of mental imagery. *Psychological Bulletin, 80,* 1–24.

Slobin, D. 1985. *The crosslinguistic study of language acquisition.* Vol. 1, *The data.* Hillsdale, N.J.: Erlbaum Associates.

Smith, E. E., and J. Jonides. 1999. Storage and executive processes in the frontal lobes. *Science, 283,* 1657–1661.

Verbal Representation

Verbal language is one of the languages of thought. It is particularly well suited for some types of thoughts—so much so, that it is at times difficult to separate the actual thought from the verbal process. This unclear boundary might give the impression that thought and verbal representation are one and the same thing. The places where verbal language fails, however, illustrate that verbal language is not the same as thought. There is no real way, for example, to describe adequately what happens when one catches a ball in midair. Surely it is possible to say that the ball was seen and the arm went up in such a way that the trajectories of the ball and the hand ultimately converged. But such a verbal description does not in any way allow one to understand how the information about the moving ball was handled by the visual system, what representations took place such that the visual information could be recoded in a motor program that would cause just the right muscles to contract, just at the correct speed and combination, in order for the ball to be caught. Even short of that, it is very hard to learn to catch a ball if you are given only words of explanation on how to do it. Imagine trying to catch a ball with your eyes closed following only verbal instructions. Imitation, in this case, is a better method. Another example is the experience, when learning a new sport like skiing or tennis, of talking to oneself about what needs to be done, being completely sure of what to do, and then doing a dreadful job at it.

Verbal language is also not particularly good at describing the visual environment. At least some visual objects are not amenable to verbal description and coding. The obvious example is color, but the difficulty does not end there. Think how poor a mental image of the Eiffel Tower a listener would construct from simply a verbal description by someone who has seen it, however good an observer and narrator the person might be. On the other hand, saying that a cat is ten times larger than a mouse does convey good information. The value of verbal language is measured by the way it represents knowledge and thought and the efficiency with which it allows the storage, manipulation, and communication of knowledge and thought. Its uniqueness has to do with the special rules by which the objects of verbal language—phonemes, graphemes, syllables, words, sentences, and even paragraphs (see Chapter 8)—can be combined to change meaning, which makes it possible for a relatively manageable number of objects to cover most knowledge that lends itself to verbal language. Equally efficiently, there is a finite number of ways by which words can be modified—morphology—which results in changes in meaning. In visual language the image of a lion may be chasing the image of an antelope, or the roles can be reversed by altering the position of the visual objects. However, there is no evidence that a limited number of elementary shapes exists (akin to phonemes in verbal language), which in different combinations can account for all visual forms, or that the visual environment can thus be parsed and rearranged to change meaning. The special process associated with verbal language, therefore, is as crucial an aspect of verbal language as the objects of thought it can represent.

Verbal languages exhibit significant variation. There is first variation dictated by modality specificity, at least that aspect of verbal language having to do with communication. For instance, verbal language can be oral, written, based on signing, or perceived through touch, as in Braille. Although the deep processes must be shared among these different modalities, as evidenced by results of developmental studies, it is clear that the sheer difference in input and output channels change important properties, such as timing and content. It is not possible, for instance, to sign around corners, in the way that is possible to use speech around corners. "Yelling" in sign language does not reach as far as yelling in speech. Therefore, it is clear that some additional content sharing is needed for one form of communication and not for the other. This, in fact, may be the main reason why the channels through which verbal language communication evolved in the human species involved sound rather than sight. Braille and standard reading are different in that they are a later acquired mechanism for representing a previously learned language in the auditory modality; in this way they are elaborations rather than variants of verbal language.

This part of the volume has three sections. Section 1, "Verbal Processes," considers neural and functional mechanisms underlying some of the rules of verbal language. The focus is not on the objects of language, on whether, say, the discussion is about food or flying an airplane, but rather about how the discussion takes place. The power of verbal language lies in its ability to change meaning by changing the temporal order of a relatively small number of sounds, the number and types of which are language dependent—different, for instance, in English and in French. There are in practice an unlimited number of new meanings that a language can accrue based on this principle—the so-called open class words. Another powerful feature of verbal language is its syntax, which again can create new meaning by word order. Meaning can be changed by adding and subtracting bits of sound, which constitutes the morphological transformation of words, and by changing prosody. We also realize that at a higher level, meaning can be manipulated by decisions about when to speak and when not to, what to say, in what order, and so on. These higher-order processes, however, may not be unique to verbal language. These features of verbal language are clearly unique and to our knowledge are only manifested in nature by the human species.

In Section 2, "Verbal Content," the issue of the objects of thought themselves is raised. How would some objects, say, foods, be organized differently from other objects, say, tools. Injury to the brain sometimes appears to affect one class of words, leaving the other classes intact. What different types of representation are there? Some, directly linked to the perceptual systems, are easily recoded in the visual, auditory, or somesthetic systems. For instance, the word "dog" conjures up in mental imagery in the listener some prototype dog or a unique exemplar—say, Lassie—with little difficulty. Other words are more abstract and do not have an obvious relationship to a sensory history, at least not with respect to external experience. The word "anger" may not be imageable in the same easy way that the word "dog" is, but certainly there are emotional (limbic) links to the word that elicit visceral sensations and can activate autonomic and somatic motor systems to act very quickly. In a real sense, words such as "anger" and "love" can be "imaged" in visceral sensory systems much like the words "carrot" and "dog" can be imaged in the visual sensory system. The idea, therefore, is that categories depend on connectivity. Questions about verbal content do not end here. So, for instance, we seek explanations for why patients with certain forms of aphasia are able to respond appropriately to the command "Open your mouth!" but not to the command "Open your fist!" Why would that be? How could this be explained solely on the basis of linguistics? The understanding of the handling by the brain of categories of objects is central to the understanding of verbal content.

In Section 3, "Verbal Variants," the issue of linguistic diversity is considered. Multilingualism figures prominently, albeit not exclusively. By multilingualism we commonly mean more than one verbal language cutting across different cultures, and, as shown more recently, cutting across genetic backgrounds, such as Chinese, English, and Navaho. But sign language, which is altogether as powerful a language of thought as any verbal language communicated orally, appears to follow many of the combinatorial rules typical of oral languages as well. Moreover, the course of sign language acquisition in the children of deaf signing parents is strikingly similar to the acquisition of oral languages by hearing babies. It would be easy to make the case that sign language is a verbal language represented and communicated in a different modality. Similarly, reading and writing visual text or Braille is another example of the mapping of a verbal language onto a different modality, visual and somesthetic, respectively, albeit a verbal language that is first acquired through the auditory system. Language variants among the verbal languages help us to understand verbal language at a deeper level, independent of the sensory-motor systems that help implement it.

Section 1
Verbal Processes

Although investigators have attempted to understand how the brain supports verbal language for over 150 years, the result has been exceptionally unrevealing. At best we have learned that, in a very general sense, injury to certain parts of the brain's left hemisphere alter verbal language function, and that the effect on language of injury in one place is different from the effect of injury in another. With better methods for identifying smaller lesions, the map relating dysfunction to brain location has continued to improve. This improvement occurs only up to a point, however, because in many cases the lesion is too small to produce consistent and reliable losses, if any. Additional help has been gained with the use of brain activation techniques—functional magnetic resonance imaging (fMRI), positron emission tomography (PET), evoked potentials mapping, magnetoencephalography, infrared mapping—to help outline the areas of the brain that participate in different aspects of language function. As might be surmised a priori, more areas are linked to language function by these imaging methods than the number of areas that, when damaged, result in language dysfunction. Most of the areas disclosed either by lesion analysis or by activation studies are areas that participate in the process of language. Some, however, address content, in that it is known that some areas of the brain participate in the representation and recognition of specific categories of objects. Why the brain is organized differently for different categories of objects—say, tools, animals, foods, and so on—is still a matter of debate, but the answers to this question cannot come from linguistic analysis alone and require knowledge concerning the evolution of the brain and learning.

Chapter 1 begins the section with an examination of what is known about the structure of the human brain that could explain the subspecialization of the brain for categories. What is likely to play a role in the answer is that areas that have separate patterns of connectivity in the extant brain, that is, to the visual system, or the limbic system, or the motor system, have evolved from ancestral forms that had equivalent patterns of connectivity. Thus experience with the environment has for a long time been segregated along separate systems. The longer this segregation has been in place, the more likely that it has been coded in the genome.

Chapter 2 constitutes a formal attempt to describe modules of language processing and their layout in the brain. The result, found by other workers as well, indicates that areas of the brain concerned with process are different from those concerned with content. The frontal lobes, in general, participate in processing, including access to knowledge, while the posterior parts of the brain represent the objects of knowledge themselves, including fragments that can be combined to access meaning. Nonetheless, it is easy to see that difficulties with language comprehension can arise from problems with access to knowledge as well as from the degradation of the representations of the objects of knowledge themselves, and that it may be difficult at times to tell the two apart.

Chapter 3 deals with syntactic processing, investigating differences in the anatomy of the system involved in some types of syntactic judgment between young adults and elderly. These differences constitute a remarkable finding. Given the fact that categories behave as if they are separate in the brain in large part because of the evolutionary experience of the species with different types of objects, it is likely that this is modified, if ever so slightly, every generation, as the environment changes and adaptation continues. Moreover, experience at the individual level may cause reorganization during a lifetime, such that the maps may be different in the old compared with the new. However, it is more difficult to conceive that the areas that mediate the implementation of the rules of language, such as syntax—verbal processes—would change. Or does the change reflect not pathological change but, rather, a situation in which areas less capable are playing a greater role because they are now needed in old age?

Chapter 4 closes the section by exploring the classic question regarding the brain's treatment of phonological versus lexical-semantic tasks leading to single-word comprehension. It has been known from lesion analysis that different parts of the brain are called upon to solve either type of task. However, the differences in timing between the two tasks cannot easily be assessed from current imaging techniques, let alone from lesion analysis. Combinations of techniques that have the ability to separate in space, on the one hand, and in time, on the other, at the correct scales, may allow for the elucidation of the temporo-spatial participation of the brain in verbal language function.

The Neuroanatomy of Categories 1

Albert M. Galaburda

Some aspects of human cognition can be understood by knowing the connectivity of the brain, and, to the extent that some of the connections find antecedents in earlier evolutionary times, some aspects of cognition can be understood in terms of evolution. These statements may be particularly relevant to the finding of categorical organization of knowledge in the brain. Modern brain mapping devices, which include positron emission tomography (PET) (see Petersen et al., 1988), functional magnetic resonance imaging (fMRI) (see Menon et al., 1992), electroencephalography (EEG) and evoked potentials (EP or ERP) (see Hillyard and Picton, 1987), magnetoencephalography (MEG) (see Yamamoto et al., 1988; Yamamoto, Uemura, and Llinas, 1992), and repetitive transcranial magnetic stimulation (rTMS) (see Mills, Murray, and Hess et al., 1987; Pascual-Leone, Gates, and Dhuna, 1991; Flitman et al., 1998), have together succeeded in implicating a larger constellation of brain regions that participate in linguistic activities than previously disclosed by the time-honored patient lesion analysis. In spite of this important achievement with the use of these new instruments, the ultimate goal of the cognitive neuroscience approach to language is to discover not just where and by which brain regions is language carried out, but also the ways by which the brain carries out language. As this challenge is likely to keep the field occupied for decades to come, a more immediate goal is to understand how the regions of the brain, thought to participate in language function, as shown coarsely by imaging instruments, map onto what is known in detail about the anatomy of the relevant brain circuits. Many of the details have not actually been learned in the human brain directly, but are extrapolations of the anatomy known about the brains of mainly nonhuman primates. This chapter outlines a model of human forebrain cortical organization that is helpful for understanding the results of mapping studies of language function, particularly where it concerns categorical knowledge. Moreover, in the spirit of the present volume, the model to be discussed is also useful to the understanding of other cognitive functions, including high-level vision and visual languages, and motor control.

The Standard Model of the Cognitive Brain

Most neurologists and cognitive scientists use a model of cortical organization that is inherited from the work of Flechsig (1876) in the nineteenth century. This model posits three general types of cerebral cortex: primary cortex, first-order association cortex, and second-order association cortex, often also referred to as integration cortex. The model is based on Flechsig's observations that the three types of cortex myelinate at different times during early brain development, with the primary cortices myelinating first and the integration cortices myelinating last. This led many to the conclusion that integration cortex is the most evolved and slowest to develop, a fact that made it a likely candidate for carrying out uniquely human behaviors such as language. Of course, evidence from work in modern developmental neurobiology indicates clearly that the rules that govern cortical development are of a different sort, and in fact there is no good evidence in support of the notion that cortical regions develop at different developmental times (Lidow, Goldman-Rakic, and Rakic, 1991). Moreover, the conclusions reached on the basis of the myelogenetic studies alone failed to take into consideration the fact that in their mature states different regions of the cortex do not exhibit the same degree of myelination (Sanides and Hoffmann, 1969). Therefore, comparing their myelination schedules as if all the cortical areas were headed toward the same point is not a meaningful comparison. Thus, for instance, if primary cortices such as Brodmann areas 4 or 17 achieve a higher density of myelination at the end of development, it is possible that they will look myelinated earlier than cortices such as limbic area 24, which even at the end achieve little myelination.

Furthermore the model fails because it does not provide sufficient detail about the further architectonic differentiation of the purported three types of cortex. Nor does it supply information about connectivity among the areas, other than to suggest that the primary cortices receive substantial input from the relay sensory nuclei of the thalamus, while association and integration cortices do not, another claim that has not been borne out by more modern connectional studies (see Jones and Powell, 1971; Berson and Graybiel, 1978; Raczkowski and Rosenquist, 1983). Nonetheless, the model does provide for interesting observations regarding the effects of brain injury on language functions. Thus, for example, injury resulting in the standard aphasic disorders involves predominantly association cortices (for example, Broca's area or Wernicke's area), whereas lesions affecting primary cortices may produce sensory perceptual anomalies without aphasia (for example, pure word deafness), and lesions affecting integration cortices may be associated with disorders affecting facts and processes that go beyond the purely linguistic domain (for example, associative agnosias).

Syndromes the Standard Model Does Not Explain

It is important to say at the start that brain injury has often unpredictable effects on behavior. This is not so much because the standard model is wrong, but rather because it is underspecified. Thus, for instance, injury to a particular portion of the cortex may produce different behaviors in different patients, and, in some cases, no behavioral anomaly altogether that can be detected by standard clinical means. Leaving aside the issue of heterogeneity of lesions (to make certain that the two lesions being compared are identical) there are several explanations for these observations, all of which lead to the conclusion that no matter what model one adopts for understanding the effects of lesions and the organization of behavior, it has to answer to the fact that there is extensive individual variability. This variability arises from genetic differences to some extent (Collins, 1985; Geschwind and Galaburda, 1985a,b,c), some of which manifest themselves as variable hand preference and brain asymmetry. For example, there is a difference in the response to brain injury and aphasia for familial right- and left-handers (Gloning, 1977). Variability may also stem from learning differences (Pascual-Leone and Torres, 1993; Karni et al., 1995; Xerri et al., 1996), between people with and without literacy (Miceli et al., 1981; Lecours et al., 1987; Castro Caldas et al., 1998), and between literate people whose first language is English or Japanese (Sasanuma, 1975).

The standard model does not adequately explain observations made on patients with frontal lobe injury. For example, if the integration cortex of the frontal lobe is uniform, why is it that lesions in the dorsomedial portion of the frontal lobe tend to produce problems with motivation for and activation of behavior (Nemeth, Hegedus, and Molnar, 1988), whereas lesions in the ventrolateral portions of the lobe interfere with the proper conduct of the behaviors themselves, of which, for instance, agrammatism (Chapter 3; Goodglass, 1997), aprosodic speech production (Ross, 1981), and phonemic paraphasias are examples (Monoi et al., 1983), and ventral frontal lesions produce difficulties with comportment (Raleigh et al., 1979; Raleigh and Steklis, 1981; Bakchine et al., 1989). Furthermore, it appears that in order for a dorsomedial lesion to produce a permanent deficit, the injury has to be bilateral, whereas the ventrolateral lesions typically produce permanent deficits from unilateral involvement only. Why would that be?

In the parietal lobe, disconnection of perisylvian cortex and/or striatum, basal ganglia, and thalamus from dorsomedial zone, such as by a lesion injuring the dorsomedial zone itself or by large deep lesions in the inferior parietal lobules interrupting the deep white matter, often produce disturbances of attention and spatial awareness (Vallar and Perani, 1986), whereas ventral lesions interfere with specific knowledge or representations (Feinberg et al., 1994; Shelton et al., 1994). Furthermore, there is nothing in the standard model to help us understand why the dorsal portions of the visual system extract such a different type of information about the visual environment from that obtained by the ventral portions, the former being concerned with spatial scanning, location, and orientation, the latter with details about visual objects, such as color, texture, and shape (Haxby et al., 1991). The temporal lobe is responsible for, in addition to the bulk of the cortical auditory system (Galaburda and Sanides, 1980; Galaburda and Pandya, 1983; Rivier and Clarke, 1997), the visual representations of object properties (Mishkin and Ungerleider, 1982), except for its most superior medial portion, adjacent to the splenium of the corpus callosum, which again appears to represent the spatial environment rather than specific objects (Epstein and Kanwisher, 1998).

Although, in a sense, the observations listed above address the issue of the cortical representation of different types of knowledge in general, whether visual, somesthetic, or auditory, some characteristics of objects addressing the notion of categories are not addressed by the standard model. Therefore, many clinical and some mapping observations using imaging devices have shown that different types of objects, belonging to separate categories, are processed using different portions of the so-called high-level, second-order association cortex (integration cortex). For instance, injury to portions of the temporal lobe result separately in difficulties processing knowledge about tools, faces, living things, animals, proper names, and so on (McKenna and Warrington, 1978; Damasio, 1990; Hillis and Caramazza, 1991). Reduction of cortical zones to a simple triad of primary, association, and integration cortices is inadequate to account for these observations from clinical neuroscience. But there is a great deal of heterogeneity within the so-called association and integration areas. Can exploration of the anatomical basis for this heterogeneity illuminate the reasons for the observed functional heterogeneity?

The Abbie-Sanides Hypothesis

In fact, any attempt to classify the cerebral cortex can be a daunting experience that will undoubtedly leave some dissatisfied. Following Flechsig, neuroanatomists like Campbell, Brodmann, von Economo and Koskinas, Sarkissov and Filimonov, and the Vogts and their large school set forth to subdivide the cerebral cortex into component areas by virtue of regional differences in cellular architecture and patterns of myelination and vascularization. Dozens of areas and in some cases hundreds of subregions could be identified, depending on the criteria used for parcellation and the detail to which the criteria were applied. The resulting maps are often unwieldy and do not usefully contribute to the solution of the problem of cognitive neuroscience examined in the present chapter: how do the data on the effects of brain injury and brain activation with respect to language and other cognitive processes map onto these detailed models of cortical parcellation? In fact, the models are even less useful than the standard Flechsig model because the additional detail obscures the correlation between behavior and brain injury or activation provided by the subdivision of the cortex into primary and association areas, without helping to explain the categorization of knowledge within the association cortices.

Abbie (1940) and subsequently Sanides (1970) provide a hierarchical model for the subdivision of the cortex into component areas, which helps to solve the problem of categories of knowledge, at least in part. This hierarchical order has a phylogenetic perspective, but it obviously makes assumptions about similarities and differences that exist between human and nonhuman primate brains, which often cannot be ascertained, at least in detail. It also makes no claims regarding ontogenetic development of areas, and, although the model makes specific claims about what new cortical areas arose in evolution from where, any attempt to link the model to knowledge about cortical development in fetal and postnatal life is bound to fail. In fact, the model is most acceptable as a descriptive program of extant cortical organization without undue reference either to brain evolution or brain development. In this sense, and in this alone, the model is useful and does help explain some of the lesion and activation data better than other cortical models available at present. The reader should keep in mind the fact that the observations that led to the model came essentially from nonhuman primate brains; nonetheless, where it has been possible to compare observations of this type to those in human brains, the data have been convergent (Galaburda and Sanides, 1980; Galaburda and Pandya, 1983).

The most primitive vertebrate brains, such as the brain of a fish, do not actually have a cerebral cortex, defined as a layered outer mantle of neurons. Moreover, a six-layered outer mantle—the isocortex or neocortex—does not appear clearly until the mammalian line, with some suggestion of its presence in some turtles. Only primates have true temporal lobes, which appear to arise from the overexpansion of the parieto-occipital regions, both ventrally and anteriorly, dragging with them the dorsal hippocampus toward its predominant position in the primate brain in the anterior medial temporal surface.

The cortex-like mantle of cells in fish, frog, and snake brains contains two distinct zones. These zones are distinguishable by the fact that one, the archicortex, which is located dorsomedially in the hemisphere, has large (long projecting and motor) neurons, while the other, the paleocortex, located ventrolaterally, has relatively small (local circuit and sensory) neurons. The dorsomedial zone receives its inputs largely from the hypothalamus, a sensor of the internal environment, and projects deeply into the subcortex, eventually innervating the muscles of locomotion. The ventrolateral zone, on the other hand, receives many inputs from the thalamus carrying information from the sense organs and hence the external environment. The output of the ventrolateral zone is via the dorsomedial zone to indirectly affect the motor system. The dorsomedial zone is preserved in mammals within the famed Papez circuit connecting hippocampus, hypothalamus, medial thalamus, and cingulate gyrus (see Veazey, Amaral, and Cowan, 1982). The dorsomedial zone is strongly bilaterally and homotopically interconnected (joining same rather than different areas across the corpus callosum) (Vogt, 1985; Koester and O'Leary, 1994). The ventrolateral zone is preserved in mammals in the insular cortex, the orbital surface of the frontal lobe, and the temporopolar cortex. This zone is only patchily connected across the corpus callosum (Yorke and Caviness, 1975; Beck and Kaas, 1994).

In mammals a large mass of six-layered cortex is interposed between the dorsomedial and ventrolateral roots. This large region of cortex can also be subdivided into a more dorsomedial portion and a more ventrolateral portion. The dorsomedial portion is still characterized by its having relatively large neurons with long subcortical and interhemispheric projections, while the ventrolateral portion contains a large contingent of thalamus-related small neurons, as well as a well-developed contingent of layer III medium-sized neurons involved in corticortical (associational) connectivity. Relatively speaking, there are large areas in the ventrolateral portions devoid of homotopic interhemispheric connections, which we have suggested is associated with asymmetry and functional independence of these areas between the hemispheres (Rosen, Sherman, and Galaburda, 1989; see also Aboitiz, 1992). In the primate brain, the ventrolateral portion is smaller than the dorsomedial portion in the frontal lobe (Sanides, 1972), but larger than the dorsomedial portion in the parietal and temporal lobes (Figure 1.1). In the frontal lobe, the dorsomedial portion and the ventrolateral portions are separated by the inferior frontal sulcus. In the parietal lobe, the two portions are separated by the intraparietal sulcus. In the temporal lobe, the collateral sulcus and rostral portion of the calcarine sulcus separate the dorsal and ventral portions. The ventrolateral portions in the frontal lobe include the inferior frontal gyrus and most of the orbital surface of the lobe (excluding the ventromedial edge of the orbital surface). In the parietal lobe, the ventrolateral portions include the inferior parietal lobule, with the angular and supramarginal gyri. In the temporal lobe, the ventrolateral portions include the superior, middle, and inferior temporal gyri, as well as the lingual and fusiform gyri, but it excludes, at least in part, the dorsal portion of the parahippocampal gyrus, which belongs instead among the dorsomedial zone together with the neighboring hippocampus.

In addition to the division of the mass of isocortex interposed between the dorsomedial and ventrolateral roots into two subregions bearing resemblance to the root areas to which they relate, each subregion can be further subdivided according to how far it is from its respective roots. Thus areas in close proximity to the roots, for instance the cingulate and parahippocampal cortices in the dorsomedial zone and the peri-insular cortex in the ventrolateral zone, tend to be relatively less cellular and less obviously six-layered. In a stepwise fashion belts of cortex surrounding the roots become more cellular and lose the distinctive features of the roots such that several steps away from the dorsomedial and ventrolateral roots respectively, cortices look more like one another than like their respective roots. Frontal areas 46, 45, and 10, for example, bear more resemblance to one another than to the cingulate and insular cortices. Likewise, it appears that these more evolved belts of cortex no longer adhere to the strict pattern of connections typical of their roots. Nonetheless, the ventrolateral-derived areas still receive thalamic inputs from sensory relay nuclei

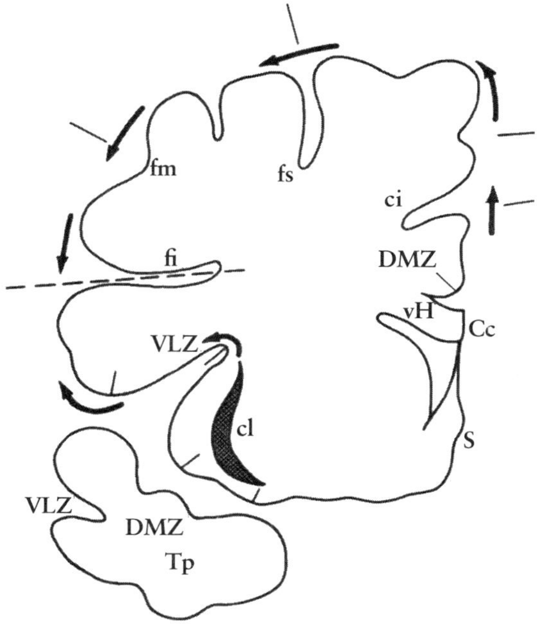

Figure 1.1. Line drawing of a cross section of the human frontal lobe to show the location of the two root zones, the dorsomedial zone (DMZ) and the ventrolateral zone (VLZ). Belts of progressive cortical specialization (separated by lines) occur away from the root zones (direction shown by arrows). The temporal pole (Tp) belongs mainly to the VLZ, but the DMZ is shown where it does occur more caudally in the temporal lobe. The hippocampal remnant (vH) lies at the location of the original DMZ (the archicortex), while the claustrum (cl) lies at the location of the original VLZ (the paleocortex). In the frontal lobe the dorsomedial and ventrolateral influences meet in the inferior frontal sulcus (fi). In the parietal lobe, they meet in the intraparietal sulcus. In the temporal lobe they meet in the collateral sulcus and rostral portion of the calcarine sulcus. Other abbreviations: Cc (corpus callosum); ci (cingulate sulcus); fs (superior frontal sulcus); fm (middle frontal sulcus); s (septum). Adapted with permission from F. Sanides, "Representation in Cerebral Cortex," in *The Structure and Function of Nervous Tissue,* vol. 5, ed. Geoffrey H. Bourne (New York: Academic Press, 1968), p. 372.

and connect with more dorsal areas to gain access to output subcortical channels (Yeterian and Pandya, 1991, 1995).

The purpose of organizing the anatomical knowledge in this fashion is to support the hypothesis that knowledge about internal and external experience could be stored and processed in these consecutive evolutionary belts of cortex such that objects with a longer shared history with the species may be stored and processed in units that are closer to the roots, while objects with a shorter shared history may be stored and processed by units that are farther away, each with its own set of input-output relationships to sense organs and motor systems. This would explain, for instance, why knowledge about animals may be processed in a part of the temporal lobe that is closer to the polar root than the region implicated in the processing of tools (see Damasio, 1996). Such an explanation would be altogether different, though not mutually exclusive, from those that invoke different brain localization on the basis of different sensory-perceptual-motor characteristics of the objects (see also Caramazza and Shelton, 1998).

The progressive belts of cortex are themselves subdivided into smaller areas, which resemble one another more than they do members of the belts closer or farther from the root. Thus, for instance, in the classic auditory region, we found three areas belonging within the same belt, which included the classical primary auditory cortex and two flanking association areas. A similarly arranged group of three was found closer to the temporal pole and another group of three farther from the temporal pole (Galaburda and Pandya, 1983). It is tempting to hypothesize that each module of three represents phylogenetically separate auditory regions with a different history regarding auditory experience and the species. What is striking in this progression from one stage to the other of modular differentiation is the fact that the so-called classic auditory areas do not appear distinctive in any other way than by being just another set of modules in this stepwise differentiation. The units within the modules retain a comparable architectonic relationship to one another and share a similar pattern of connections irrespective of whether the module in question is close or far from the root cortex in the temporal pole (Galaburda and Pandya, 1983). Viewed as a whole these observations allow one to say that the standard primary and association areas describing the organization of the visual, somesthetic, and auditory cortices (for example, 17, 18, and 19; 3, 1, and 2; and 41, 42, and 22 of Brodmann respectively) are but one of a series of evolutionarily hierarchical stages of sensorimotor processing. Furthermore, it is possible to conceive of the cortex as a superimposition of hierarchical modules based on their evolutionary age, which might then be used to explain phenomena such as categorical knowledge based on the shared evolutionary relationship that has existed in the brain with specific kinds of objects.

A Program for Categorical Knowledge

What the model that has been outlined above predicts is a categorically based knowledge system relating to the original organization of the forebrain cortex as well as to a superimposed set of subdivisions that arose later, when the mammalian cortex became increasingly specialized. The primeval vertebrate brain contained a dorsomedial module that responded to internally generated signals reflecting, for instance, changes in blood glucose, temperature, and hormonal levels, which led to direct activation of externally oriented attentional mechanisms and muscles of locomotion. On the other hand, a ventrolateral module received detailed information regarding specific visual, auditory or somesthetic objects in the external environment, which was needed in order to determine whether they arose from suitable food, reproductive, and other survival-relevant targets. The more evolved brain present in extant mammals, including humans, continues this original arrangement. It is only more capable of directed attention and exploration of the environment, and of planning for future exploration and attention. It is also presumably more capable of perceiving, representing, categorizing, and remembering a much larger assortment of objects from experience. One could add that some of these objects have not changed much over the history of the species, and are to an extent represented in a more hard-wired fashion in old sensorimotor modules; others, which change from generation to generation, and even during the life of the individual (sometimes quite quickly), make use of similarly organized modules, which however retain more plasticity and are newer in phylogenetic arrival.

The model would thus predict that the generation of activity, including preparation for and long-term planning of action, would arise from derivatives of the frontal lobe associated with the dorsomedial system. This in fact appears to be the case. Activation of the brain in relation to the preparation for movement involves frontal cortex located in the dorsomedial portions of the hemisphere (Decety et al.,

1994; Kawashima, Roland, and O'Sullivan, 1994; von Giesen et al., 1994; Deiber et al., 1996), and injury to this region, particularly when bilateral, results in severe and long-lasting deficits in planning and activation for action, such as akinesia and mutism (Freemon, 1971; Gugliotta et al., 1989). The so-called supplementary motor aphasia and related transcortical motor aphasia, characterized by extreme paucity in linguistic behavior, arises from dorsomedial lesions in the frontal lobe or injury to its connections to the striatum and the perisylvian (ventrolateral) language areas (Freedman, Alexander, and Naeser, 1984; Gold et al., 1997). Conversely, lesions in the ventrolateral portions of the frontal lobe, although they do not interfere with the will to engage in linguistic behavior, severely impair the ability to generate normal language, with specific problems with phonological and syntactic processing (Goodglass, 1997; see also Chapter 3). Lesions affecting the inferior surface of the frontal lobe, closer to the ventrolateral root, affect social communication and other behaviors that disclose the emotional state of the individual (Hornak, Rolls, and Wade, 1996). Thus patients show exaggerated or inappropriate displays of emotion and disinhibition.

In the parietal and occipital lobes, dorsal lesions interfere with the patient's attention to peripheral stimuli and produce a tendency to ignore peripheral space in favor of analyzing details in central and close intrapersonal space, even to the point of overfocus on parts of objects rather than on whole objects (Michel and Eyssette, 1972; Denny-Brown, 1977; Juergens, Fredrickson, and Pfeiffer, 1986; Verfaellie, Rapcsak, and Heilman, 1990; Rizzo, 1993). Ventral lesions instead affect the analysis of central and close intrapersonal space, whereby the affected patient may be unable to make comments about his or her own body (Roeltgen, Sevush, and Heilman, 1983; De Renzi and Lucchelli, 1988). Furthermore, lesions in the ventrally located occipitotemporal regions interfere with the ability to understand and describe visual objects presented in central vision (Albert et al., 1979; Riddoch and Humphreys, 1987). Of great interest is the discovery of a region in the dorsal portion of the parahippocampal gyrus caudally at the level of the splenium of the corpus callosum, which belongs to the dorsomedial zone that has migrated to the temporal lobe, which appears to process place rather than the objects in it (Epstein and Kanwisher, 1998).

The entire superior temporal gyrus belongs to the ventrolateral zone and analyzes the "object" properties of auditory signals rather than their spatial location, the cortical localization of which is unknown. There is a region caudal to the cingulate gyrus in the medial parietal lobe (thus a part of the dorsomedial zone) with strong connections to the superior temporal gyrus (Pandya and Yeterian, 1990), which is ideally situated to deal with auditory-directed attention and may also play a role in sound localization. Functional information regarding this region, however, is lacking.

Modules at a given distance from the root in the auditory system have a specific connectional relationship with modules at the same distance from the root in the visual and somesthetic modalities and frontal lobe regions (Pandya and Yeterian, 1990). In other words, not only are there self-contained modules within each modality, with thalamic inputs and access to the motor system, but modules of equivalent evolutionary age in different modalities are uniquely connected to one another. This is compatible with a system whereby it is possible not only to represent different types of information in given modules but also to establish intermodal association among the modules. This function would be considered important in order, say, to name an object presented visually or to know something about its function or its history.

Concluding Remarks

The human brain, like other primate brains, contains a large number of neocortical areas that differ in their cellular organization (cytoarchitecture) and connectivity. It is possible to relate these areas to regions already present in the brains of primitive vertebrates, which belong to two primordial types. One of these may be designed to respond to internal changes, which leads the animal to explore the environment in search of desirable targets. The other may be designed for assessing details about the target properties, among other reasons to ensure that they are indeed desirable, and for manipulating them.

The large expanse of cortex situated between these two cortical roots in primates is further subdivided into zones that may be designed to carry out specialized exploration of and attention to the environment in response to internal stimuli and drives, on the one hand, and specialized analysis and manipulation of objects in the environment, on the other. Attention to speech and speech itself may be thought of as special cases of this dichotomy. Furthermore, the further subdivision of the cortex into sensorimotor processing modules at varying distances from the root zones, and therefore presumably having different evolutionary ages and shared evolutionary histories with the environment, is compatible with the notion that knowledge in the brain will be processed in different modules on the basis of the evolutionary relationship that exists between a particular knowledge category and the brain.

The Flechsig model of primary, association, and integration areas is wrong. It suggests that integration cortex is the most evolved form of cortex, while the primary cortex is the least evolved. This is contrary to the notion that, in part, evolution leads to specialization. The primary cortex is the most specialized of the cortices in the forebrain, as evidenced by its discarding all other properties in favor of a single property, say hearing, or vision, or pyramidal versus stellate neurons. The integration cortex is the least specialized, containing multiple types of neurons connected most broadly. In further support of this claim, integration cortices are located closest to the root cortices (also known as limbic cortices).

To the extent one travels along the integration cortices away from their roots, one is able to see a stepwise, modular differentiation of zones with discrete input and output relationships. Each of these subsystems is postulated to represent a bit of the evolutionary history between the evolving human and its environment. Such a scheme could support observations in clinical cases of categorical knowledge segregated anatomically in the so-called integration cortices. However, although this scheme provides a general blueprint for categorical knowledge, it is important to note that development and learning, particularly pathology of development (for example, developmental dyslexia) and extreme variants in learning (for example, sign language in congenitally deaf signers), are capable of wreaking havoc with this scheme, producing striking changes in the structural-functional maps.

References

I am grateful to Michael P. Alexander for his valuable comments on the manuscript.

Abbie, A. A. 1940. Cortical lamination of the Monotremata. *Journal of Comparative Neurology, 72,* 428–467.

Aboitiz, F. 1992. Brain connections: Interhemispheric fiber systems and anatomical brain asymmetries in humans. *Biol. Res., 25,* 51–61.

Albert, M. L., Soffer, D., Silverberg, R., and Reches, A. 1979. The anatomic basis of visual agnosia. *Neurology, 29,* 876–879.

Bakchine, S., Lacomblez, L., Benoit, N., Parisot, D., Chain, F., and Lhermitte, F. 1989. Manic-like state after bilateral orbitofrontal and right temporoparietal injury: Efficacy of clonidine. *Neurology, 39,* 777–781.

Beck, P. D., and Kaas, J. H. 1994. Interhemispheric connections in neonatal owl monkeys (Aotus trivirgatus) and galagos (Galago crassicaudatus). *Brain Res., 651,* 57–75.

Berson, D. M., and Graybiel, A. M. 1978. Parallel thalamic zones in the LP-pulvinar complex of the cat identified by their afferent and efferent connections. *Brain Res., 147,* 139–148.

Caramazza, A., and Shelton, J. R. 1998. Domain-specific knowledge systems in the brain: The animate-inanimate distinction. *Journal of Cognitive Neuroscience, 10,* 1–34.

Castro Caldas, A., Petersson, K. M., Reis, A., Stone-Elander, S., and Ingvar, M. 1998. The illiterate brain: Learning to read and write during childhood influences the functional organization of the adult brain. *Brain, 121,* 1053–1063.

Collins, R. L. 1985. On the inheritance of direction and degree of asymmetry. In *Cerebral lateralization in nonhuman species,* ed. S. D. Glick, 41–71. New York: Academic Press.

Damasio, A. R. 1990. Category-related recognition defects as a clue to the neural substrates of knowledge. *Trends in Neuroscience, 13,* 95–98.

Damasio, H., Grabowski, T. J., Tranel, D., Hichwa, R. D., and Damasio, A. R. 1996. A neural basis for lexical retrieval. *Nature, 380,* 1–12.

Decety, J., Perani, D., Jeannerod, M., Bettinardi, V., Tadary, B., Woods, R., Mazziotta, J. C., and F. Fazio. 1994. Mapping motor representations with positron emission tomography. *Nature, 371,* 600–602.

Deiber, M. P., Ibanez, V., Sadato, N., and Hallett, M. 1996. Cerebral structures participating in motor preparation in humans: Positron emission tomography study. *Journal of Neurophysiology, 75,* 233–247.

Denny-Brown, D. 1977. Spasm of visual fixation. In *Physiological Aspects of Clinical Neurology,* ed. F. C. Rose, 43–75. Oxford: Blackwell Scientific Publications.

De Renzi, E., and Lucchelli, F. 1988. Ideational apraxia. *Brain, 111,* 1173–1185.

Epstein, R., and Kanwisher, N. 1998. A cortical representation of the local visual environment. *Nature, 392,* 598–601.

Feinberg, T. E., Schindler, R. J., Ochoa, E., Kwan, P. C., and Farah, M. J. 1994. Associative visual agnosia and alexia without prosopagnosia. *Cortex, 30,* 395–411.

Flechsig, P. 1876. *Die Leitungsbahnen in Gehirn und Rückenmark des Menschen auf Grund entwicklungsgeschichtlicher Untersuchungen.* Leipzig: W. Engelmann.

Flitman, S. S., Grafman, J., Wasserman, E. M., Cooper, V., O'Grady, J., Pascual-Leone, A., and Hallett, M. 1998. Linguistic processing during repetitive transcranial magnetic stimulation. *Neurology, 50,* 175–181.

Freedman, M., Alexander, M. P., and Naeser, M. A. 1984. Anatomic basis of transcortical motor aphasia. *Neurology, 34,* 409–417.

Freemon, F. R. 1971. Akinetic mutism and bilateral anterior cerebral artery occlusion. *J. Neurol. Neurosurg. Psychiatry, 34,* 693–698.

Galaburda, A. M., and Pandya, D. N. 1983. The intrinsic architectonic and connectional organization of the superior temporal region of the rhesus monkey. *Journal of Comparative Neurology, 221,* 169–184.

Galaburda, A., and Sanides, F. 1980. Cytoarchitectonic organization of the human auditory cortex. *Journal of Comparative Neurology, 190,* 597–610.

Geschwind, N., and Galaburda, A. M. 1985a. Cerebral lateralization. Biological mechanisms, associations, and pathology: I. A hypothesis and a program for research. *Archives of Neurology, 42,* 428–459.

——— 1985b. Cerebral lateralization. Biological mechanisms, associations, and pathology: II. A hypothesis and a program for research. *Archives of Neurology, 42,* 521–552.

——— 1985c. Cerebral lateralization. Biological mechanisms, associations, and pathology: III. A hypothesis and a program for research. *Archives of Neurology, 42,* 634–654.

Gloning, K. 1977. Handedness and aphasia. *Neuropsychologia, 15,* 355–358.

Gold, M., Nadeau, S. E., Jacobs, D. H., Adair, J. C., Rothi, L. J., and Heilman, K. M. 1997. Adynamic aphasia: A transcortical motor aphasia with defective semantic strategy formation. *Brain Lang., 57,* 374–393.

Goodglass, H. 1997. Agrammatism in aphasiology. *Clinical Neuroscience, 4,* 51–56.

Gugliotta, M. A., Silvestri, R., De Domenico, P., Galatioto, S., and Di Perri, R. 1989. Spontaneous bilateral anterior cerebral artery occlusion resulting in akinetic mutism: A case report. *Acta Neurol.* (Naples), *11,* 252–258.

Haxby, J. V., Grady, C. L., Horwitz, B., Ungerleider, L. G., Mishkin, M., Carson, R. E., Herscovitch, P., Schapiro, M. B., and Rapoport, S. I. 1991. Dissociation of object and spatial visual processing pathways in human extrastriate cortex. *Proceedings of the National Academy of Sciences USA, 88,* 1621–1625.

Hillis, A. E., and Caramazza, A. 1991. Category-specific naming and comprehension impairment: A double dissociation. *Brain, 114,* 2081–2094.

Hillyard, S. A., and Picton, T. W. 1987. Electrophysiology of Cognition. In *Handbook of Physiology: The Nervous System,* ed. F. Plum, 519–584. Baltimore: American Physiological Society.

Hornak, J., Rolls, E. T., and Wade, D. 1996. Face and voice expression identification in patients with emotional and behavioral changes following ventral frontal lobe damage. *Neuropsychologia, 34,* 247–261.

Jones, E. G., and Powell, T. P. 1971. An analysis of the posterior group of thalamic nuclei on the basis of its afferent connections. *Journal of Comparative Neurology, 143,* 185–216.

Juergens, S. M., Fredrickson, P. A., and Pfeiffer, F. E. 1986. Balint's syndrome mistaken for visual conversion reaction. *Psychosomatics, 27,* 597–599.

Karni, A., Meyer, G., Jezzard, P., Adams, M. M., Turner, R., and Ungerleider, L. G. 1995. Functional MRI evidence for adult motor cortex plasticity during motor skill learning. *Nature, 377,* 155–158.

Kawashima, R., Roland, P. E., and O'Sullivan, B. T. 1994. Fields in human motor areas involved in preparation for reaching, actual reaching, and visuomotor learning: A positron emission tomography study. *Journal of Neuroscience, 14,* 3462–3474.

Koester, S. E., and O'Leary, D. D. 1994. Axons of early generated neurons in cingulate cortex pioneer the corpus callosum. *Journal of Neuroscience, 14,* 6608–6620.

Lecours, A. R., Mehler, J., Parente, M. A., et al. 1987. Illiteracy and brain damage—1. Aphasia testing in culturally contrasted populations (control subjects). *Neuropsychologia, 25,* 231–245.

Lidow, M. S., Goldman-Rakic, P. S., and Rakic, P. 1991. Synchronized overproduction of neurotransmitter receptors in diverse regions of the primate cerebral cortex. *Proceedings of the National Academy of Sciences USA, 88,* 10218–10221.

McKenna, P., and Warrington, E. K. 1978. Category-specific naming preservation: A single case study. *Journal of Neurology, Neurosurgery and Psychiatry, 41,* 571–574.

Menon, R. S., Ogawa, S., Kim, S. G., Ellermann, J. M., Merkle, H., Tank, D. W., and Ugurbil, K. 1992. Functional brain mapping using magnetic resonance imaging: Signal changes accompanying visual stimulation. *Invest. Radiol. 27* Suppl. 2, S47–53.

Miceli, G., Caltagirone, C., Gainotti, G., Masullo, C., Silveri, M. C., and Villa, G. 1981. Influence of age, sex, literacy, and pathologic lesion on incidence, severity, and type of aphasia. *Acta Neurol. Scand., 64,* 370–382.

Michel, F., and Eyssette, M. 1972. [Ocular ataxia and visuomotor ataxia in bilateral lesions of the parieto-occipital junction: Balint's syndrome, Holmes' syndrome and related syndromes]. *Rev. Otoneuroophtalmol., 44,* 177–186.

Mills, K. R., Murray, N. M., and Hess, C. W. 1987. Magnetic and electrical transcranial brain stimulation: Physiological mechanisms and clinical applications. *Neurosurgery, 20,* 164–168.

Mishkin, M., and Ungerleider, L. G. 1982. Contribution of striate inputs to the visuospatial functions of parieto-preoccipital cortex in monkeys. *Behav. Brain Res., 6,* 57–77.

Monoi, H., Fukusako, Y., Itoh, M., and Sasanuma, S. 1983. Speech sound errors in patients with conduction and Broca's aphasia. *Brain Lang., 20,* 175–194.

Nemeth, G., Hegedus, K., and Molnar, L. 1988. Akinetic mutism associated with bicingular lesions: Clinicopathological and functional anatomical correlates. *Eur. Arch. Psychiatry Neurol. Sci., 237,* 218–222.

Pandya, D., and Yeterian, E. 1990. Architecture and connections of cerebral cortex: Implications for brain evolution and function. *Neurobiol. Higher Cog. Function, 29,* 53–84.

Pascual-Leone, A., Gates, J. R., and Dhuna, A. 1991. Induction of speech arrest and counting errors with rapid-rate transcranial magnetic stimulation. *Neurology, 41,* 697–702.

Pascual-Leone, A., and Torres, F. 1993. Plasticity of the sensorimotor cortex representation of the reading finger in Braille readers. *Brain, 116,* 39–52.

Petersen, S. E., Fox, P. T., Posner, M. I., Mintun, M., and Raichle, M. E. 1988. Positron emission tomographic studies of the cortical anatomy of single-word processing. *Nature, 331,* 585–588.

Raczkowski, D., and Rosenquist, A. C. 1983. Connections of the multiple visual cortical areas with the lateral posterior-pulvinar complex and adjacent thalamic nuclei in the cat. *Journal of Neuroscience, 3,* 1912–1942.

Raleigh, M. J., and Steklis, H. D. 1981. Effect of orbitofrontal and temporal neocortical lesions of the affiliative behavior of vervet monkeys (Cercopithecus aethiops sabaeus). *Exp. Neurol., 73,* 378–389.

Raleigh, M. J., Steklis, H. D., Ervin, F. R., Kling, A. S., and McGuire, M. T. 1979. The effects of orbitofrontal lesions on the aggressive behavior of vervet monkeys (Cercopithecus aethiops sabaeus). *Exp. Neurol., 66,* 158–168.

Riddoch, M. J., and Humphreys, G. W. 1987. A case of integrative visual agnosia. *Brain, 110,* 1431–1462.

Rivier, F., and Clarke, S. 1997. Cytochrome oxidase, acetylcholinesterase, and NADPH-diaphorase staining in human supratemporal and insular cortex: Evidence for multiple auditory areas. *Neuroimage, 6,* 288–304.

Rizzo, M. 1993. "Balint's syndrome" and associated visuospatial disorders. *Baillieres Clin. Neurol., 2,* 415–437.

Roeltgen, D. P., Sevush, S., and Heilman, K. M. 1983. Pure Gerstmann's syndrome from a focal lesion. *Archives of Neurology, 40,* 46–47.

Rosen, G. D., Sherman, G. F., and Galaburda, A. M. 1989. Interhemispheric connections differ between symmetrical and asymmetrical brain regions. *Neuroscience, 33,* 525–533.

Ross, E. D. 1981. The aprosodias: Functional-anatomic organization of the affective components of language in the right hemisphere. *Archives of Neurology, 38,* 561–569.

Sanides, F. 1970. Functional architecture of motor and sensory cortices in primates in the light of a new concept of neocortex evolution. In *The Primate Brain,* ed. C. R. Noback and C. Montagna, 137–208. New York: Appleton-Century-Crofts.

——— 1972. Representation in the cerebral cortex and its areal lamination patterns. In *The Structure and Function of Nervous Tissue,* ed. G. H. Bourne, 330–453. New York: Academic Press.

Sanides, F., and Hoffmann, J. 1969. Cyto- and myeloarchitecture of the visual cortex of the cat and of the surrounding integration cortices. *J. Hirnforsch, 11,* 79–104.

Sasanuma, S. 1975. Kana and Kanji processing in Japanese aphasics. *Brain Lang., 2,* 369–383.

Shelton, P. A., Bowers, D., Duara, R., and Heilman, K. M. 1994. Apperceptive visual agnosia: A case study. *Brain Cogn., 25,* 1–23.

Vallar, G., and Perani, D. 1986. The anatomy of unilateral neglect after right-hemisphere stroke lesions. A clinical/CT-scan correlation study in man. *Neuropsychologia, 24,* 609–622.

Veazey, R. B., Amaral, D. G., and Cowan, W. M. 1982. The morphology and connections of the posterior hypothalamus in the cynomolgus monkey (Macaca fascicularis). II. Efferent connections. *Journal of Comparative Neurology, 207,* 135–156.

Verfaellie, M., Rapcsak, S. Z., and Heilman, K. M. 1990. Impaired shifting of attention in Balint's syndrome. *Brain Cogn., 12,* 195–204.

Vogt, B. A. 1985. Cingulate cortex. In *Cerebral Cortex,* ed. A. Peter and E. G. Jones, 89–149. New York: Plenum Press.

von Giesen, H. J., Schlaug, G., Steinmetz, H., Benecke, R., Freund, H. J., and Seitz, R. J. 1994. Cerebral network underlying unilateral motor neglect: Evidence from positron emission tomography. *J. Neurol. Sci., 125,* 29–38.

Xerri, C., Coq, J. O., Merzenich, M. M., and Jenkins, W. M. 1996. Experience-induced plasticity of cutaneous maps in the primary somatosensory cortex of adult monkeys and rats. *J. Physiol. Paris, 90,* 277–287.

Yamamoto, T., Uemura, T., and Llinas, R. 1992. Tonotopic organization of human auditory cortex revealed by multi-channel SQUID system. *Acta Otolaryngol., 112,* 201–204.

Yamamoto, T., Williamson, S. J., Kaufman, L., Nicholson, C., and Llinas, R. 1988. Magnetic localization of neuronal activity in the human brain. *Proceedings of the National Academy of Sciences USA, 85,* 8732–8736.

Yeterian, E. H., and Pandya, D. N. 1991. Corticothalamic connections of the superior temporal sulcus in rhesus monkeys. *Exp. Brain Res., 83,* 268–284.

Yeterian, E. H., and Pandya, D. N. 1995. Corticostriatal connections of extrastriate visual areas in rhesus monkeys. *Journal of Comparative Neurology, 352,* 436–457.

Yorke, C. H., Jr., and Caviness, V. S., Jr. 1975. Interhemispheric neocortical connections of the corpus callosum in the normal mouse: A study based on anterograde and retrograde methods. *Journal of Comparative Neurology, 164,* 233–245.

The Neurological Organization of Some Language-Processing Constituents

2

Edgar Zurif

My colleagues and I study aphasia to learn how the system for understanding natural language is neurologically organized. Our work is informed by a functional analysis of the normal system—a description of some of its components (broadly, those having to do with syntactic and semantic processing) and of the way in which these components, or modules, interact. This much is standard. Also standard: we take the specific deficits following focal brain damage to be explicable in terms of disruptions to one or more of these components.

What sets us apart from some other researchers, however, are the kinds of details that enter into our componential analysis and that support our inferences concerning "functional lesions." The difference turns on the way in which we isolate modules. Unlike other approaches, we do not license processing modules solely on the basis of formal linguistic theory. We do not distinguish, say, between a syntactic processing constituent and a semantic processing constituent simply because the representational formats they operate on are different. Rather, we seek evidence for the uniqueness of processing constituents in terms of their real-time fixed and mandatory operating characteristics.

The point here is that modules and their representations constitute evanescent, intermediate stages in the chain of comprehension; they are, therefore, most directly revealed by measurements taken during the brief course of their operation. And in line with this notion, we chart "functional lesions" in terms of alterations to their operating characteristics. In effect, we seek a functional layout of the comprehension system that is elaborated in real-time terms. This is one feature of our research program.

Another feature turns on neurological matters. In the first instance, we try to provide evidence that the effects of focal brain damage distinguish between modules, sparing one, disrupting another. In this way we check whether our theory is neurologically defensible. But we also seek data on the neuroanatomical layout of the system—on how the modules are geographically distributed.

Our connection to neuroanatomy is based on the fact that the aphasic syndromes we study—Broca's and Wernicke's for the most part—are distinguishable both clinically and with respect to lesion site. So, clinically, we can contrast, among many other things, the nonfluent telegraphic speech of Broca's aphasic patients and the fluent, rather empty speech of Wernicke's aphasic patients (Goodglass and Kaplan, 1972). And neuroanatomically, we can contrast the two syndromes along an anterior-posterior axis. Although variable, the generally large left inferior frontal cortical lesions associated with Broca's aphasia cluster about a modal site that is quite different from that for Wernicke's aphasia. For the latter, the greatest involvement appears to be confined to more posterior regions, implicating especially the posterior superior portion of temporal cortex. (For details see Benson, 1985; Vignolo, 1988; Naeser et al., 1989; Alexander et al., 1990.)

As will be seen, we capitalize on this difference. We show that the region associated with Broca's aphasia is crucial for some early syntactic business, but not for a later semantic operation. And we show just the opposite involvement for the region associated with Wernicke's aphasia.

Neuroanatomical Dissociations with Respect to Syntactic Processing

Syntactically Licensed Dependency Relations

The starting point here is that most aphasic patients have sentence-level comprehension impairments, particularly for noncanonical structures. Noncanonical structures are those in which the nounphrase (NP) preceding the verb is mapped not as the agent of the action, but rather as its theme (the entity acted upon). Such structures, it is claimed (see Chomsky, 1981), involve a particular kind of dependency relation. Consider, for example, the sentence, "It was the boy whom the girl chased." To interpret this sentence, the constituent "the boy" must be understood to be the direct object of the verb "chased" even though it is near the beginning of the sentence instead of after the verb. This is accountable by representing the direct object as having been "moved" from its position within the phrase headed by the verb. The claim is that the moved constituent (or "antecedent," as it is also termed) leaves an abstract trace in the vacated position and that it forms a dependency relation with the trace for the purpose of interpretation. In the example given, the constituent "the boy" gets assigned its role of "chasee" only indirectly, only by being coindexed to this abstract trace: it was (the boy)$_i$ whom the girl chased (t)$_i$. In effect, "the boy" is encountered before the verb but interpreted after it, at the trace position.

Within this theoretical framework, the Broca's patients' comprehension problem for noncanonical sentences has been described as an inability to represent traces and, in consequence, as an inability to assign thematic roles to moved constituents (see Grodzinsky, 1990; Hickok, Zurif, and Conseco-Gonzalez, 1993; Mauner, Fromkin, and Cornell 1993). The matter gets more complicated, however. Movement and syntactic dependencies involving traces exist even in canonical structures wherein the agent precedes the action. (It was the girl$_i$ who (t)$_i$ chased the boy.) And for structures of this sort, Broca's patients show good comprehension. Why should this be? Why should they understand canonical better than noncanonical forms when both involve movement?

The explanation given is that even for canonical structures—even for structures they understand—their comprehension is abnormally based on nongrammatical heuristics. An example is the agent-first strategy rooted to linear order (in contrast to grammatical hierarchization) and based on the statistical likelihood that agents precede themes in sentences. Assigning agency to the first encountered (unassigned) NP works for canonical structures that maintain this order even in the face of movement. But it does not work for noncanonical structures. (See Grodzinsky, 1990, 2000, for a detailed discussion of this matter.)

Comparable analyses have not appeared for Wernicke's patients. Although these patients, too, have considerable difficulty understanding noncanonical constructions, their problem does not appear to be so syntactically focused as it is in Broca's aphasia. It seems also to require a consideration of semantic factors. This is shown, for example, by the errors patients make in sentence-picture matching tasks: Wernicke's patients often choose semantically inappropriate foils (see Caramazza and Zurif, 1976; Heilman and Scholes, 1976), whereas Broca's display only syntactically based errors, that is, reversals in the assignment of agent and theme (see Caramazza and Zurif, 1976; Ansell and Flowers, 1982; Caplan and Futter, 1986; Wulfeck, 1988).

Syntactic Knowledge versus Syntactic Processing

The Broca's syntactic problem does not seem to reflect a loss of syntactic knowledge. For one thing, some Broca's patients have been observed to carry out quite complex syntactic judgments even though lacking the ability to exploit their grammatical sensitivity for comprehension purposes (Linebarger, Schwartz, and Saffran, 1983). Admittedly, this evidence is far from solid (Zurif and Grodzinsky, 1983; Grodzinsky and Finkel, 1998). But there is another, more persuasive argument against a knowledge limitation, namely, that the Broca's comprehension problem has sometimes been found to be relieved by relaxing various task demands—by repeating sentences and delivering them more slowly. So the knowledge seems to be there; the problem seems to be in accessing it. Accordingly, we have sought to account for the Broca's limitation in terms of a disruption to localizable processing resources necessary for implementing syntactic knowledge in real time. There are several steps to this account.

Lexical Activation

The first step has to do with lexical activation patterns quite apart from syntactic considerations. The data here are from priming experiments wherein lexical decisions are normally faster for target words when they are immediately preceded by semantically associated words than when preceded by unrelated words. This pattern is taken to indicate that the preceding word—the priming word—has been activated and that this activation, having spread within a semantic network including the target, has lowered the target's recognition threshold. But this pattern does not hold for Broca's patients. They do not show the normal pattern of faster word recognition in semantically facilitating contexts (Milberg and Blumstein, 1981; Prather, Zurif, Stern, and Rosen, 1992). But they are not completely insensitive to prime-target relations either. Rather, they show automatic priming in a temporally protracted way—they show a slower-than-normal activation pattern (Prather, Zurif, Stern, and Rosen, 1992; Prather, Zurif, Love, and Brownell, 1997).

Wernicke's patients, by contrast, show a roughly normal lexical activation pattern (Milberg and Blumstein, 1981; Swinney, Zurif, and Nicol, 1989).[1] And this sets up the next step, which has been to chart the way in which these different activation patterns play out at the sentence level, particularly with respect to the syntactic dependencies between moved constituents and their traces.

Gap-filling

A pertinent fact in this respect is that traces—or the empty positions (the gaps) indexed by traces—have real-time processing consequences. I refer to "gap-filling," the demonstration (based on priming patterns) that moved constituents or antecedents are reactivated at gaps—that intrasentence dependency relations involving antecedents and gaps are actually established as comprehension unfolds in real time (see Swinney and Fodor, 1989).

This effect has been observed many times and most often via a paradigm called cross-modal-lexical-priming (CMLP). In this paradigm a subject listens to and tries to understand a normally spoken sentence; moreover, while listening, the subject is also required to make a lexical (word/nonword) decision to a letter string (a "probe") flashed briefly on a computer monitor. The probe serves to indicate what words are activated at any particular time during the processing of the sentence. In this circumstance it is shown that a probe word related to the moved constituent gets primed not only immediately after the constituent is heard but again at the gap indexed by the trace. In effect, the moved constituent, by being activated when it is first heard and then by being *re*activated at the gap, serves as a prime for the probe in two locations. (See Swinney et al., 1996.)

As an example of how this works, consider the (notated) sentence, "The audience liked (the wrestler)$_i^a$ that the parish priest^b condemned (t)$_i^c$ for foul language" and its associated probes, "fighter" and "cleaner." "Fighter," of course, is related to the moved constituent "the wrestler," and "cleaner" is the control probe unrelated to any word in the sentence. A crucial fact is that the two probes are matched for reaction time as tested in a word list format in which lexical decisions are charted for individual words isolated from any sentence context. So, if while the sentence is being presented, lexical decisions take less time for the related probe "fighter" than for the control probe "cleaner," it can be inferred that the constituent "the wrestler" has been activated to serve as the prime for "fighter." As shown by the superscripts in the example, priming is usually examined just after hearing the antecedent (position a), at a pregap baseline position (position b), and at the gap indexed by the trace (position c). The baseline is important. It allows the experimenter to distinguish structurally governed reactivation at the gap site from any residual activation due simply to the earlier appearance of the antecedent. Accordingly, in the example, "fighter" is seen to prime (again, by contrast to "cleaner") at positions a and c, but not at position b. We therefore infer the existence of gap-filling—the *re*activation of the displaced constituent "the wrestler" at the trace position.

Gap-filling is an operation that must be implemented under strict time constraints—for relative clauses, the moved constituent must be reactivated as soon as the gap is encountered. After all, unlike lexical items, gaps do not provide a stable phonological form to serve temporally extended processing. What is more, slower-than-normal lexical activation may also diminish working memory capacity—that is, the capacity to keep the moved constituent in some sort of temporary memory buffer so that it *can* be reactivated. So given the patients' inability to make lexical information available in the normal time frame, we supposed that the syntactic reflex of gap-filling would be especially vulnerable for Broca's patients. And, indeed, this turned out to be the case. Just as Broca's patients fail to activate lexical information normally, so too do they fail to *re*activate lexical information at the normal time in the processing sequence—in time, that is, to fill gaps left by constituent movement (Swinney et al., 1996; Zurif et al., 1993).

Moreover, this failure applies only to the Broca's patients. Wernicke's patients, in line with their normal lexical activation patterns, show gap-filling in the normal manner (Swinney et al., 1996; Zurif et al., 1993). This Broca-Wernicke difference with respect to gap-filling has been observed in two experiments—one using canonical (subject-relative) sentences of the sort that Broca's patients, but not Wernicke's patients, routinely understand (Zurif et al., 1993); the other using noncanonical (object-relative) sentences that both groups have problems understanding (Swinney et al., 1996). Accordingly, Broca's patients do not form syntactic dependency relations, even for sentences that they can understand. Likely they rely on nongrammatical strategies as described earlier. In contrast, Wernicke's patients do implement syntactic dependencies in real time, even for sentences they do not understand.

Clearly, we have isolated an intermediate processing product, the sparing or disruption of which cannot be inferred just by examining comprehension end points.

Functional Neuroanatomy: First Pass

So far I have presented evidence that damage to the left inferior frontal brain region associated with Broca's aphasia disrupts the real-time formation of syntactic dependency relations in a manner that posterior damage associated with Wernicke's aphasia does not. I have also presented evidence to suggest that the failure of this syntactic operation following left anterior damage can be linked to a rather elemental disruption of lexical activation. And from the perspective of this connection, we begin to see that the brain region implicated in Broca's aphasia need not be the locus of syntactic representations per se, but instead might be involved only insofar as it provides the general resources that sustain lexical information activation.

I have suggested that these resources are necessary for the normal speed of activation (and reactivation) of information. But there are other possibilities. The resources might have to do with establishing absolute activation levels (Milberg et al., 1995)—lower levels easily being reflected as slower-than-normal activation rise times. Or they might have to do with memory storage, even if only as an indirect consequence of the burden imposed upon storage by slower-than-normal lexical activation. Another possibility is that the brain area associated with Broca's aphasia sustains elementary activation parameters and working memory separately. But all of these possibilities have a point in common: in each, a syntactic limitation stateable in the abstract terms of linguistic theory can be linked to changes in localizable processing resources—resources that depend upon the integrity of anterior but not posterior cortical regions.

Neuroanatomical Dissociations with Respect to Semantic Processing

Actually, little is known about the functional commitment of the left posterior cortical region associated with Wernicke's aphasia. Clinical and experimental observations, mostly at the word level, suggest that Wernicke's aphasic patients have a semantic impairment not observed in Broca's aphasics (see, for example, Goodglass and Kaplan, 1972). But it is clear that Wernicke's patients also have sentence comprehension problems that are not accountable by reference to single-word comprehension levels.

Accordingly, we have been trying to explore the Wernicke's problem—and thereby a function of left posterior cortex—at the level of *combinatorial* semantic operations. This level incorporates considerations of both lexical semantics and syntactic composition. It is the level at which both kinds of information are brought into correspondence to create the interpretation of a sentence. The operation that we have been focusing upon is one that mediates this correspondence.

Aspectual Coercion

This mediating operation is termed "aspectual coercion" (Moens and Steedman, 1987; Pustejovsky, 1995; Jackendoff, 1997). It is purely semantic in nature (that is, it is not syntactically encoded) and its purpose is to make elements within a verb phrase agree in their intrinsic temporal constraints.

Consider the contrast between "The girl slept until dawn" and "The girl jumped until dawn." The interpretation of the first of these two sentences is obtained straightforwardly via simple syntactic composition. "The girl" (subject) is performing an activity "sleep" for the period of time indicated by the phrase "until dawn." Interpretation is syntactically transparent. However, this is not the case for the second of the two sentences. The interpretation we retrieve from this sentence is that the girl jumped *repeatedly* until dawn. And this meaning does not come either from "jump" or from "until dawn"; nor is it signaled by any morpho-syntactic means. Yet the sense of repetition cannot be avoided—a phenomenon that, following Jackendoff (1997), we refer to as "enriched composition."

Different explanations have been offered for this phenomenon. Jackendoff (1997) and Pustejovsky (1995) have both opted for generative systems wherein lexical entries with detailed internal structures can generate different senses when combined with one another. Others (for example, Klein and Sag, 1985) have attributed (via a "type-shifting" operation) a derived status to the iterative versions of lexical entries. Importantly, however, both explanations converge on the distinction drawn here between syntactically transparent sentences and sentences requiring enriched composition: both treat aspectual coercion as a nonsyntactic phenomenon requiring some sort of semantic operation.[2]

Real-time Processing

Our first step was to isolate this combinatorial semantic operation during the course of normal sentence processing. We have recently completed an on-line study of aspectual coercion in which college-age subjects were tested on sentences of the following sort: "The little girl dived in the pool until the teacher told her to eat if she wanted to keep her strength up" versus "The little girl dogpaddled in the pool until the teacher told her . . ." As with the earlier example, the first sentence requires enriched composition; it must be interpreted to involve a repetition of dives. The second sentence, by contrast, does not require the notion of repetition—"dogpaddle" is lexically codified as an ongoing process, so word meanings can be combined in a syntactically transparent way.

To isolate the enriched composition operation required in the first sentence, we used a dual-task interference paradigm. In this situation, a subject listens to a sentence over earphones and at one point, while listening to the sentence, must make a lexical decision for a visually presented letter string. This paradigm, like the CMLP paradigm we use for our syntactic work, is cross-modal. But the two differ in a very important respect. In CMLP, the visual probe word is associated with—and is primed by—a word in the sentence (the moved constituent). By contrast, in the dual task interference situation, the probe is *not* related to anything in the sentence. Rather in the latter paradigm, the lexical decision task and the primary task of trying to understand the sentence are assumed to *compete* for resources. Accordingly, if sentence comprehension requires an extra operation of enriched composition, the secondary lexical decision task should have fewer available resources and take longer to perform, compared with when comprehension is syntactically transparent.

In our use of the paradigm, we placed the probe 250 msec after the temporally bounding word (or phrase if necessary)—specifically, 250 msec after "until" in each of the above sentences. We chose this temporal point because semantic processes seem to be active then (Shapiro and Levine, 1990; McElree and Griffith, 1995). And we chose correctly. Gaining data from neurologically intact young adults, we discovered that the decision times for probes associated with "enriched" sentences were greater than for probes associated with syntactically transparent sentences. In effect, we discovered the "cost" of an independent nonsyntactic compositional process—a process rooted to a generative lexicon (Piñango, Zurif, and Jackendoff, 1999).

Semantic Composition in Aphasia

We have yet to carry out a comparable on-line study with aphasic patients. We do, however, have some off-line data. Specifically, we have some data on aphasic comprehension that directly implicate the enriched versus syntactically transparent distinction and, what is more, do so in a manner that begins to suggest a double dissociation—a specific semantic role for left posterior cortex that can be set against the syntactic role earlier charted for left anterior cortex.

The study is ongoing. Here are some of its details. The task requires patients to answer a binary-choice question for each sentence presented. For example, for the sentence, "The tiger jumped for an hour," we contrast "Did the tiger jump only one time?" (the incorrect choice) with "Did the tiger jump time and time again?" (the correct choice). This, of course, is an example of a sentence requiring enriched composition. Its syntactically transparent counterpart is "The tiger jumped over the tree," and again, the contrast is between "Did the tiger jump only one time?" and "Did the tiger jump time and time again?" In this way, we contrast an enriched versus a syntactically transparent condition by using the same verb placed in two different contexts.

To date we have tested three Broca's patients and three Wernicke's patients. And the data are impressively straightforward. The Broca's patients performed well on both the transparent and the nontransparent sentences. The Wernicke's patients did well only on the transparent sentences; indeed, they had more than twice the number of errors for the syntactically nontransparent sentences than for their transparent counterparts (Piñango and Zurif, 1998).

It is a slim data base, but an encouraging one for the various notions expressed here. The Broca's patients' ability to deal with the requirement of semantic composition is to be expected. These patients have a sentence comprehension problem only in the total absence of semantic constraints, not when more semantic work is required. This makes sense given that the Broca's problem seems to be with the speed of information activation: since semantic composition is temporally less demanding than syntactic gap-filling (see McElree and Griffith, 1995), a delay in the availability of lexical information sufficient to disrupt the syntactic reflex need not also affect the semantic operation.

As for Wernicke's patients, the data begin to explain their variable sentence-level semantic problem. The data suggest that at least some of this variability may be accounted for in terms of whether sentence interpretation can be carried out in a syntactically transparent fashion or whether it requires the extra step of semantic combination. The Wernicke's comprehension seems to be particularly vulnerable in the latter circumstance—that is, for sentences requiring the extra computation associated with enriched composition.

Conclusion: A Second Pass at Functional Neuroanatomy

It has become increasingly clear that the brain area associated with Broca's aphasia is crucial for at least one early-stage syntactic operation. Thus many of the sentence-level comprehension problems found in Broca's aphasia can be viewed as reflections of the failure to form the linked-element syntactic structures that support semantic inference.

But the system of semantic inference, itself, does not seem affected after left inferior frontal brain damage. Rather the semantic system seems to rely on the integrity of posterior brain regions—particularly the posterior superior temporal area associated with Wernicke's aphasia. Moreover, our data suggest that at least one part of this posterior semantic system has to do with compositional operations—operations that come into play at the syntactic-semantic interface when interpretation is not syntactically transparent. Again, the data are scanty on this point. But they encourage us to continue to study the semantic system within its proper ecological niche, that is, in terms of the operations involved in combining word meanings into contextualized interpretations.

Notes

The writing of this chapter and much of the research reported in it were supported by NIH grants DC02984, DC03660, and DC00081.

1. The fact that Wernicke's patients show the normal pattern of faster word recognition in semantically facilitating contexts should not be interpreted as indicating that these patients are entirely normal in accessing word meaning. Although these data suggest normal initial contact with lexical representations, they do not rule out the possibility of "course-coding" (Beeman et al., 1994) and therefore of a less-than-normally precise apprehension of a word's meaning.
2. Aspectual coercion is not the only form of enriched composition. There appear to be a variety of such cases that, together, cannot be dismissed as a series of exceptions to syntactic transparency. Rather, these cases point to a phenomenon that must somehow be accommodated at the syntax-semantics interface.

References

Alexander, M., Naeser, M. A., and Palumbo, C. L. 1990. Broca's area aphasias: Aphasia after lesions including the frontal operculum. *Neurology, 40,* 353–362.

Ansell, B., and Flowers, C. 1982. Aphasic adults' use of heuristic and structural linguistic cues for analysis. *Brain and Language, 26,* 62–72.

Beeman, M., Friedman, R., Grafman, J., Perez, E., Diamond, S., and Lindsay, M. 1994. Summation priming and coarse semantic coding in the right hemisphere. *Journal of Cognitive Neuroscience, 6,* 26–45.

Benson, D. F. 1985. Aphasia. In *Clinical neuropsychology,* vol. 2, ed. K. Heilman and E. Valenstein. New York: Oxford University Press.

Caplan, D., and Futter, C. 1986. Assignment of thematic roles by an agrammatic aphasic patient. *Brain and Language 27,* 117–135.

Caramazza, A., and Zurif, E. B. 1976. Dissociation of algorithmic and heuristic processes in language comprehension: Evidence from aphasia. *Brain and Language, 3,* 572–582.

Chomsky, N. 1981. *Lectures on government and binding.* Dordrecht: Foris.

Goodglass, H., and Kaplan, E. 1972. *The assessment of aphasia and related disorders.* Philadelphia: Lea and Febiger.

Grodzinsky, Y. 1990. *Theoretical perspectives on language deficits.* Cambridge: MIT Press.

——— 2000. The neurology of syntax. *Behavioral and Brain Sciences, 23*(1).

Grodzinsky, Y., and Finkel, L. 1998. The neurology of empty categories: Aphasics' failure to detect ungrammaticality. *Journal of Cognitive Neuroscience, 10,* 281–292.

Heilman, K., and Scholes, R. 1976. The nature of comprehension errors in Broca's conduction and Wernicke's aphasic patients. *Cortex, 12,* 258–265.

Hickock, G., Zurif, E. B., and Canseco-Gonzalez, E. 1993. Structural description of agrammatic comprehension. *Brain and Language, 45,* 371–395.

Jackendoff, R. 1997. *The architecture of the language faculty.* Cambridge: MIT Press.

Klein, E., and Sag, I. 1985. Type-driven translation. *Linguistics and Philosophy, 8,* 163–202.

Lineberger, M., Schwartz, M., and Saffran, E. 1983. Sensitivity to grammatical structure in so-called agrammatic aphasics. *Cognition, 13,* 361–393.

Mauner, G., Fromkin, V., and Cornell, T. 1993. Comprehension and acceptability judgments in agrammatism: Disruption in the syntax of referential dependency and the two-chain hypothesis, *Brain and Language, 45,* 340–370.

McElree, B., and Griffith, T. 1995. Syntactic and thematic processing in sentence comprehension: Evidence for a temporal dissociation. *Journal of Experimental Psychology: Learning, Memory, and Cognition, 21,* 134–157.

Milberg, W., and Blumstein, S. 1981. Lexical decision and aphasia: Evidence for semantic processing. *Brain and Language, 14,* 371–385.

Milberg, W., Blumstein, S., Katz, D., Gershberg, E., and Brown, T. 1995. Semantic facilitation in aphasia: Effects of time and expectancy. *Journal of Cognitive Neuroscience, 7,* 33–50.

Moens, M., and Steedman, M. 1987. Temporal ontology in natural language. *Proceedings of the 25th ACL meeting.* Stanford University, Stanford, Calif.

Naeser, M. A., Palumbo, C., Helm-Estabrooks, N., Stiassny-Eder, D., and Albert, M. 1989. Severe non-fluency in aphasia: Role of the medial subcollosal fasciculus and other white-matter pathways in recovery of spontaneous speech. *Brain, 112,* 1–38.

Piñango, M. M., Zurif, E. B., and Jackendoff, R. 1999. Real time processing implications of enriched composition at the syntax-semantics interface. *Journal of Psycholinguistic Research, 28,* 395–414.

Piñango, M. M., and Zurif, E. B. 1998. The cortical layout of language. Manuscript. Brandeis University.

Prather, P., Zurif, E. B., Stern, C., and Rosen, T. J. 1992. Slowed lexical access in non-fluent aphasia. *Brain and Language, 43,* 336–348.

Prather, P., Zurif, E. B., Love, T., and Brownell, H. 1997. Speed of lexical activation in nonfluent Broca's aphasia and fluent Wernicke's aphasia. *Brain and Language, 59,* 391–411.

Pustejovsky, J. 1995. *The generative lexicon.* Cambridge: MIT Press.

Shapiro, L., and Levine, B. 1990. Verb processing during sentence comprehension in aphasia. *Brain and Language, 38,* 21–47.

Swinney, D., and Fodor, J. A., eds. 1989. Special issue on sentence processing. *Journal of Psycholinguistic Research, 18*(1), 1–85.

Swinney, D., Zurif, E. B., and Nicol, J. 1989. The effects of focal brain damage on sentence processing: An examination of the neurological organization of a mental module. *Journal of Cognitive Neuroscience, 1,* 25–37.

Swinney, D., Zurif, E. B., Prather, P., and Love, T. 1996. Neurological distribution of processing resources underlying language comprehension. *Journal of Cognitive Neuroscience, 8,* 174–184.

Vignolo, L. 1988. The anatomical and pathological basis of aphasia. In *Aphasia,* ed. F. C. Rose, R. Whurr, and M. A. Wyke. London: Whurr.

Wulfeck, B. 1988. Grammaticality judgments and sentence comprehension in agrammatic aphasia. *Journal of Speech and Hearing Research, 31,* 72–81.

Zurif, E. B., and Grodzinsky, Y. 1983. Sensitivity to grammatical structure in agrammatic aphasics: A reply to Linebarger, Schwartz, and Saffran. *Cognition, 15,* 207–213.

Zurif, E., Swinney, D., Prather, P., Solomon, J., and Bushell, C. 1993. An online analysis of syntactic processing in Broca's and Wernicke's aphasia. *Brain and Language, 45,* 448–464.

Brain Organization for Syntactic Processing 3

David Caplan, Nathaniel Alpert, and Gloria Waters

The ability to assign the syntactic structure of a sentence and to use it to determine the semantic relationships between the words in the sentence (the sentence's propositional content) is central to normal comprehension of language. The syntactic structure of a sentence is the principal determinant of how the meanings of the words in a sentence are related to each other (Chomsky, 1965, 1981, 1986, 1995), and there is near universal agreement that, when normal language users understand sentences, they construct syntactic structures as part of this process (Frazier and Rayner, 1982; Bates et al., 1982; Bates, Friederici, and Wulfeck, 1987; Clifton and Ferreira, 1987; Frazier, 1987a,b, 1989, 1990; Bates and MacWhinney, 1989; MacWhinney, 1989; McClelland, St. John, and Taraban, 1989; Frazier and Clifton, 1989, 1996; Just and Carpenter, 1992; Trueswell, Tanenhaus, and Kello, 1993; MacDonald, Pearlmutter, and Seidenberg, 1994; Pearlmutter and MacDonald, 1995). In this chapter we review studies in our lab using positron emission tomography (PET) that investigate the neural basis for this function.

Methods

All studies reported here used the plausibility judgment task. In this task, the subject either read or listened to a sentence and made a speeded decision as to whether it was plausible (made sense) or not. In the activation condition, sentences that are syntactically more complex were presented; in the baseline condition, sentences that are less complex were presented. In all experiments, implausible sentences were rendered implausible by virtue of an incompatibility between the animacy or humanness features of a noun phrase and the requirements of a verb, as in the example *The book enjoyed the boy.* Therefore, plausibility judgments did not depend upon subjects searching semantic memory for obscure facts but could be made on the basis of readily available semantic information.

In all experiments, sentences were blocked by syntactic type, as is required by the PET technique. To reduce the possibility that subjects might habituate to more complex structures or develop nonsyntactic strategies to make judgments regarding the status of a sentence in these blocks, we varied the animacy of nouns in grammatical positions in the sentences. The more and less complex sentences contained the same words and expressed the same content, so that differences in lexical items and propositional meaning were not responsible for any regional cerebral blood flow (rCBF) effects. All nouns were common and were preceded by definite articles so as to make the same referential assumptions in the more and less complex syntactic conditions. The point of implausibility was varied throughout the implausible sentences of each syntactic type to force subjects to read or listen to each sentence in its entirety to make a judgment that it was plausible. Implausibility points were slightly earlier on average in the more complex sentences, biasing against the simple forms benefiting from the use of a strategy that judges a sentence to be acceptable when a certain point in the sentence had passed. All experiments in the PET scanner were preceded by behavioral testing in the psychology lab to ensure that there was behavioral evidence in the form of longer reaction times (RTs) and sometimes more errors that the more complex sentences were indeed more complex, and these measurements were repeated in the PET environment to be sure that these differences obtained there.

Subjects in all experiments were strongly right-handed and had no first-degree left-handed relatives. All had normal vision and hearing, and no history of neurological or psychiatric disease.

PET techniques were ones in widespread use. PET data were acquired on a General Electric Scanditronix PC4096 15-slice whole-body tomograph in its stationary mode in contiguous slices with center-to-center distance of 6.5 mm (axial field equal to 97.5 mm) and axial resolution of 6.0 mm FWHM, with a Hanning-weighted reconstruction filter set to yield 8.0 mm in-plane spatial resolution. Subjects' heads were restrained in a custom-molded thermoplastic face mask, and aligned relative to the cantho-meatal line, using horizontal and vertical projected laser lines. Subjects inhaled $^{15}O\text{-}CO_2$ gas by nasal cannulae within a face mask for 90 seconds, reaching terminal count rates of 100,000 to 200,000 events per second. Each PET data acquisition run consisted of twenty measurements, the first three of 10 seconds' duration and the remaining seventeen of 5 seconds' duration each. Scans 4–16 were summed after reconstruction to form images of relative blood flow. The summed images from each subject were realigned using the first scan as the reference using a least-squares fitting technique (Alpert et al., 1996). Spatial normalization to the coordinate system of Talairach and Tournoux (1988) was performed by deforming the contour of the 10 mm parasagittal PET slice to match the corresponding slice of the reference brain (Alpert et al., 1993). Following spatial normalization, scans were filtered with a two-dimensional Gaussian filter, full width at half maximum set to 20 mm. Data were analyzed with SPM95 (Friston et al., 1991, 1995; Worsely et al., 1992).

Experiments with Young Subjects Using Relative Clauses

In the first set of experiments, we contrasted more complex subject-object (SO) sentences (for example, *The juice that the child spilled stained the rug*) with less complex object-subject (OS) sentences (for example, *The child spilled the juice that stained the rug*). There is considerable behavioral evidence that SO sentences are more demanding of processing resources than OS sentences (Waters, Caplan, and Hildebrandt, 1987; King and Just, 1991). The higher demands made by the SO sentence are thought to be related to maintaining the head noun of a relative clause in memory while the relative clause is bring structured, computing the syntactic structure of the relative clause, relating the head noun of the relative clause to a syntactic position in the relative clause, relating the head noun of the relative clause to its position as the subject of the main clause, and interpreting the resulting syntactic structure semantically (Just and Carpenter, 1992; Gibson, 1997).

Eight male subjects (ages 19–28) participated in Experiment 1a (Stromswold et al., 1996). Behavioral results (visual presentation) are shown below:

	Subject object	Object subject
Mean RT (msec)	4,230	3,719

PET results for Experiment 1a, indicating areas of increased rCBF, were:

Location	Max Z-score	Number of pixels	Location (X,Y,Z)
Broca's area pars opercularis	2.7	131	–46, 5, 9.8, 4.0

There was an increase in rCBF in the pars opercularis of Broca's area when PET activity associated with OS sentences was subtracted from that associated with SO sentences.

Experiment 1b (Caplan, Alpert, and Waters, 1998) was a replication of this study with eight female subjects, aged 21–31. Behavioral results (visual presentation):

	Subject object	Object subject
Percentage correct	90.5	94.4
Mean RT (sd) in msec	2,886 (1,119)	2,548 (1,011)

PET results:

Location	Max Z-score	Number of pixels	Location (X,Y,Z)
Medial frontal gyrus	3.8	131	10, 6, 52
Cingulate gyrus	3.5	173	–2, 6, 40
Broca's area, pars opercularis	3.0	47	–42, 18, 24

There again was an increase in rCBF in the pars opercularis of Broca's area when PET activity associated with OS sentences was subtracted from that associated with SO sentences. There was also activation in the medial frontal and cingulate gyri.

Experiment 2 (Caplan, Alpert, and Waters, 1999) was a replication of this study with auditory presentation. Sentences in condition 1 consisted of cleft-object sentences (for example, *It was the juice that the child enjoyed*), and sentences in condition 2 consisted of cleft-subject sentences (for example, *It was the child that enjoyed the juice*). We used cleft-object and cleft-subject sentences instead of the subject-object and object-subject sentences used in the previous research because preliminary testing of SO and OS sentences presented auditorily failed to demonstrate differences in RTs for end-of-sentence plausibility judgments. This is probably because the demands made by the embedded clause in SO sentences are over by the end of the sentence, when the judgment is made. The cleft-object and cleft-subject sentences make the same contrast between object and subject relativization that the contrast between SO and OS sentences makes.

Sixteen subjects, eight male and eight female, ages 22–34, were tested in Experiment 2. Behavioral results (auditory presentation):

	Cleft object		Cleft subject	
	Plausible	Implausible	Plausible	Implausible
Mean percentage errors/subject	18.1	7.5	14.7	7.6
Mean RT (sd) in msec	3,635 (255)	3,717 (268)	3,465 (277)	3,545 (202)

PET results:

Location	Max Z-score	Number of pixels	Location (X,Y,Z)
Medial frontal gyrus	4.0	317	–2, 18, 48
Superior parietal lobe	3.3	97	–18, –48, 44
Broca's area pars triangularis	3.1	48	–52, 18, 24

There was an increase in rCBF in the pars triangularis of Broca's area when PET activity associated with cleft-subject sentences was subtracted from that associated with cleft-object sentences. There was also activation in the medial frontal gyrus and in the left superior parietal area.

Experiment 3 (Caplan et al., 2000) investigated the possibility that the increases in rCBF in Broca's area in Experiments 1 and 2 were due to increased rehearsal associated with the more complex sentences. Broca's area is involved in rehearsal (Démonet et al., 1996), so this possibility must be considered. To address this issue, we repeated Experiment 1 under conditions of concurrent articulation. Concurrent articulation engages the articulatory loop and prevents its use for rehearsal (Baddeley, Thomson, and Buchanan, 1975). If the rCBF increase in Broca's area continued to be found under these conditions, it was highly likely that it would be due at least in part to abstract psycholinguistic operations, not just to more rehearsal associated with the more complex sentences.

Eleven subjects, five male and six female, aged 19–35, were tested in Experiment 3. Behavioral results (written presentation with concurrent articulation):

	Object subject		Subject object	
	Plausible	Implausible	Plausible	Implausible
Mean percentage errors/subject	7.8	7.8	18.3	12.2
Mean RT (sd) in msec	4,373 (1,215)	4,237 (1,176)	5,168 (1,683)	5,215 (1,685)

PET results:

Location	Max Z-score	Number of pixels	Location (X,Y,Z)
Broca's area (Brodmann 45)	3.6	112	–46, 36, 4
Left thalamus (centromedian nucleus)	3.4	62	–14, –20, 4
Cingulate gyrus (Brodmann 31)	3.4	158	–10, –36, 40
Medial frontal gyrus (Brodmann 10)	3.2	113	0, 56, 8

There was an increase in rCBF in the pars opercularis of Broca's area when PET activity associated with OS sentences was subtracted from that associated with SO sentences. There were also increases in rCBF in the dorsomedial nucleus of the left thalamus, the posterior cingulate, and the medial frontal gyrus.

These four experiments all showed activation in Broca's area associated with more complex relative clauses. This activation persisted under concurrent articulation conditions. This suggests that Broca's area is the primary locus of some aspect of syntactic processing associated with structuring relative clauses that is more resource-demanding in object- than in subject-relativized structures. No other language regions were activated in these experiments. CBF was also increased in medial frontal lobe structures in several experiments, and in the centromedian nucleus of the left thalamus in the articulatory suppression experiment, possibly the result of a non-domain-specific arousal and directed attention associated with increases in mental effort (Posner et al., 1987, 1988).

Experiments with Young Subjects Using Active and Passive Sentences

Experiment 4 studied the rCBF changes associated with making judgments about passive versus active sentences. Passive sentences are more complex syntactically than active sentences because their structure is more elaborate and the relationship between thematic roles and grammatical positions is noncanonical for English. To control for length, we used both full passive sentences *(The car was admired by the boy)* and truncated passives *(The car was admired)* to compare with the active sentences *(The boy admired the car)*. The sentences were presented auditorily. Behavioral results for Experiment 4 (auditory presentation):

	Active		Passive	
	Plausible	Implausible	Plausible	Implausible
Mean RT in msec taken from end of sentence or point of anomaly	560	809	617	1,051

RTs were longer for passive than for active sentences. However, there were no reliable differences in rCBF associated with processing these two types of sentences. The implication of this study, in combination with the previous ones, is that all syntactic contrasts do not provoke the same patterns of rCBF increases. This suggests a different internal organization of language-devoted cortex for different syntactic operations.

Experiments with Elderly Subjects Using Relative Clauses

In the final experiment (Caplan, Waters, and Alpert, under review), we replicated the Stromswold et al. (1996) and Caplan, Alpert, and Waters (1998) experiment with thirteen elderly subjects, aged 61–70. Behavioral results for Experiment 5 (written presentation) were:

	Subject object		Object subject	
	Plausible	Implausible	Plausible	Implausible
Mean percentage errors/subject	7.9	16.2	7.9	7.0
Mean RT (sd) in msec	4,877(1,859)	5,279(1,867)	4,485(1,619)	4,716(1,772)

PET results:

Location	Max Z-score	Number of pixels	Location (W,Y,Z)
Inferior parietal lobe (area 40)	3.77	127	−54, −32, 32
Superior frontal gyrus	3.10	73	−22, 56, 8

Unlike the young subjects studied in Stromswold et al. (1996) and Caplan, Alpert, and Waters (1998, 1999), there was no increase in rCBF in Broca's area, but rather in the inferior parietal lobe. There was also an increase in rCBF near the midline of the superior frontal gyrus.

Discussion

The results of these studies reveal localized increases in rCBF in a variety of locations when subjects made judgments about the plausibility of syntactically more complex sentences with object-relativized relative clauses compared with when they made such judgments about syntactically less complex sentences with subject-relativized relative clauses. These increases in rCBF can be divided into several groups:

1. Increases in rCBF in Broca's area. This was found in all experiments with young people. It suggests that this region is the primary site of some aspect(s) of processing relative clauses in this population. The relevant aspects are unknown but are likely to be related to maintaining the head noun of a relative clause in a working memory system while its role in the relative clause (and possibly in the main clause) is established.

2. Increases in rCBF in other "language" areas and not in Broca's area. This was seen in elderly subjects, suggesting a reorganization of the brain for this aspect of syntactic processing as a function of age. It should be noted that the elderly subjects performed more slowly and less accurately than the young subjects, and that this different localization may reflect differences in syntactic processing ability, not age per se. This will require additional experimentation with subjects matched for one of these factors who vary on the second.

3. Increases in rCBF in midline frontal and thalamic structures. This was found in Experiments 1b (written presentation, young females), 2 (auditory presentation, young males and females), 3 (written presentation with concurrent articulation, young males and females), and 5 (written presentation, elderly males and females). This activation has been attributed to non-domain-specific functions such as arousal and deployment of attention. Of note is that it was often found in more superior structures in these studies than has been the case in previous work, raising questions about its interpretation.

4. Other increases in rCBF. There was one other increase in rCBF in the high parietal lobe in Experiment 2 that is unaccounted for.

5. No increases in rCBF. We found that contrasting active and passive sentences was not associated with reliable changes in rCBF despite the presence of behavioral effects in this experiment.

Overall, these results suggest a brain organization for syntactic processing in which:

1. Different syntactic structures activate brain regions in different ways; compare the difference between relative clauses and the active/passive contrast.

2. There is a preferred site for some aspects of syntactic processing. In young subjects, this appears to be Broca's area for some aspect of the processing of relative clauses.

3. This preferred site may differ in different groups of subjects. For the processing of relative clauses, this site appears to vary as a function of age and/or processing efficiency, but not as a function of sex in young subjects. Whether other factors such as handedness affect it is unknown.

4. Regions of the brain involved in arousal, attention, and motivation sometimes become active during more complex syntactic processing.

These conclusions are highly tentative, and require more research to validate or modify. The research does, however, demonstrate that activation studies of syntactic processing using highly structured materials can yield interpretable results that can form the basis for theory development in this area.

References

This work was supported by grants from NIH (DC02146 and AG09661).

Alpert, N., Berdichevsky, D., Weise, S., Tang, J., and Rauch, S. 1993. Stereotactic transformation of PET scans by nonlinear least squares. In *Quantifications of brain functions: Tracer kinetics and image analysis in brain PET,* ed. K. Uemura, 459–463. Amsterdam: Elsevier Science Publishers, B.V.

Alpert, N. M., Berdichevsky, D., Levin, Z., Morris, E. D., and Faschman, A. J. 1996. Improved methods for image registration. *NeuroImage, 3,* 10–18.

Baddeley, A. D., Thomson, N., and Buchanan, M. 1975. Word length and the structure of short-term memory. *Journal of Verbal Learning and Verbal Behavior, 14,* 575–589.

Bates, E., and MacWhinney, B. 1989. Functionalism and the competition model. In *A Cross-Linguistic Study of Sentence Processing,* ed. B.M.a.E. Bates, 3–73. Cambridge: Cambridge University Press.

Bates, E., McNew, S., MacWhinney, B., Devescovi, A., and Smith, S. 1982. Functional constraints on sentence processing. *Cognition, 11,* 245–299.

Bates, E., Friederici, A., and Wulfeck, B. 1987. Comprehension in aphasia: A cross-linguistic study. *Brain and Language, 32,* 19–67.

Caplan, D., Alpert, N., and Waters, G. S. 1998. Effects of syntactic structure and propositional number on patterns of regional cerebral blood flow. *Journal of Cognitive Neuroscience, 10,* 541–552.

——— 1999. PET studies of syntactic processing with auditory sentence presentation. *NeuroImage, 9,* 343–351.

Caplan, D., Alpert, N., Waters, G. S., and Olivieri, A. 2000. Activation of Broca's area by syntactic processing under conditions of concurrent articulation. *Human Brain Mapping, 9,* 65–71.

Caplan, D., and Waters, G. In press. Verbal working memory and sentence comprehension. *Behavioral and Brain Sciences.*

Caplan, D. Waters, G. S., and Alpert, N. Under review c. Localization of syntactic comprehension by positron emission tomography in elderly subjects.

Chomsky, N. 1965. *Aspects of the theory of syntax.* Cambridge: MIT Press.

——— 1981. *Lectures on government and binding.* Dordrecht: Foris.

——— 1986. *Knowledge of language.* New York: Praeger.

——— 1995. *Barriers.* Cambridge: MIT Press.

Clifton, C., and Ferreira, F. 1987. Modularity in sentence comprehension. In *Modularity in knowledge representation and natural-language understanding,* ed. J. L. Garfield, 277–290. Cambridge: MIT Press.

Démonet, J. F., Fiez, J. A., Paulesu, E., Peterson, S. E., and Zatorre, R. J. 1996. PET Studies of Phonological Processing: A Critical Reply to Poeppel. *Brain and Language, 55,* 352–379.

Frazier, L. 1987a. Sentence processing: A tutorial review. In *Attention and performance XII: The psychology of reading,* ed. M. Coltheart, 559–586. London: Lawrence Erlbaum Associates.

——— 1987b. Theories of sentence processing. In *Modularity in knowledge representation and natural-language understanding,* ed. J. Garfield, 291–307. Cambridge: MIT Press.

——— 1989. Against lexical generation of syntax. In *Lexical representation and process,* ed. W. Marslen-Wilson, 505–528. Cambridge: MIT Press.

——— 1990. Exploring the architecture of the language-processing system. In *Cognitive models of speech processing: Psycholinguistic and computational perspectives,* ed. G. T. M. Altmann, 409–433. Cambridge: MIT Press.

Frazier, L., and Clifton, C. 1989. Successive cyclicity in the grammar and the parser. *Language and Cognitive Processes, 4,* 93–126.

——— 1996. *Construal.* Cambridge: MIT Press.

Frazier, L., and Rayner, K. 1982. Making and correcting errors during sentence comprehension: Eye movements in the analysis of structurally ambiguous sentences. *Cognitive Psychology, 14,* 178–210.

Friston, K. J., Frith, C. D., Liddle, P. F., and Frackowiak, R. S. J. 1991. Comparing functional (PET) images: The assessment of significant change. *Journal of Cerebral Blood Flow and Metabolism, 11,* 690–699.

Friston, K. J., Holmes, A. P., Worsley, K. J., Poline, J. B., Frith, C. D., and Frackowiak, R. S. J. 1995. Statistical parametric maps in functional imaging: A general approach. *Human Brain Mapping, 2,* 189–210.

Gibson, E. 1997. Syntactic complexity: Locality of syntactic dependencies. Manuscript.

Just, M. A., and Carpenter, P. A. 1992. A capacity theory of comprehension: Individual differences in working memory. *Psychological Review, 99*(1), 122–149.

King, J., and Just, M. A. 1991. Individual differences in syntactic processing: The role of working memory. *Journal of Memory and Language, 30,* 580–602.

MacDonald, M. C., Pearlmutter, N. J., and Seidenberg, M. S. 1994. Lexical nature of syntactic ambiguity resolution. *Psychological Review, 101,* 676–703.

MacWhinney, B. 1989. Competition and connectionism. In *A Cross-Linguistic Study of Sentence Processing,* ed. B.M.a.E. Bates, 422–457. Cambridge: Cambridge University Press.

McClelland, J. L., St. John, M., and Taraban, R. 1989. Sentence comprehension: A parallel distributed processing approach. *Language and Cognitive Processes, 4,* 287–336.

Pearlmutter, N., and MacDonald, M. 1995. Individual differences and probabilistic constraints in syntactic ambiguity resolution. *Journal of Memory and Language, 34*(4), 521–542.

Posner, M. I., Inhoff, A. W., Friedrich, F. J., and Cohen, A. 1987. Isolating attentional systems: A cognitive-anatomical analysis. *Psychobiology, 15*(2), 107–121.

Posner, M. I., Peterson, S. E., Fox, P. T., and Raichle, M. E. 1988. Localization of cognitive operations in the human brain. *Science, 240,* 1627–1631.

Stromswold, K., Caplan, D., Alpert, N., and Rauch, S. 1996. Localization of syntactic comprehension by positron emission tomography. *Brain and Language, 52,* 452–473.

Talairach, J., and Tournoux, P. 1988. *Coplanar stereotaxic atlas of the human brain.* New York: Thieme Medical Publishers.

Trueswell, J. C., Tanenhaus, M. K., and Kello, C. 1993. Verb-specific constraints in sentence processing: Separating effects of lexical preference from garden-paths. *Journal of Experimental Psychology: Learning, Memory, and Cognition, 19,* 528–553.

Waters, G., Caplan, D., and Hildebrandt, N. 1987. Working memory and written sentence comprehension. In *Attention and Performance XII,* ed. M. Coltheart, 531–555. London: Erlbaum.

Worsley, K. J., Evans, A. C., Marrett, S., and Neelin, P. 1992. A three-dimensional statistical analysis for rCBF activation studies in human brain. *Journal of Cerebral Blood Flow and Metabolism, 12,* 900–918.

Spatial and Temporal Dynamics of Phonological and Semantic Processes

4

Jean-François Démonet and Guillaume Thierry

Progress in our understanding of the neural counterparts of cognitive entities depends not only on refined functional anatomy but also on precise recording of the time-course of neural activities throughout the neural ensembles that are recruited during any cognitive function. Recent improvements in the sensitivity and resolution of functional neuroimaging techniques allow us to gather reliable spatial and temporal information on neural activities associated with cognitive processes. Here, as an illustration of such a multimodality approach to a tentative neurophysiology of cognition, we present two studies of the phonological and lexical semantic processes involved in single-word language comprehension tasks. The results were obtained via two different techniques. Positron emission tomography (PET) provided anatomical localizations of across-task changes in neural activities (Démonet et al., 1992, 1994a,b), while multichannel mapping of EEG event-related potentials (ERPs) showed the temporal dynamics of language-related neural activities in each task and ERP distribution over different locations on the scalp (Thierry, Doyon, and Démonet, 1998).

Task Design

Whereas the techniques in the two experiments differed very much in terms of signal characteristics, the language tasks were kept constant, conducted in small groups of right-handed, highly educated normal volunteers. Monitoring auditory tasks were chosen so that subjects remained deeply engaged in the tasks that they were given. These consisted in an auditory, nonverbal task using pure tones and two verbal tasks in which emphasis was put on either phonological or lexical semantic processes, respectively.

In all three tasks, stimuli were digitized, delivered binaurally, consisted of 30 percent of targets among distractors, and were monitored by right fingers clicking on computer buttons.

In the phonological task (the "Phoneme" task), subjects were presented with multisyllable pseudo-words and were asked to press a designated button whenever they detected the presence of the phoneme /b/ if and only if it was preceded by the phoneme /d/ in a previous syllable, such as in /redozabu/. The majority of the distractors involved either /d/ but not /b/ ("dx" type) or /b/ but not /d/ before ("xb" type) and the rest were fillers with neither /d/ nor /b/ ("xx" type).

The structure of the lexical semantic task (the "Word" task) paralleled that of the phonological task but involved adjective-noun pairs. Subjects had to click on the "target" button when hearing names of small animals if and only if they were preceded by positively denotating adjectives (for example, "kind mouse"). Three types of distractors were presented: positive-big, negative-small, and negative-big.

Although these two language tasks had several features in common (twofold and sequential criterion for target identification, working memory and attentional resource requirements), they were designed in order to tease apart as much as possible two different modes of language stimuli processing. The phonological task might be viewed as a phonological awareness task. It was expected to lead subjects to use a parsing strategy in which the phonemic and syllabic structure of the stimuli would be worked out in detail. On the contrary, the lexical semantic task was meant to require only superficial and automatic access to phonological representations upon lexical identification of words. Attentional resources, it was thought, would mainly be devoted to analyzing the meaning of the heard words.

The choice of these tasks was also guided by neuroanatomical considerations. From lesion-based studies, it has been suggested (Cappa, Cavalotti, and Vignolo, 1981) that aphasic patients presenting with predominantly phonemic disorders suffered from lesions located close to the left sylvian fissure, whereas patients showing mostly lexical semantic symptoms tend to present lesions located in the inferior part of the left temporal or left parietal lobes. Using functional imaging, we addressed whether such a differential topography might also be observed in normal subjects while performing language tasks in which either phonological or lexical semantic processes would predominate.

The PET Study

The PET study was conducted with nine volunteers using the Oxygen 15 method, and the analysis of variations in regional cerebral blood flow (rCBF) was performed with SPM software from Frackowiak and Friston (1994).

The analysis of error rates and reaction times in subjects showed that the phonological task, though correctly performed in all subjects, gave rise to more false positives and prolonged processing times (Figure 4.1) than the other two tasks.

Because integration of radioactivity counts over a 60 sec period is needed, the PET technique does not allow the analysis of the neural activities related to each type of stimulus that was identified in the task design. This technique only permits global comparisons across tasks to assess whether local increases of rCBF occurred while subjects underwent a given task, compared with another.

Despite this limitation in the time domain, these comparisons showed that different patterns of rCBF increase were generated by each of the two language tasks, respectively (Figure 4.2). In accordance with lesion-based studies, the phonological task yielded activations localized in the vicinity of the left perisylvian areas. The lexical semantic task activated a more widespread pattern involving the middle and inferior temporal and the inferior parietal (angular gyrus) regions together with localizations that were not predicted by the lesion-based model, namely the left superior prefrontal, the posterior cingulate, and the right inferior parietal regions.

This complex pattern of activation associated with our lexical semantic task was further confirmed by an analysis of the same results based on a correlational analysis (Démonet, Wise, and Frackowiak,

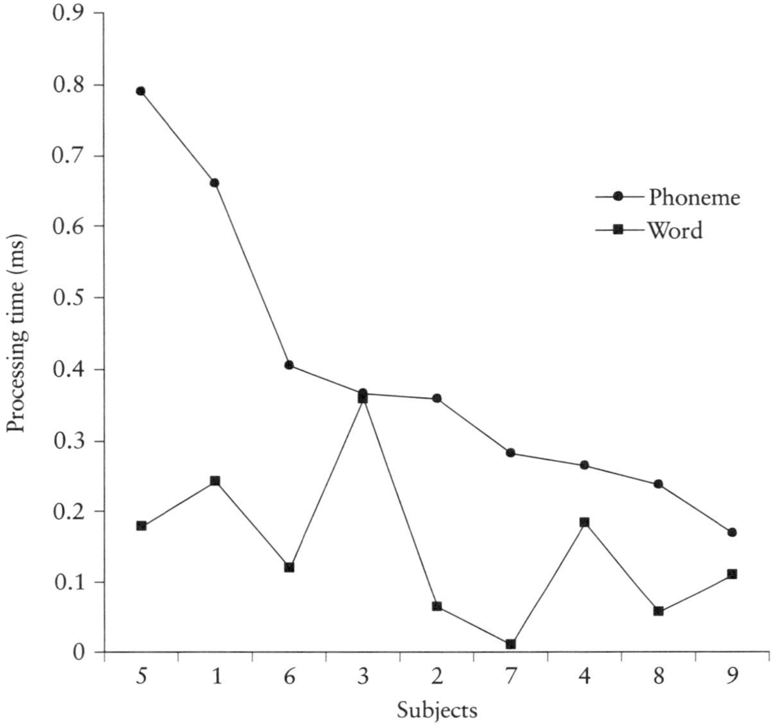

Figure 4.1. Processing times assessed for each subject in the Phoneme task and in the Word task (see Démonet et al., 1992, for details). The processing time was significantly longer in the Phoneme task than in the Word task, and especially so in the slowest subjects for the Phoneme task.

1993) and by other studies using either PET (such as Vandenberghe et al., 1996) or fMRI (such as Binder et al., 1997).

Activations in the periphery of the left sylvian fissure in our phonological task were replicated in a further study (Démonet et al., 1994b) and proved to be congruent with several studies devoted to the functional anatomy of phonological processes (for a critique, discussion, and review, see Poeppel, 1996, and Démonet et al., 1996). Of particular interest for the significance of our results is their high degree of convergence with those described by Paulesu, Frith, and Frackowiak (1993) in a study of phonological working memory. A small left-sided perisylvian network involving Wernicke's area, the supramarginal gyrus, and Broca's area was identified as the neural counter-

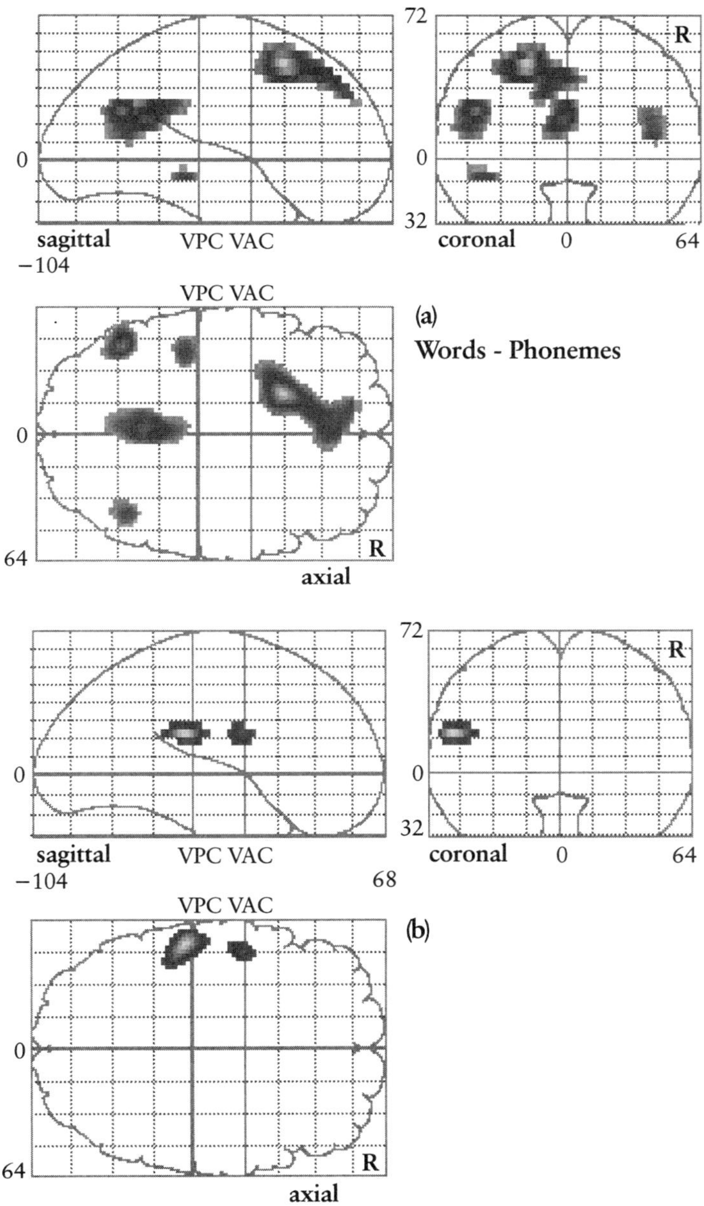

Figure 4.2. PET study. SPM maps of significant ($p < .001$ after correction for multiple comparisons) increases of blood flow in the Word task compared with the Phoneme task (Figure 4.2a), and conversely (Figure 4.2b). Pixels are depicted in glass-views of a standardized brain space (Talairach and Tournoux, 1988).

parts of the "articulatory loop" in Baddeley's model (1986). More precisely, the inferior part of the left supramarginal gyrus was activated in Démonet et al. (1994a) in a location (x, y, z = –52, –26, 20) that is very close to that described by Paulesu, Frith, and Frackowiak (1993) (x, y, z, = –44, –32, 24) as a focus corresponding to short-term phonological storage. This supports our view that a strong component of working memory is present in our phonological task. In this framework, short-term maintenance of phonemes or syllables is probably crucial to achieve this task, and this might correspond to quite a precise localization in the left supramarginal gyrus.

In a correlational analysis of rCBF changes in the lexical semantic task (Démonet, Wise, and Frackowiak, 1993), we proposed, by analogy with our viewpoints on phonological tasks, that the activation of the left angular gyrus we found in this task might, at least in part, represent a similar short-term memory storage process related to lexical items. This would represent an equivalent to the phonological storage taking place in the left supramarginal gyrus.

The ERP Study

Using the same tasks, the ERP portion of our work allowed us to analyze the respective neural correlates of different types of stimuli within each task in terms of temporal dynamics and distribution over the scalp.

Because of their similarities in structure, the two language tasks may be accomplished using the same, rather obvious, strategy. This strategy consists in detecting only stimuli containing the phoneme /d/ or a positive adjective and in rejecting other stimuli, that is, those containing either the phoneme /b/ or the name of a small animal in their final part. We therefore labeled these stimuli ("dx" and "db" types, or "positive-big" and "positive-small" types) "hold," since, upon detection of the conditioning item, they require further maintenance of the heard sequence that will be loaded into the working memory system. On the contrary, the "xb" and "xx" pseudo-word or both the "negative" word stimuli may both be designated as "release" stimuli, since the absence of the conditioning item would preclude these stimuli's meeting the target criteria. Consequently their identification as "nontarget" stimuli does not require further processing, and their analysis may be halted.

The ERP study was carried out with twelve volunteers on a 32-electrode Neuroscan© system with continuous EEG sampled at 500 Hz and post-hoc 40 Hz low-pass filtering. After elimination of eye-blink artifacts, motion artifacts, and erroneous trials, at least thirty exemplars of each stimulus type and for each task formed the averaged ERP data recorded over 1800 msec epochs. Error rates and reaction times were similar to those observed in the PET study.

The analysis of the grand average of ERPs in the two language tasks led to the identification in both cases of typical auditory late components N1-P2, as well as further specific events that we characterized as split points, since they consisted of divergence between ERPs respectively elicited by "hold" and "release" stimuli, in each task (Figure 4.3). "Hold" stimuli elicited a shift toward negative potentials, whereas "release" stimuli tend to elicit positive shifts. This divergence seems to correspond to an ERP correlate of the decision taken by the subjects on whether or not a given stimulus should be further processed and maintained in the working memory system as a potential target, that is, whether a conditioning item (phoneme /d/ or positive adjective) was detected by subjects or not.

Although this pattern of divergence was clearly observed in both tasks, this phenomenon differed from one language task to another in two ways. First, the split points differed in latency. Second, the distribution over the scalp of the release-hold differences was completely different (Figure 4.3).

Because of the different timing of ERPs in the phonological and the semantic tasks, direct, between-task comparisons appeared of marginal relevance, unlike in the PET study. In turn, the within-task contrasts between release and hold ERPs turned out to be of crucial interest.

The mean duration of the first two syllables of the pseudo-words was shorter (512 msec) than that of the adjective (684 msec). Despite this, the typical latency of the split recorded over fronto-central electrodes in the phonological task (782 msec) occurred *well after* the end of the trace of these first two syllables upon which subjects were to make their decision. In contrast, the lexical semantic split was observed on fronto-central electrodes at 654 msec, that is 30 msec *before* the mean end of the acoustic traces of adjectives. This cross-over tem-

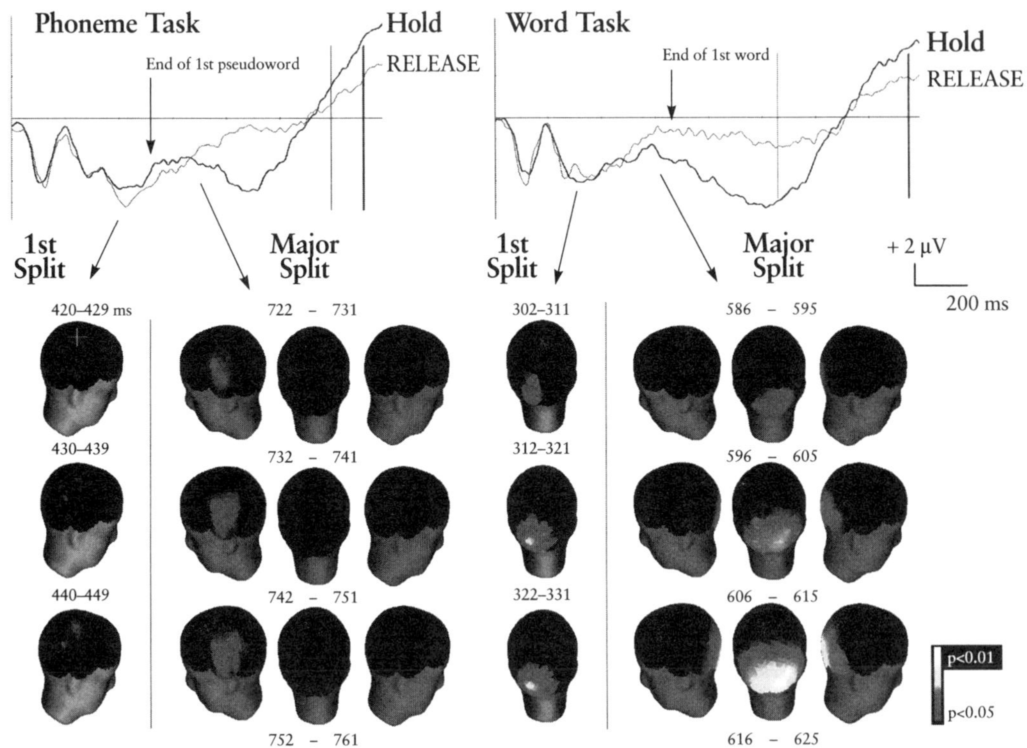

Figure 4.3. Grand average of ERPs recorded over the fronto-central electrodes of potentials respectively elicited by hold and release stimuli in the Phoneme and the Word tasks (top) and interpolated mapping of the difference (paired *t*-tests) between Hold and Release following split points.

poral pattern suggests that, in accordance with our theoretical views, the phonological task was performed in a sequential, step-by-step, parsing mode. This sequential processing is much slower than the probabilistic, nonexhaustive way of processing lexically valid items in the semantic task (Marslen-Wilson and Tyler Komisarjevsky, 1980), so that semantic features of the heard words can be accessed quickly, ensuring faster processing in this task.

After the split points between hold and release stimuli, sustained divergences between ERPs were observed in both tasks for more than 200 msec. Differences between these potentials were computed and their distribution over the scalp was studied via t-maps interpolated between the electrodes. In the phonological task, the divergence first appeared and remained predominant over left-sided central electrodes, the maximum difference being centered on the T7 electrode. This is congruent with the left-sided perisylvian foci of activation in our PET study. In the lexical semantic task, the divergence first occurred on the posterior O1 electrode and quickly spread toward the homologous O2 electrode, with further spreading to the entire set of posterior electrodes in both hemispheres. This bilateral and posterior distribution of ERP differences is compatible with the presence of activation foci in the left and right angular gyri in our PET study, although it does not account for the remaining aspects of the complex pattern observed in the left hemisphere.

In sum, the split phenomenon observed in both tasks is likely to relate, on the one hand, to common attentional and problem-solving mechanisms based on the maintenance of potential targets in working memory and the release of attention for irrelevant distractors, and, on the other hand, to language-specific modulations of this basic algorithm induced by the lexical status of the processed stimuli. Pseudo-words yield a slow, sequential process probably operated in the left hemisphere, via a perisylvian "articulatory loop." This mode of language processing is related to phonological awareness strategies that normal subjects may resort to when learning new words. Real-word processing corresponds to a faster, automatized, and probabilistic mode of processing, relating to long-lasting exposure to lexical items that permits quick access to semantic representations.

Conclusion

These studies represent only a preliminary illustration of a multimodal neuroimaging approach to cognitive processes. By seeking anatomical and temporal indexes of the neural activities subserving two major modes of oral language comprehension, we gathered functional information whose different components complement one another but lack overlap in terms of time or space resolution. It is hoped that, given promising developments of new techniques such as event-related fMRI, resolution in both time and space will come from the same data set or that analysis of ERP sources can be merged with magnetic resonance data as future tools for the physiology of cognition.

References

Baddeley, A. D. 1986. *Working memory.* Oxford: Oxford University Press.

Binder, J. R., Frost, J. A., Hammeke, T. A., Cox, R. W., Rao, S. M., and Prieto, T. 1997. Human brain language areas identified by functional magnetic resonance imaging. *J. Neuroscience,* Jan. 1, *17* (1), 353–362.

Cappa, S. F., Cavalotti, G., and L. A. Vignolo. 1981. Phonemic and lexical errors in fluent aphasia: Correlation with lesion site. *Neuropsychologia, 19,* 171–177.

Démonet, J.-F., Chollet, F., Ramsay, S., Cardebat, D., Nespoulous, J. L., Wise, R., Rascol, A., and Frackowiak, R. S. J. 1992. The anatomy of phonological and semantic processing in normal subjects. *Brain, 115,* 1753–1768.

Démonet, J.-F., Fiez, J. A., Paulesu, E., Petersen, S. E., and R. J. Zatorre. 1996. PET studies of phonological processing: a critical reply to Poeppel. *Brain and Language, 55,* 352–379.

Démonet, J.-F., Price, C., Wise, R., and Frackowiak, R. S. J. 1994a. Differential activation of right and left posterior sylvian regions by semantic and phonological tasks: A positron emission tomography study in normal human subjects. *Neuroscience Letters, 182,* 25–28.

——— 1994b. A PET study of cognitive strategies in normal subjects during language tasks: Influence of phonetic ambiguity and sequence processing on phoneme monitoring. *Brain, 117,* 671–682.

Démonet, J.-F., Wise, R., and Frackowiak, R. S. J. 1993. Language functions explored in normal subjects by positron emission tomography: A critical review. *Human Brain Mapping, 1,* 39–47.

Frackowiak, R. S. J., and K. J. Friston. 1994. Functional neuroanatomy of the human brain: Positron emission tomography—a new neuroanatomical technique. *Journal of Anatomy, 184,* 211–225.

Marslen-Wilson, W., and L. Tyler Komisarjevsky. 1980. The temporal structure of spoken language understanding. *Cognition, 8,* 1–71.

Paulesu, E., Frith, C. D., and Frackowiak, R. S. J. 1993. The neural correlates of the verbal component of working memory. *Nature, 362,* 342–345.

Poeppel, D. 1996. A critical review of PET studies of phonological processing. *Brain and Language, 55,* 317–351.

Talairach, J., and Tournoux, P. 1988. *Co-planar stereotaxic atlas of the human brain.* New York: Thieme Medical Publications.

Thierry, G., Doyon, B., and Démonet, J.-F. 1998. Spatio-temporal dynamics of auditory language processing. Cognitive Neuroscience Society, Annual Abstract Program, Supplement of the *Journal of Cognitive Neuroscience,* Abstr. 69.

Vandenberghe, R., Price, C., Wise, R., Josephs, O., and Frackowiak, R. S. 1996. Functional anatomy of a common semantic system for words and pictures. *Nature,* Sept. 19, *383* (6597), 254–256.

Discussion: Section 1

Localization

STEPHEN KOSSLYN: What is the alternative to strict localization?

DAVID CAPLAN: In general or for these data?

KOSSLYN: For these data.

CAPLAN: I suppose that the alternative is that there is a distributed system that involves all of the perisylvian cortex; that within that system there is an area that becomes more specialized—the preferred site of processing—but when it is otherwise occupied it cannot do that processing. Now, what does that mean mathematically; or, how could that possibly work? Well, since this discussion is supposedly among friends, let me go off on a limb, and someone can saw it off behind me. I am not necessarily enthusiastic about all connectionist modeling, but if you are thinking of alternatives to a localizing system, I guess one thinks about connectionist modeling. In many of these connectionist systems with hidden units, the hidden units tend to organize, at least partially. Even though there is a clear sense in connectionist systems that all hidden units are involved in a representation, some representations tend to activate parts of the net more than others. This is to say that some representations have greater effects on synaptic strengths, or connectional strengths, in some parts of the net than in other parts. It is the only thing that I can think of that might be analogous to a distributed system with some specialization in the brain.

Specific Task versus Complexity to Explain Differences

ALFONSO CARAMAZZA: It was not clear to me what your conclusion was. Do the experiments you report actually have anything to do with syntax? Or, do the results instead have to do just with processing complexity, memory load, length of sentences, and so on? There are many things that are manipulated in your experiments. And those of us who are a little bit outside the area do not know which of these are significant.

CAPLAN: I think the answer that I would give to that question is that syntax is not all of a piece. For those of you who do not deal with language at all, this might take a little explaining. Syntax is basically the set of relationships between words in a sentence that are given by the organization of the categories to which they belong. You may have noticed that in the examples that I put up, I sometimes change the words in sentences. For instance, the first set of sentences were about tenants and leaks and landlords and irrigation. But when I showed a syntactic tree, the words in the tree were not about tenants and leaks and irrigation; they were about something else. But the relationships between those words were the same. And those relationships were given by the categories to which the words belonged, noun, verb, adjective, noun-phrase, relative clause, and so on. Those hierarchically organized sets of categories can define any number of relationships. For instance, in the example that I gave with a relative clause, what is relevant is what node immediately dominates another.

I think that for many psychologists, especially aphasiologists working on this problem since the 1980s (or, 1976, when Alfonso [Caramazza] and Edgar [Zurif] first published a paper that suggested that syntactic operations could be disturbed in isolation, there has been a tendency to lump all of the syntactic relationships, and the processes that must go on in producing them and comprehending them, together into one kind of isolated functional domain. But for anybody who has studied linguistics, it is clear that they are all quite different. Linguists have been concerned about all of these small distinctions for a long time. Thus I think that the active-passive contrast I have been examining depends on which side of the telescope you look through. Looked at through the side of the telescope linguists use, it is quite a different contrast from the relative clause difference.

Then, what is the difference? Is it length? Is it the particular nature of the syntactic representations? You could suggest a variety of differences. One that is potentially interesting is that the active-passive relationship, despite the fact that some linguists represent it in terms of traces and kinds of syntactic operations, could also be represented totally lexically. The relative clause structure is not a lexical structure. It is given by the presence of relative pronouns and word order in the sentence. And so it cannot be activated purely lexically, not in the same way that an active-passive relationship can. It is conceivable that that makes a difference. One could come up with many other differences, which could be explored. I do not know if that is a complete answer.

ALBERT GALABURDA: Stephen?

KOSSLYN: I found this morning's session extremely interesting. But sometimes I wonder a tiny bit whether we are looking not just at trees, but actually at the bark, and whether we could take a step back and ask about the forest. One of the themes of the meeting is to try to look for commonalities and differences among the kinds of representations that are used in verbal languages and nonverbal languages. Listening to you, I noticed that maybe working memory might have something to do with many of the phenomena. I mean that working memory might be involved in whatever these traces are. So I wondered about the role of working memory in language. I wondered about what kinds of representations will be used in working memory. Edgar talked about something very abstract for the trace, an unconscious abstract representation, which might be interesting to try to explore. And then I could not help but notice in your slides, David [Caplan], that maybe even images, something visual, might be going on in the representation of language. I wondered whether the panelists from this morning's session could take a big step backward and try to get a larger perspective on what was said, in terms of what might be relevant to the languages of the brain. Could I start with Al [Galaburda]?

GALABURDA: Let me just add to your list, "attention load." Certainly one of the areas where we saw activation in the parietal lobe could respond differentially to different attentional requirements for different kinds of speech processing.

But to return to your "step back" question, what appears to me to come out of our discussions this morning is that in principle there seem to be two types of language systems: first, those that are very close to the input and output channels, which seem to be concerned with representing language before or after meaning (respectively). These areas are located in relation to the primary auditory cortex in hearing subjects and around primary motor cortex for motor control of tongue, palate, larynx, and so on. They are concerned with the processes of language. Second, on the other hand, the content of language is not comparably localized and involves large areas of the cortex, including prefrontal cortex, anterior temporal cortex, parietal cortex, which depend on hard-wired relationships and learning histories. Most of aphasiology, I believe, and even most of what linguists are concerned with, relates to process and not content.

BARBARA GROSZ: I wanted to add an amendment to Stephen's question. I was struck in many of the talks, but especially in the last one, by the fact that all the examples were in English. I wondered what happened if one looked at other languages. In particular, it was the comments about traces versus pronouns that caught my attention. So, if one looks at languages like Japanese, which do not use pronouns in the same way as English, what happens there? I wonder whether there are aphasics who speak other languages in whom there is perhaps more dependency on morphology.

JEAN-FRANÇOIS DÉMONET: Yes, of course, because of time constraints I could not go into more detail about the implications of verbal working memory and how it is related to the findings I presented. In the phonological task I have used, it is obvious that verbal working memory is strongly involved. In fact, the results I just showed you are strikingly similar to those obtained by Paulesu using a proper verbal working memory experiment and an activation PET study. For instance, the coordinated activation in the supramarginal gyrus is exactly the same in the two studies. It is clear that there is a very strong involvement of verbal working memory in the phonological task, but probably also in the lexical-semantic task. However, the way verbal working memory was involved in the two tasks was obviously different. Broca's area was activated in both cases, whereas the left supramarginal gyrus was activated only in the phonological task. I think that a very consistent finding after meta-analysis of many activation studies is that processes are common among many tasks, much more so than representations.

Process/Content

DÉMONET: I am sorry for Alfonso [Caramazza], but in general we end up with results that show that activation foci are much more related to processes than to cognitive representation, what we mean by cognitive representations. This agrees with Al Galaburda's distinction between process and content language areas.

FROM THE FLOOR: Is this then a statement about the limitations of your technique? Or are you saying that these techniques are not useful for addressing questions about what objects are being manipulated? It seems to me that you have raised a fundamental point, then. Many of us, including me, who are outside of the area of neuroimaging, looked at this technique as a great new tool for answering questions not only about the processes that are involved but about the objects that are being manipulated.

But it seems to me that what you are claiming now is that there may be a very serious limitation to how we interpret these kinds of data. I am not saying that the limitation cannot be overcome with analysis, time, and so on, but certainly it is something that you have to keep in mind in interpreting the various results that are being presented, since we could be looking not so much at things such as semantics or lexical, but at something else instead. If this is the case, then the ball is back in your court. Can you design experiments that are going to allow us to take these things apart so we can learn about, say, this commonalities of imagery and language and whatever else?

DÉMONET: To say the least, I think that the classical subtraction ways of analyzing the data are very primitive, and we really want to attempt a far more detailed and refined analysis of our data.

JACQUES MEHLER: I was wondering whether or not we are not jumping a level when we try to discuss the results of all of these very interesting contributions about which we heard this morning. We had quite considerable descriptions of linguistic structure, on the one hand, and beautiful data about brain activation, on the other. Then people try to link brain activation directly to linguistic structure. However, who has talked about the kinds of tasks the subjects are accomplishing? And how do we know, for instance, that these different tasks actually tap substantial, interesting levels of processing? I shall give just two examples: one is whether we have explored in activation studies what happens if we block anomalous sentences into homogenous presentations and use that as the subtraction. Or if we block sentences such as those David showed us. Maybe they do not make a difference, but to be sure, maybe they should be part of the design. We do this in experimental psychology when we try to assess sentence processing.

Another question is whether it is really the case that an awareness task in phonology actually taps into phonologic processes. Do you really think that when you listen to me, you try to guess whether I am saying a B before a D or D before a B? Is this process of guessing part of the phonologic apparatus? We have had this friendly discussion with Jean-François [Démonet] many times. I agree that it is interesting that when you do phonological awareness problem-solving tasks you get some kind of activation, and when you do lexical problem-solving tasks you get a different kind of activation. But, that these tasks address phonological representation or lexical representation is something that we still need to prove.

CAPLAN: Could I comment on that? I think that Jacques is exactly right. And it bears on the question that Alfonso was asking about representations versus processing. I do not think we know how much these tasks affect our results. But we think we know that they do affect our results. There was a paper published in *Science* in 1996 from the Carnegie-Mellon group, looking at syntactic processing. They used sentences very similar to the type that we used, with only slight differences. But it may be those slight differences that are the driving force behind the differences in activation. When very similar subtractions were performed, the authors described activation in Broca's area, in Wernicke's area, and, to a lesser degree, in the right hemisphere homologs of Broca's and Wernicke's areas.

In subjects' task, rather than have them make sentence acceptability judgments, subjects read a sentence and then answered a visually presented question about whether a statement corresponded to what was in the sentence. Both of these tasks have some memory load, but there is a slightly different memory load in the Carnegie-Mellon experiment. It is a very small difference, but perhaps not so small in cognitive terms. This clearly relates to the issue raised several times already about process versus representation. We do not know the answers to these questions, but I suppose that one way to think about them is that if you get convergence across a whole variety of tasks when you are looking at a particular representation, then you are more likely looking at where that representation is. If you get convergence across a whole variety of representations when you are looking at a particular task, then you are seeing the localization of the task. But we are a long way from really knowing that this is even possible to show.

Section 2
Verbal Content

Some of the most remarkable observations in all of clinical neurology have been made on aphasic patients who show difficulties handling information on one category of objects. Some, for instance, seem to have lost their ability to say anything about tools; others draw a blank when questioned about living things. As it happens, the lesions that produce loss of one type of knowledge are in different locations than those that produce loss of another type. More recently, brain activation studies have underscored the fact that slightly different components of the semantic system are activated when a subject is asked to process the information of one category as compared with another. This should not be surprising, at least intuitively, since if one can engage in metacognitive exercises whereby one can segregate the objects of the world into categories, at some neural level this segregation must also take place. What is more interesting is that modules participating in the processing of one category are often quite far away on the cortical surface from modules participating in the processing of another category. Aside from this discovery, most of the information we have to date about the participation of brain regions in language function has to do with language processes rather than language content.

The notion of language content is not simple and straightforward. There is perceptual content and conceptual content. There is action and intentionality. In Chapter 5, Pierre Jacob asks, first, whether the content of mental representation is capable of generating or changing observed behavior. Second, if we step aside from the issue of causality, what is the link between mental content and behavior? The second question can be answered in neural terms, at least in part. Assuming that content is represented in the brain in certain areas, or in certain combinations of areas, or in particular ways of activating a particular area, and that motor programs are represented in another part of the brain, or parts, and so on, then all one needs for the neural model is to establish that there exist neural connections—axons—that link these two types of areas. Causality is another question altogether, since the demonstration of connectivity does not address this issue in the least. In fact, the activation of two or three or four brain areas during the performance of a task cannot address causality either. Even with the advent of timed measurements of activation, all one can comment on is the directionality of information flow, and not causality. Thus if area A activates before area B, this may be the result of area C, the cause, activating A and B in that sequence. However, the situation is not hopeless. If one can determine that, say, the disappearance of mental representation R abolishes action M, and that the disappearance of region r, which mediates mental representation R, causes dysfunction of region m, which is part of the system that contains the motor programs for action M, we are on our way to demonstrate a causal relation. This type of evidence has been gathered most often from patients with brain lesions. More recently, through the use of transcranial magnetic stimulation, using parameters that suppress the activity of a given brain area, it has been possible to study the causal role of that area in the performance of a particular task. It is clear at the neural level that causality requires connectivity, although causality and connectivity are not identical.

An important question remains as to how the brain came to be organized differently for processing different categories of objects. Chapter 7, by Alfonso Caramazza, tackles this question. His posture on this issue is strongly evolutionary as opposed to developmental, and he uses clinical examples to support his position. It is not difficult to accept the proposition that evolution plays a large role in categorical knowledge. For instance, in the frog, which may be thought to have the prototypical early vertebrate brain, information from the olfactory system connects to very different portions of the brain from information coming in through the eyes or from the visceral organs through the hypothalamus. Already in the frog information is discretely and widely segregated. However, there is also evidence that development can wreak havoc with these maps. It has been shown, for example, that subjects with early-acquired blindness activate the visual cortex when they read Braille, and that suppression of the visual cortex interferes with accuracy of Braille reading. Neurosurgeons mapping the motor system in order to spare as much useful cortex as possible during removal of a tumor or an epileptic focus have found motor representations in the dorsal parietal lobe. Illiterate subjects who suffer injury to the right hemisphere are as a rule more anomic than literate subjects, indicating that learning about the world through reading forces a more important participation of the left hemisphere in semantic organization. Experience, then, is likely to play a role in the mapping of knowledge in the brain.

In verbal language, content can sometimes be packed into a single word, as in yelling "Fire!" in a crowded theater. At other times many words strung together are needed, as in reading a whole Agatha Christie novel before being sure "who dunnit." Chapter 8, by Barbara Grosz, analyzes content at the level of discourse. Little has been written in the neurological literature about discourse and its brain underpinnings. As mentioned above, the focus has been on areas of the brain that mediate verbal processes, on the one hand, and those that mediate verbal content, on the other, but the latter at the single-word level. Yet clinicians are familiar with patients who either stop talking (and thinking?), or whose discourse becomes strikingly curtailed in length. There are other patients whose discourse is abnormal because there is loss of individual content words. So, for instance, patients with Alzheimer's disease may talk incessantly but convey very little information, because they talk, usually inadequately, around words that they cannot conjure up. The former type of patient, in contrast, just doesn't say much. We see this in patients with lesions (usually bilateral) dorsally placed in the frontal lobes. It is of interest, and probably important to realize, that these patients not only say little, but also do little and, many believe, think little. Patients with Broca's aphasia, who also have frontal lobe lesions, usually in the ventral premotor and prefrontal areas, also produce curtailed (and agrammatical) discourse. But in these patients one has the distinct impression that thinking is not curtailed, and certainly, to the extent that they can overcome the handicap of their right-sided motor paralysis, their actions are not curtailed. Patients with Parkinson's disease also exhibit limited verbal and motor expression. The verbal and motor activities not only are curtailed in length, but are very slow and effortful—exhausting sometimes—and there is some evidence that thinking suffers from the same difficulties. Finally, there is a large group of patients whose thinking is disorganized and aimless, whose actions are poorly planned and often inappropriate, and who at the same time may exhibit abnormal levels and types of motor activity. One sees this phenomenon in patients with injury in the more rostral portions of the frontal lobes, the so-called prefrontal cortex, or in patients who show dysfunction in these regions even in the absence of structural damage, such as bipolar patients and patients with obsessive-compulsive disorders.

Except for the case of Broca's aphasia, where the problem is strictly restricted to the mechanics of language and speech processing, these examples produce problems that are not just limited to verbal discourse and instead affect all aspects of a patient's mental and neurological functioning. It seems reasonable to conclude as a first pass that discourse, in addition to relying on linguistic mechanisms, depends very importantly on metalinguistic mental processes, and that the frontal lobes, especially the dorsolateral prefrontal cortex, are required for its proper expression.

The phrase "Washington, D.C." refers to a place that is in the same geographic location no matter who thinks it or says it. This is in contrast to the word "here," the content of which depends on where the thinker or speaker of the word is located. "Here" means Washington, D.C., only when the speaker or thinker is in Washington, D.C. The content nature of words like "here"—indexical words—and related concepts—deferential concepts—are the focus of concern of François Recanati in Chapter 6. There are least two meanings to the word "content," and, Recanati argues, only one of these can explain the behavior—either thinking or acting—of the thinker or actor. One form of "content" is much more relative than the other, and one has to wonder about how the brain handles this difference. One possibility is that the two forms of "content" differ in their connectivity to perceptual systems.

Can Mental Content Explain Behavior? 5

Pierre Jacob

Some representations are mental; others are not. A road sign, a map, and the utterance of a sentence of a natural language are nonmental representations. All representations, whether mental or nonmental, have contents. Some have a conceptual content; others have a nonconceptual content. For example, motor representations, sensory experiences, perceptual representations, and mental images have nonconceptual contents. To restrict myself to mental sensory experiences in the visual modality, visual experiences and visual mental images have pictorial nonconceptual content. Among an individual's mental representations, thoughts and propositional attitudes have conceptual contents. And so do an individual's utterances, which, as just noted, are nonmental representations.

No doubt there are many important differences between conceptual and nonconceptual content. In this chapter, however, I will disregard the many significant differences between the varieties of mental contents and instead ask a general question about the explanatory role of content: can mental content explain an individual's intentional behavior? Is the content of an individual's mental representation one of the causally efficacious properties of the individual's representation in the process whereby it contributes to the production of the individual's intentional behavior?

Not everything an individual does is produced by the content of some of the individual's mental representations. Only an individual's *intentional* behavior is. The fact that I snore and vomit—if and when I do—is not something that can be explained by the contents of some of my mental representations. Nor is it intentional behavior. Suppose, however, that I move my right hand to the vicinity of a glass containing water and located a few inches from my chest. Suppose I grasp it, move it to my lips, and drink water from it. What I did when I grasped the glass and drank water from it *is* intentional behavior. And it can be explained by the fact that I believed that the glass in front of me contained water and I wanted a sip of water. Furthermore, I will assume that my belief that the glass in front of me contained water is some state of my nervous system. So I assume that my brain state has several nonsemantic neurophysiological properties. But it also has content or, as I shall say, it has a semantic property. The question I want to raise is the following: can the semantic property of my belief—what I believe—be a causally efficacious property of my brain state? If many of the neurophysiological properties of my brain state are causally efficacious in the process whereby I grasp the glass with the fingers of my right hand, can the semantic property of my brain state be causally efficacious too?

The Argument against the Causal Efficacy of Content

Many philosophers, whom I shall label intentional irrealists, would respond negatively to this question. On their view, content cannot be a causally efficacious property of an individual's mental representation. I think the argument for their view can be put in the following way:

1. A decent causal explanation of why some cause *c* produced some effect *e* must refer to some causally efficacious property of *c* in the process whereby *c* caused *e*.
2. Only *c*'s intrinsic properties (or properties that supervene on *c*'s intrinsic properties) are causally efficacious in the production of *e*.
3. A representation's content (or meaning) is one of its extrinsic historical properties.
4. Therefore: the content of an individual's mental representation *R* is not causally efficacious in the process whereby *R* contributes to the production of the individual's (intentional) behavior.

Although I think the premises are true, I don't accept the conclusion.[1] In what follows I will say why I think the premises are true and why I think the conclusion does not follow.[2]

I will assume that in the nonpsychological sciences, it is widely assumed that causal relations hold between events, as when one says that the short circuit caused the fire or the collision between a meteorite and the earth caused the extinction of dinosaurs. *c* caused *e*. In the psychological domain, we may say that my belief *c* caused my bodily motion *m*. A cause, however, has many different properties, not all of which may equally be causally efficacious. Causal efficacy is not fairly distributed among the properties of a cause. In order to show this last point, I will borrow a famous example from Fred Dretske (1988).

The Meaningful Sound

Let *c* be some upper sound produced by a soprano on a particular occasion, for example, Renata Tebaldi singing a particular air of *Traviata* at a particular time *t*. Let it also be the third note of the scale. Suppose *c* broke a window at $t + 1$. Call *e* the breaking of the window. *c* caused *e*. Suppose *c* had a meaning. Call it *F*. Did *c* cause *e* by virtue of being *F*? Was *c*'s being *F* causally efficacious in the process whereby *c* caused *e*? No, it wasn't. Why not? Because if *c* had had another meaning or if *c* had had no meaning at all, it might still have produced *e;* it might still have broken the window. What was causally efficacious in the process of window breaking was *c*'s having an acoustic property, *K*, not *c*'s being *F*. If *c* had not been *K*, it might not have broken the window. The reason *c*'s being *K* was causally efficacious in breaking the window is that the causal relation between *c* and *e* can be subsumed under a nomic correlation between the fragility of the windowpane and *c*'s being *K*. But there is no such correlation between the fragility of the glass and *c*'s being *F*.

This example shows, I think, two things. First, it shows that not all the properties of cause *c* can be causally efficacious in the process whereby *c* produces *e*—something which is presupposed or implied by the first premise. Furthermore, unlike the acoustic property *K* of the sound, its meaning *F* is not one of its intrinsic properties. The acoustic property *K* is an intrinsic property of the sound in the sense that the sound would not be the sound it is if it lacked property *K*. Arguably, *event c,* which consists of the producing of a given sound, would not be the same event if the sound lacked its meaning. But there is, I think, a sense in which the sound—unlike the event of producing the sound—would be same sound if it had the same acoustic property *K* and if it lacked semantic property *F*. But the sound would not be the same sound if it had semantic property *F* and another acoustic property *K**. Unlike the sound's acoustic property *K*, its meaning *F* derives from Giuseppe Verdi's intentions. *F* is therefore a historical extrinsic property of the sound.[3] Granted, the sound itself was chosen by Verdi. But its being *K*, unlike its being *F*, did not depend on Verdi's intentions. Verdi gave the sound its meaning; he did not make up the musical scale.

On my view, there is a difference between the meaning of a sound produced by a singer and the mental content of a human being's brain state, for example, Verdi's musical intention. The latter is primitive (or original); the former is derivative upon the latter. Generally speaking, the meanings of nonmental representations are derivative on the meanings of mental representations. In spite of this difference, though, mental content too is a historical extrinsic property, not an intrinsic property, of an individual's brain state. It depends on correlations between an individual's brain, on the one hand, and properties instantiated in the individual's environment, on the other. This is the substance of the third premise. To further establish the plausibility of premises (2) and (3), I'll now borrow an example from Dan Dennett (1987). But I'll exploit it in a Dretskean non-Dennettian way.

The Vending Machine

Let *S* be a French vending machine emitting soft drinks upon receiving French coins worth 5 French francs. Call *m S*'s output at *t,* namely the delivery of a drink via the opening of a valve in *S* at *t*. Call *c* a particular 5-franc coin inserted in *S*'s slot at *t* – 1. The insertion of coin *c* caused *m,* the delivery of the drink. Now, *c* has intrinsic physical properties *P: c* is a metal disk with a characteristic mass, a characteristic physical and chemical composition, a characteristic diameter, and so on. And *c* has a monetary value: it is worth 5 French francs. Call *c*'s monetary value *V*. What conferred *V* onto *c* is the fact that *c* stood in some appropriate historical relation to a person working for the French Treasury Department who imprinted onto it the requisite "autograph." To see how extrinsic the relation that conferred *V* onto *c* is, let *c** be another metal disk that is physically and chemically indistinguishable from *c* because it instantiates *P* too. If *c**, however, did not stand in the required historical relation to the hands of the right people working for the French Treasury Department, then in spite of the fact that *c** is *P*, still *c** would lack *V*. To say that *V* is a historical extrinsic property of *c* is to say that *c*'s being *V* does not supervene on *c*'s being *P*.

No doubt the insertion of *c* in *S*'s slot at $t - 1$ produced *m*, the delivery of a drink, at *t*. Had some other physical object lacking *P* been inserted in *S*'s slot, it would not have produced *m*. And no doubt *c* is *V*. But the question I want to ask is: was *V* causally efficacious in the process whereby the insertion of *c* caused *m*? Was the fact that *c* was *V* causally responsible for the opening of a valve in *S* that in turn freed a drink? I want to say: no, the fact that *c* was *V* was not causally efficacious in the process of valve opening that in turn delivered a drink. The vending machine does not really detect monetary value *V*. What it is sensitive to is not instantiations of *V*, but instantiations of *P*. The opening of the valve in *S* is nomically correlated with property *P* of *c*, not with property *V*. As philosophers say, property *V* is "epiphenomenal" in the mechanism by which the insertion of *c* produces *m*.

So, *if c*'s being *V*—if the monetary value of a metal disk—is a relevant model of how an individual's brain state instantiates mental content, then what I believe when I believe that the glass in front of me contains water does not causally explain at all what I do when I move my right hand to the vicinity of the glass, grasp the glass with the fingers of my right hand, move it to my lips, and drink water from it. This in a nutshell is conclusion (4), that is, the conclusion drawn by intentional irrealists from premises (1)–(3). Again, I accept the premises. Am I then not forced to accept the conclusion? The rest of this chapter is an attempt to show why not.

Why the Conclusion Does Not Follow from the Premises

The vending machine is a physical device that responds to inputs of a specified kind by producing a characteristic output: it emits a drink upon receiving metal disks with intrinsic physical property *P* and extrinsic property *V*. The question we asked was: is *c*'s being *V* causally efficacious in the mechanism whereby a valve opens in *S* and a drink is emitted? Does the fact that *c* is *V* explain *m*, *S*'s delivery of a drink? Let's say that this is a question about the *mechanism* of valve opening in *S*. We were, I claim, forced to admit that only property *P* of *c* is causally efficacious in the mechanism of valve opening in *S*. Property *V* of *c* is not.

Notice, however, that strictly speaking, the question about the mechanism is *not* a question about *S*'s *behavior*. It is a question about the production of physical motion *m*. How can this be? Isn't *S*'s behavior simply *m*, that is, the delivery of a drink? I want to suggest that no, physical motion *m*—the delivery of a drink—is *not* quite the same thing as *S*'s behavior. *S*'s behavior is a process, one constituent of which is *m*—the delivery of a drink—and another constituent of which is the cause of *m*, namely, the insertion of coin *c*. Indeed, on what I shall call the *componential* view of behavior (championed by Dretske 1988 and which I accept),[4] it is a conceptual mistake to confuse the output of behavior with behavior itself: as much so as to confuse a constituent of something (for example, an event) with what it is a constituent of (a process or a sequence of events). *S*'s behavior is the process whereby the insertion of coin *c* in *S*'s slot at $t - 1$ produces *m*, the delivery of a drink at *t*. The very fact that *m* cannot happen at the very instant at which *c* is being inserted shows that there are two distinct events: the insertion of *c* in *S*'s slot and then the production of *m*. Thus *S*'s behavior is a sequence of events that are related to one another as a cause to its effect. Hence *S*'s behavior could be symbolized thus: $[c \rightarrow m]$.

From now on, I will assume that the componential conception of behavior is on the right track and that *S*'s behavior is distinct from its output, *m*, the delivery of a drink. If so, I can now say why I think conclusion (4) does not follow from premises (1)–(3). What reflection on the vending machine example shows is that extrinsic property *V* of *c* is not causally efficacious in producing physical motion *m* in *S*. The economic value of coin *c* is not causally efficacious in the emission of a drink via the mechanism of valve opening in *S*. Nothing has been said yet about explaining *S*'s behavior. By parity of reasoning, what follows from premises (1)–(3) is *not* that the content of an individual's representation *R* is not causally efficacious in explaining the individual's behavior, which could be symbolized thus: $[R \rightarrow m]$. Rather, what follows from premises (1)–(3) is that the content of an individual's representation *R* is not causally efficacious in the production of some of the individual's physical motion, *m* (where again *m* is a constituent of the individual's behavior).

Since I assume that behavior is not just physical motion, I will now argue that there is a sense in which explaining *S*'s behavior is not the same thing as explaining the production of *S*'s physical motion *m*. What I earlier called the question about the mechanism was the question: what property of inserted coin *c* is causally efficacious in the mechanism of valve opening which yields a drink? Consider now a different question: why is it that every time a metal disk *c* with property *P* is inserted in *S*'s slot, *S* does *m*, that is, *S* emits a drink? Why do instances of the former regularly produce instances of the latter? This is a question about the structure of *S*'s behavior in the following obvious sense: what we want to know now is why *S*'s behavior is a process of a certain type. Why does *S*'s behavior consist of the insertion of metal disks of type *c* followed by events of type *m*, emissions of a drink? Why does *S*'s behavior consist in the production of *m* by *c*? Why is *S*'s behavior constituted by the coordination between *c* and *m* rather than between *c* and something else?

Notice that, unlike the question about the mechanism, the question about the structure of *S*'s behavior is a *historical* question. The question is: how did it come about that insertions of coins of type *c* regularly produce events of type *m*? And the expected answer to this historical question about the structure of *S*'s behavior is going to refer to a *selective* process. Furthermore, I want to suggest that perhaps *c*'s having extrinsic property *V* does explain, after all, the structure of *S*'s behavior: perhaps *c*'s being *V* explains the coordination between *c* and *m*.

Let us suppose first that, thanks to the efforts of the French Treasury Department, instantiations of property *V* are reliably correlated with instantiations of property *P*. The general answer to the historical question about the structure of *S*'s behavior will go like this: *c* has been coordinated with *m* because metal disks of type *c* with property *P* were chosen (or selected) by a human engineer as causes of *m*, the opening of a valve in *S* emitting drinks. The correlation is not perfect: occasionally, the insertion of a counterfeit—a coin that is not really worth 5 French francs—gets the machine to deliver a drink. But it is good enough. Presumably, the cost of designing a more sensitive vending machine is not worth the effort. Notice that a counterfeit must have intrinsic property *P*, even though it does not instantiate extrinsic property *V*.

Now, suppose that for some reason at time *t*, the head of the French Treasury Department decides to change the intrinsic properties of coins worth 5 French francs. After *t*, then, there is no reliable correlation between instantiations of intrinsic property *P* and instantiations of extrinsic property *V*: metal disks with property *P* no longer instantiate property *V*. After *t*, property *V* is to be instantiated by metal disks with intrinsic property *P**. If this were so, then insertion of metal disk *c* having property *P* in *S*'s slot would *not* cause *m* anymore. After *t*—assuming that the price of drinks remains fixed over the change of decision—French engineers must design new vending machines such that insertion of metal disks *c** with intrinsic property *P** (not *P*) in their slots will cause *m*, the delivery of a drink.

If so, then it's fair to say that some metal disks with property *P** have been selected in the process of production of *m*, because they instantiate extrinsic property *V*. Likewise, before the decision to change the intrinsic properties of coins, metal disks *c* having property *P* were selected as causes of *m* because they then instantiated extrinsic property *V*. Had they not instantiated property *V*, they would not have been selected as causes of *m* in the first place. So I do want to claim that extrinsic property *V* does after all explain the structure of *S*'s behavior. It does explain why coins with intrinsic property *P* were selected as causes of *m*.

Concluding Remarks

To sum up, the vending machine shows three things. First, it shows that the delivery of a drink, *m*, is not the same thing as *S*'s behavior.

Second, it shows that we can distinguish two kinds of causal explanations: the ahistorical explanation of the mechanism whereby *c* causes *m* and the historical explanation of why *c* was recruited as a cause of *m*. Third, it shows that *c*'s being *P* is involved in the mechanism whereby *c* causes *m*, and *c*'s being *V* explains why *c* was recruited as a cause of *m*. Of course, coins with property *V* were selected as causes of *m* by human engineers with propositional attitudes (intentions, beliefs, and desires). So the selection process was an *intentional* process. I have simplemindedly (I confess) assumed that the causal efficacy of *c*'s being *V* in the explanation of the structure of *S*'s behavior is a relevant model of the causal efficacy of mental content in the explanation of an individual's intentional behavior. It is incumbent upon anybody who makes such an assumption to show two things. The first is to argue that the content of an individual's mental representation *R* can indeed explain the recruitment of *R* as a cause of some physical motion *m* of some of the individual's bodily parts. The second is to argue that the selection process whereby *R* was selected as a cause of *m* is a nonintentional process.

I will merely ask you to imagine a prey, which I'll call *D* (for deer), executing some flight motion *m* at *t*. I grant that the prey's behavior is not voluntary behavior, because it is instinctive. However, I will assume that it is intentional, because the flight motion is caused by some internal representation. I will now argue that we can at least ask three different questions about *D*'s flight motion *m*.

First, we can ask: why does *D* produce *m* at *t*? Answer: because at *t* – 1, *D* detected predator *P* in the vicinity. Call *c* *D*'s internal state whereby *D* dectected its predator. The presence of predator *P* prompted *D* to enter *c* at t – 1, which in turn caused *m* at *t*.

Second, we can ask the ahistorical question: what is the internal mechanism whereby *c* in *D* causes *m*? General answer: motor neurons in *D*'s motor cortex are wired to fire upon receiving inputs from sensory neurons in *D*'s visual (or olfactory) system. And the former in turn govern muscle contraction in *D*'s limbs. Presumably, the fact that *c* represents or reliably indicates the presence of predator *P* is not part of the answer to the question of the mechanism whereby *c* causes *m*.

Finally, consider the historical question: how did it come about that every time *D* is in state *c*, *D* does *m*? Why does it do *m* rather than something else? Why was *c* recruited as a cause of *m*, *flight* movement, rather than *fight* movement *m′* or *no* movement at all? The answer, I think, to this last question would come in two steps. First, *c* was recruited as a cause of *m* (flight movement) in *D* by natural selection. I assume that natural selection is a *non*intentional selection process. In the competition for survival between ancestors of preys of type *D* and other animals that were preys of ancestors of predator *P*, natural selection favored the former because they had a coordination between *c* and *m*. Preys of ancestors of *P* that lacked a coordination between *c* and *m* did not survive and went extinct. Second, natural selection would *not* have recruited *c* as a cause of *m* in ancestors of *D* if *c* had *not* been correlated with the presence of predator *P*. In other words, I claim, *c* would not have been turned into a cause of *m* by natural selection if it had not been a reliable *indicator* of the presence of a predator.

Like property *V* of coins, the *content* of a prey's perceptual state *c*—its being a reliable indicator of predators—is a historical extrinsic property. It too, I suggest, plays a causal role in the historical explanation of the structure of the prey's behavior: it contributes to explaining why *c* was coordinated with flight motions *m* in the presence of predator *P*. Unlike the monetary value of coins, however, the content of the prey's brain state turns on natural selection, which is a nonintentional selection process.

Notes

1. Unlike many philosophers, I think content can explain some of the things an individual does. It is an open question whether Davidson's (1980) anomalous monism allows content to explain intentional behavior. Eliminative materialists such as Quine (1960), Churchland (1984), and Stich (1983) explicitly deny it. So does Dennett (1987), according to whom there cannot be semantic engines. And so does Fodor (1987), who thinks that syntactic, not semantic, properties of mental symbols can be causally efficacious.
2. This argument makes use of the contrast between a thing *x*'s intrinsic and extrinsic properties. Although the contrast is notoriously hard to capture, it is, I believe, useful. Intuitively, a property is intrinsic only when its being instantiated by *x* at time *t* does not depend on anything other than *x* at *t*. It is extrinsic if it is not intrinsic.

3. The extrinsicness of meaning has been emphasized notably by Putnam (1975).
4. See Jacob (1997), chap. 8.

References

Churchland, Paul M. 1984. *Matter and consciousness.* Cambridge: MIT Press.

Davidson, Donald. 1980. *Essays on actions and events.* Oxford: Clarendon Press.

Dennett, Daniel C. 1987. Evolution, error, and intentionality. In *The intentional stance,* by Daniel C. Dennett. Cambridge: MIT Press.

Dretske, Fred. 1988. *Explaining behavior.* Cambridge: MIT Press.

Fodor, Jerry A. 1987. *Psychosemantics.* Cambridge: MIT Press.

Jacob, Pierre. 1997. *What minds can do.* Cambridge: Cambridge University Press.

Putnam, H. 1975. The meaning of 'meaning.' In *Philosophical papers,* vol. 2, by H. Putnam. Cambridge: Cambridge University Press.

Quine, Willard Van Orman. 1960. *Word and object.* Cambridge: MIT Press.

Stich, Steve. 1983. *From folk psychology to cognitive science.* Cambridge: MIT Press.

Deference and Indexicality

6

François Recanati

Two Dimensions of Content

The content of a representation (be it a concept, a thought, a word, or an utterance) is what it is a representation of. The content of my concept of tiger is the species *tiger,* the content of my concept of Cicero is Cicero. Similarly, the content of my thought, or statement, that Cicero is a famous Roman orator is the state of affairs consisting of Cicero and the property of being a famous Roman orator.

But there is a complication. Suppose I heard of Tully in high school, without ever realizing that Tully is Cicero. I believe that there are two persons, Cicero and Tully, who both were Roman orators. Consider my belief that Cicero is a Roman orator and my belief that Tully is a Roman orator. Do they have the same content? Yes, if the content of a representation is what it is a representation of. For (1) the only difference between the two beliefs is the fact that the concept of Cicero occurs in one while the concept of Tully occurs in the other, and (2) both concepts are concepts of the same individual.

The problem with this answer is that there is another notion of content that seems equally legitimate. Arguably, two beliefs have different contents if their input-output connections are different. Suppose I believe that Cicero did, while Tully did not, denounce Catiline. Then my belief that Cicero was a Roman orator will prompt the inference that a Roman orator denounced Catiline; not so with my belief that

Tully was a Roman orator. This difference in inferential potential shows that the two beliefs somehow differ in content.

In the familiar terminology derived from Frege (1970 [1892]), we can say that there are two dimensions of content: *what* is represented (the reference) and *how* it is represented (the "mode of presentation"). In the Cicero/Tully case, the reference is the same, but the modes of presentation are different. The reference is what is relevant for evaluating a representation as correct or incorrect: it is by comparing the representation with what it is a representation of that we come to be able to evaluate it. In contrast, the mode of presentation—the way the reference is thought of—is relevant for explaining (and predicting) behavior, including linguistic and mental behavior.

Modes of Presentation as Mental Files

What are modes of presentation? How are they individuated? If concepts are construed as mental files, as I think they should be, it will be tempting to equate the mode of presentation with the information (or perhaps misinformation) contained in the file. Thus my Cicero-file and my Tully-file refer to the same individual, but contain different pieces of (mis)information concerning that individual: in contrast to my Tully-file, my Cicero-file contains something to the effect that he denounced Catiline.

But this qualitative construal of modes of presentation is not ultimately satisfactory. The criterion for distinctness of modes of presentation, as stated by Schiffer (1978) after Frege, is:

> *(Frege's Constraint)*
> If it is possible for a rational subject S to believe at the same time of a given object *a* both that it is F and that it is not F, then there are two distinct modes of presentation of *a*, m and m′, such that S believes of *a* under m that it is F and under m′ that it is not F.

Now for it to be *possible* to believe without irrationality that *a* is F and that it is not F, it is sufficient to have two distinct mental files for *a*, even if the two files contain the same information (for example, that *a* was a Roman orator). It follows that modes of presentation are not to be identified with the informational content of the mental file, but rather with the mental file itself.

Egocentric Files

One important type of case, much discussed in the recent literature on modes of presentation, concerns indexical concepts like *here, now, this man, myself,* and so on. What is it to think of an object under such a mode of presentation? What is it to think of myself as *myself,* and not, say, as *François Recanati?* What is it to think of a place as *here?* To think of a pen as *this pen?* Answer: these modes of presentation are "egocentric files," that is, special files that serve as a repository for information *gained in a certain way*—typically through perception (Evans, 1982; Perry, 1993; Recanati, 1993). The "self" file serves as a repository for information gained in the first-person way (for example, through proprioception); the "here" file serves as a repository for information gained about a place by virtue of occupying that place and being in a position to perceive what is going on there. Demonstrative files ("this man") also depend upon perception. In order to entertain a thought in which one of these modes of presentation occurs, one must be suitably related to the reference: one must be related to it so as to be able to gain information from it in the proper way.

Types and Tokens

The relational constraint I have just mentioned is a constraint on the context in which a certain type of mode of presentation can occur. All modes of presentation of the "here" type constrain the context in which they can be entertained: the context must be such that the thinker is located at a certain place, which place is the reference of the "here"-mode of presentation. This suggests the following overall picture. There are mental symbols (types) that are very much like the words "I," "here," and so on. They can be appropriately tokened only in a context that satisfies certain constraints. When the constraints are satisfied, a reference is determined, and the symbol (token) expresses a genuine mode of presentation, that is, a mode of presentation *of* something. The symbols therefore have two semantic properties: *qua* tokens (if the context is appropriate) they have a reference that they present in a certain way. *Qua* types, however, they have a "character," a constant meaning that corresponds to the constraint itself and determines the way in which the reference, if any, is presented. That constant meaning can be described as a function from (appropriate) contexts to the referential contents assumed by the symbols in those contexts.[1]

Perception and Communication

All the ways of gaining information associated with egocentric files are perceptual ways of gaining information. But perception is not the only mode of acquisition of information: communication is another. Are there modes of presentation that depend on communication in the same way in which egocentric files depend on perception?

The natural answer is: no. Communication is parasitic on perception, in the sense that the information transmitted through communication must ultimately have been acquired through perception. It is also parasitic in another sense: the addressee must be able to grasp the information thus transmitted, and that means that the information in question must be information she *might* have acquired through perception (even if, as a matter of fact, she acquired it through communication). The conceptual repertoire that communication exploits must therefore be the same repertoire that we put to use in perception.

But the natural answer is not the only possible answer. In what follows I suggest that there is a special, communication-based mode of presentation that plays quite a central role in our mental lives precisely because it enables us to go beyond our private conceptual repertoire.

Deference as Meta-representation

A woman goes to the doctor, who tells her that she has arthritis. She believes what the doctor tells her. A number of representations are involved in this simple exchange. The doctor, after clinical examination, comes to entertain the thought: "She has arthritis." He expresses that thought by telling her: "You have arthritis." The woman then comes to believe something that might be expressed by the sentence: "I have arthritis."

It seems, at this stage, that the woman has acquired the belief that she has arthritis. But suppose, as Burge did in the famous article in which this example was introduced, that the woman has no idea (or only a very vague idea) what arthritis is. Suppose she lacks the concept of "arthritis." Does she really believe that she has arthritis? Does she not, rather, believe that she has *some ailment called "arthritis"* (Donnellan, 1993)? This view seems more in line with the notion that whatever is actually communicated must be within the addressee's ken and could not exceed his or her conceptual repertoire.

On the suggested view, then, it is misleading to say that the woman comes to think "I have arthritis" as a result of the doctor's utterance. She does not actually believe that. Even if she goes about repeating "I have arthritis," and that sentence expresses the proposition that she has arthritis, still that is not what she believes in the proper sense of the term (Sperber, 1997). What she believes would be more faithfully expressed by a metalinguistic sentence: "I have an ailment called (by the doctor) 'arthritis.' " It follows that there is a divergence between the content of the utterance, which depends on social factors (namely, the conventions in force in the public language) and the content of the underlying mental representation. The mental representation is metalinguistic while the public representation is not.

Another Approach to Deference

In contrast to that metalinguistic approach, the view I am going to argue for does not rest on a distinction between the content of the public utterance and the content of the underlying mental representation. On my view, one and the same proposition, namely the proposition that the woman has arthritis, is both the content of the woman's utterance and the content of her belief. (It is also, of course, the content of the doctor's utterance and the content of the doctor's belief.)

At this point a difficulty immediately arises. How could the woman believe she has arthritis? In order to believe that she has arthritis, she must entertain a mental representation whose content is the proposition that she has arthritis. Now such a representation must contain a constituent (a concept) whose content is arthritis, and we have granted that the woman does not possess the concept of arthritis!

This difficulty is not as dramatic as it seems. It is true that, if the woman is to believe that she has arthritis, she must entertain a mental representation whose content is the proposition that she has arthritis. It is true also that such a representation must contain a concept whose content is arthritis. But "a concept whose content is arthritis" is *a* concept of arthritis, it is not *the* concept of arthritis—that concept which the woman lacks. When we say that the woman "does not possess the concept of arthritis," we are not talking of any old concept whose content is arthritis: we are referring to a specific concept endowed not only with a certain reference (arthritis) *but also with a certain character.*[2] The woman does not possess that concept, but she possesses another concept of arthritis. The concept of arthritis she possesses is a *deferential* concept, that is, the sort of concept which people who use a public word without fully understanding it typically entertain (Recanati, 1997). The difference between the woman's belief and the doctor's (or between the woman's belief and her utterance) is therefore not a difference at the content level but a difference in character or mode of presentation.

The Deferential Operator

Qua types, indexical symbols have a character, a constant meaning that determines both their reference (in context) and the way the reference is presented. That constant meaning is a function from contexts to contents. My hypothesis is that there is, in the mental repertoire, a "deferential operator" that enables us to construct deferential concepts with a semantics analogous to that of indexical concepts.

The deferential operator $R_x(\sigma)$ applies to (the mental representation of) a public symbol σ and yields a complex representation $R_x(\sigma)$—a deferential concept—which has both a character and a content. The character of $R_x(\sigma)$ takes us from a context in which there is a competent user x of σ, to a certain content, namely the content which σ has for x, given σ's own character. What is special with the deferential concept $R_x(\sigma)$ is that its content is determined "deferentially," via the content that another cognitive agent, somehow given in the context, attaches or would attach to σ in the context of utterance.

The deferential operator is the mental equivalent of quotation marks in written speech. It is metalinguistic in the sense that it involves a mention of the symbol σ and a tacit reference to its use by the cognitive agent x (which can be a community as well as an individual). But that metalinguistic aspect is located in the character of the deferential concept: the content of that concept is the same as the content of the symbol σ when used by x.

Take our "arthritis" case. When the woman who does not know what arthritis is says "I have arthritis," she does not entertain "the" concept of arthritis, as the doctor does when he tells her, "You have arthritis." They entertain different mental representations, involving different concepts. In the woman's belief a deferential concept occurs, namely: R_{doctor} *(arthritis)*. But the content of that concept is the same as the content of the doctor's concept of arthritis—indeed the woman's deferential concept is parasitic on the doctor's concept and automatically inherits its referential content, by virtue of the mechanics of the deferential operator. That referential content—arthritis—is thought of metalinguistically as "what the doctor calls *arthritis,*" but the woman's thought is fundamentally about arthritis, not about the word "arthritis." If I am right, the difference between the doctor's concept of arthritis and the woman's is similar to that between "I" and "you" in their respective utterances "You have arthritis" and "I have arthritis": "I" and "you" refer to the woman under different modes of presentation. Similarly, the doctor's concept of arthritis and the woman's deferential concept R_{doctor} *(arthritis)* both refer to arthritis, under different modes of presentation.

Conclusion: Deference as Social Indexicality

On the view I have sketched, deferential concepts are like indexical concepts, but instead of depending on perception they depend on communication. An indexical type of mode of presentation constrains the context of its tokenings: it demands that the subject who entertains the mode of presentation be directly related to the reference so as to be able to gain information from it in perception. Similarly there is a deferential type of mode of presentation which demands that the subject who entertains a mode of presentation of that type (a deferential concept) be indirectly related to the reference, via a chain of informants, so as to be able to gain information from it in communication.

Notes

1. In what follows I will use "content" always in the sense of "referential content," as opposed to "character."
2. On the character/content distinction, see Kaplan (1989).

References

Burge, T. 1979. Individualism and the mental. *Midwest Studies in Philosophy, 4,* 73–121.

Donnellan, K. 1993. There is a word for that kind of thing: An investigation of two thought experiments. *Philosophical Perspectives, 7,* 155–171.

Evans, G. 1982. *The varieties of reference,* ed. J. McDowell. Oxford: Clarendon Press.

Frege, G. 1970 (1892). On sense and reference. In *Translations from the philosophical writings of Gottlob Frege,* ed. P. Geach and M. Black, 2nd ed., 56–78. Oxford: Clarendon Press.

Kaplan, D. 1989. Demonstratives. In *Themes from Kaplan,* ed. J. Almog, H. Wettstein, and J. Perry, 481–563. New York: Oxford University Press.

Perry, J. 1993. *The problem of the essential indexical and other essays.* New York: Oxford University Press.

Recanati, F. 1993. *Direct reference: From language to thought.* Oxford: Blackwell.

——— 1997. Can we believe what we do not understand? *Mind and Language, 12,* 84–100.

Schiffer, S. 1978. The basis of reference. *Erkenntnis, 13,* 171–206.

Sperber, D. 1997. Intuitive and reflective beliefs. *Mind and Language, 12,* 67–83.

How Is Conceptual Knowledge Organized in the Brain? Clues from Category-Specific Deficits

7

Alfonso Caramazza

The patterns of spared and impaired functions that result from brain damage can be used to infer the structure of cognitive systems in the brain. The logic of this approach is straightforward: We infer the functional and neural separability of a mechanism assumed to be necessary for the performance of a task if it can be damaged independently of other processes. This logic can be extended to differences in performance for types of stimuli. For example, the selective deficit in recognizing faces may be used to infer the existence of a mechanism specialized in processing faces. However, this observation does not unequivocally support the inference of a distinct processing mechanism for face recognition. It could be argued that faces differ from other objects not in terms of the processing mechanism they engage but only in levels of processing complexity. And indeed it has been proposed that prosopagnosia is the result of a general perceptual processing deficit that manifests itself more intensely in difficult perceptual discrimination tasks such as face perception (see Bruce and Humphreys, 1994). As this example illustrates, we cannot interpret the occurrence of a disproportionate deficit for a class of objects as unambiguous proof for the existence of a dedicated mechanism for those objects. However, we would have a far stronger case if along with the selective deficit of a class of objects we could document the existence of the reverse dissociation—namely, the selective sparing of the class of objects that was supposedly thought to be more difficult to process (see Moscovitch, Winocur, and Behrmann, 1997, for an example in the case of face perception). The existence of a double dissociation for two types of stimuli makes the "processing difficulty" argument for the observed dissociations far less plausible (Shallice, 1979).

There are many other dissociations of deficits for stimulus types that have invited the inference of distinct processing mechanisms. Some of these are less controversial than others. The dissociation in processing objects versus words is generally accepted to indicate the existence of distinct processing mechanisms for the recognition of objects and words, respectively. Similarly uncontroversial is the dissociation in processing low- and high-frequency words, which is uniformly interpreted as reflecting degrees of processing difficulty and not the existence of distinct processing mechanisms. Far more controversial is the interpretation of the dissociation between words and nonwords in reading (and writing). Some theorists have argued that the double dissociation in reading words and nonwords signals the existence of independent lexical and nonlexical processing mechanisms (see, for example, Coltheart, 1985). Other theorists have proposed reading models that supposedly can accommodate the double dissociation without postulating distinct mechanisms for the two types of stimuli (see Plaut et al., 1996). Similarly controversial are the double dissociations for words of different grammatical classes. There are a number of reports of double dissociations in producing nouns versus verbs and content versus function words (see Caramazza, 1997, for review). However, the interpretation of these dissociations as reflecting the existence of distinct processing mechanisms (or distinct neural structures) for different grammatical classes remains highly controversial. Also controversial is the interpretation of semantic category-specific deficits. Nonetheless, their existence provides a window into the organization of conceptual knowledge in the brain.

Semantic Category-Specific Deficits

In a series of seminal papers, Warrington and her collaborators (Warrington, 1981; Warrington and McCarthy, 1983; Warrington and

Shallice, 1984) documented several cases of selective naming difficulties for specific semantic categories. The clearest cases involved the category of "living things" which was disproportionately impaired in some cases[1] (Warrington and Shallice, 1984) and largely spared in others (Warrington and McCarthy, 1983). Since the publication of these cases, there have been many other reports of category-specific deficits, usually reporting a broad-based dissociation between living and nonliving things. Most of these cases involved the disproportionate impairment of the category of living things (see Gainotti et al., 1995, for review). But there have also been reports of more fine-grained dissociations. Patients have been described who were severely impaired in processing animals but not other living things, such as fruits and vegetables, or artifacts (for example, Caramazza and Shelton, 1998; Hart and Gordon, 1992). For example, patient EW (Caramazza and Shelton, 1998) named correctly all fruits and vegetables (24/24) and 92 percent (98/106) of the artifacts but was only able to

Table 7.1

Living		Nonliving	Examples of case reports
Animate	Inanimate		
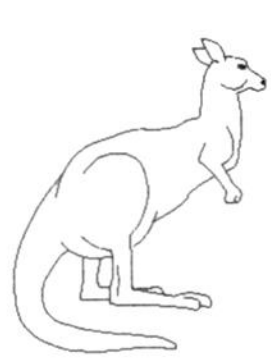	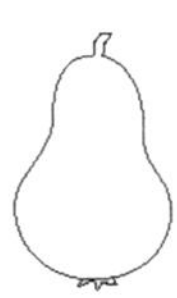	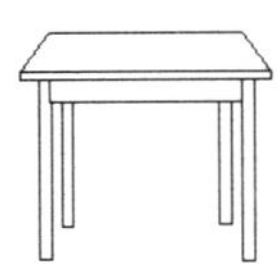	
✓	✓		Warrington & Shallice (1984) Silveri & Gainotti (1988)
		✓	Warrington & McCarthy (1983) Sacchett & Humphreys (1992)
✓			Hart & Gordon (1992) Caramazza & Shelton (1998)
	✓	✓	Hillis & Caramazza (1991)
	✓		Hart, Berndt, & Caramazza (1985) Farah & Wallace (1992)
✓		✓	Not observed

✓ = Disproportionate impairment

name correctly 34 percent (16/47) of the animal pictures. The reverse dissociation has also been reported. Hillis and Caramazza (1991) describe a patient who was impaired with all categories but animals. And there are also reports of patients with impairment restricted to the category of fruits and vegetables (Hart, Berndt, and Caramazza, 1985; Farah and Wallace, 1992). A summary of the major dissociations reported to date is shown in Table 7.1. In Table 7.2 are shown examples of the definitions produced in response to named animals and other objects by a patient (JJ: Hillis and Caramazza, 1991) with selective sparing of animate objects. These definitions illustrate the striking difference in processing ability for objects in the spared and impaired categories: JJ produced highly explicit, correct definitions for animals, but ambiguous or incorrect definitions for inanimate objects.

What do these dissociations reveal about the organization of conceptual knowledge in the brain? Do they reflect the existence of specialized mechanisms for the recognition and storage of specific semantic categories? Or do they merely reflect differences in processing complexity across categories or some other noncategorical principle of organization? With one exception, current explanations of category-

Table 7.2 Examples of JJ's definitions of animate and inanimate objects

Animate objects	
Heron	"This bird has a long neck and legs. It lives near water. Stands in the water . . . very tall—maybe 6 feet. Not brown, but white and blue perhaps."
Lion	"A large animal, about 4 feet tall, maybe taller at the shoulders: it has a long body and very large paws, and stands on all four legs. It has a monstrous head with which it growls; and it has a mane—a large body of hair. It lives in Africa."
Inanimate objects	
Bench	"A device you sit on, about 12 inches high with 4 legs. It revolves you around while sitting. Can be made of metal or wood."
Celery	"Very white bodied meat . . . soft . . . easy to eat."

Source: Hillis and Caramazza, 1991.

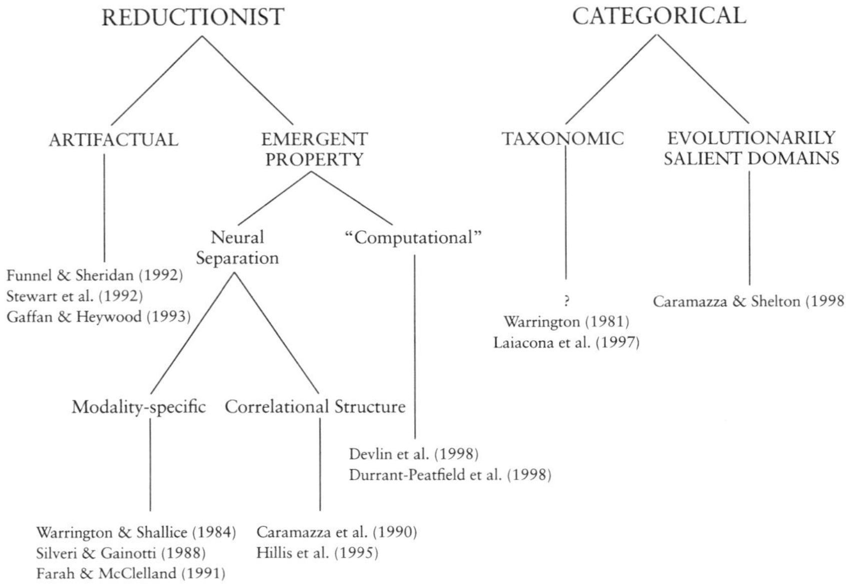

Figure 7.1

specific deficits have adopted a reductionist perspective, appealing to some or other noncategorical principle to explain the disorder. Some have appealed to the relative importance of the visual properties of objects in distinguishing among members of a semantic category; others have appealed to the relative strengths of correlations between visual and functional properties in different categories. A schematic representation of the various explanations of semantic category-specific deficits is shown in Figure 7.1.[2]

The most important distinction among the various accounts of category-specific deficits is between categorical and reductionist explanations. This distinction reflects the divide between two radically different views about the structure of human cognition—the view that the human mind is a collection of special-purpose devices each dedicated to a specific, narrowly defined purpose (for example, face perception) versus the view that the mind is a seamless, general-purpose computational device that is used for learning such diverse things as language, chess, and arithmetic. The former view is open to the possibility that there are distinct neural mechanisms for the perception and storage of different semantic categories; the latter is committed to interpreting category-specific effects as emergent properties of the (sensory/motor) structure of the members of semantic categories.[3]

Categorical Accounts

Two types of categorical organization of conceptual knowledge can be envisioned: taxonomic organization and evolutionarily defined domains. One could imagine that conceptual knowledge is organized taxonomically in such a way that each semantic category is represented/processed by a distinct neural mechanism. Such a proposal would be of little value, however, in the absence of an explicit formulation of what constitutes a semantic category. Is "animal" a semantic category for the purposes of this theory? And what about "mammal," "ferocious animal," "furniture," and "objects typically found on a writing desk"? Are any of these semantic categories the right size for the theory? To my knowledge no one has proposed that conceptual knowledge is organized taxonomically and, thus, this view will not be discussed further.[4] I turn instead to the only explicitly categorical theory of the organization of conceptual knowledge in the brain.

Caramazza and Shelton (1998) have argued that conceptual knowledge is organized in broad domains that reflect evolutionarily salient distinctions—the "domain-specific knowledge" hypothesis. This hypothesis provides a principled answer to the question of what constitutes a semantic category for the purposes of organization of conceptual knowledge in the brain. The claim is based on the assumption that evolutionary pressures resulted in dedicated neural mechanisms for processing specific kinds of objects, leading to the categorical organization of knowledge about those objects (see, for example, Gelman, 1990; Premack, 1990). The original proposal distinguished among the domains of animate objects, plant life (fruits and vegetables), and artifacts. However, a more complete list would probably include the domain of conspecific concepts, that is, concepts belonging to the same classes (see Shelton, Fouch, and Caramazza, 1998). A plausible argument can be made that evolutionary pressures led to specific adaptations for recognizing and responding to conspecifics, animals, and plant life (and perhaps artifacts). The fitness value for these adaptations is uncontroversial. For example, conspecifics are a source of nurturance and protection, animals are potential predators, and plants are a source of food and medicine. The ability to quickly and accurately categorize objects in these categories has obvious survival and reproductive value. The evolutionary adaptations for recognizing conspecifics, animals, and plant life (and perhaps artifacts) provide the skeletal framework around which to organize the rich perceptual, conceptual, and linguistic knowledge we have of these categories of objects. Because of this organization, brain damage can result in category-specific deficits for each of these evolutionarily defined domains of knowledge.[5]

Reductionist Accounts

Reductionist accounts of category-specific deficits can be divided into those that would dispense with the phenomenon as an artifact of uncontrolled accidental variables associated with the impaired categories and those that explain the effect as an emergent property of noncategorical attributes of the members of the categories—the "artifactual" and the "emergent property" accounts, respectively. A number of investigators have argued that the selective impairment of the category of living things may simply reflect the fact that these items tend to be unfamiliar, infrequent, and visually complex relative to other categories of objects (Funnell and Sheridan, 1992; Stewart, Parkin, and Hunkin, 1992; Gaffan and Heywood, 1993). Although it is not improbable that some putative category-specific effects can be explained by appeal to these extraneous factors, it is certainly not the case that all such effects can be so easily dismissed. A number of studies have shown that category-specific deficits persist even when familiarity, frequency, and visual complexity are tightly controlled (for example, Hart and Gordon, 1992; Laiacona, Barbarotto, and Capitani, 1993; Caramazza and Shelton, 1998; Lambon Ralph et al., 1998; Moss et al., 1998; Samson, Pillon, and De Wilde, 1998). And in any case, the artifactual account cannot explain the cases of selective sparing of the supposedly difficult categories (for example, Hillis and Caramazza, 1991).

The emergent property accounts of category-specific deficits can be further divided into those that explain the phenomenon by appeal to the way in which conceptual knowledge is organized in the brain and those that appeal to the computational and structural properties of semantic categories—the "neural specialization" and the "computational" accounts, respectively. The neural specialization theories argue that conceptual knowledge is organized in the brain in such a way that selective damage to particular brain areas will result in a category-like effect even though knowledge is not organized categorically. Of these theories, the one that has received the most attention is the sensory/functional theory (SFT) (Warrington and Shallice, 1984; see also Silveri and Gainotti, 1988; Farah and McClelland, 1991; Hart and Gordon, 1992; De Renzi and Lucchelli, 1994; Gainotti and Silveri, 1996).

SFT assumes that conceptual knowledge is organized into modality-specific subsystems. The major subsystems are the visual and the functional/associative components. The visual subsystem stores information about the visual characteristics of objects (for example, tables have legs) and the functional/associative ("functional" for short) subsystem stores information about the uses of objects, where they might be found, and other nonsensory properties (for example, lions are carnivores). The theory also argues that the meaning of living things depends far more on visual properties than it does on functional knowledge, while the meaning of nonliving things depends more on their functional than on their visual attributes. Thus damage to the visual knowledge subsystem will result in disproportionate impairment for the category of living things, while damage to the functional knowledge subsystem will result in disproportionate impairment for the category of nonliving things. Furthermore, since category-specific deficits are supposed to arise from the selective damage of specific subtypes of knowledge—visual for living things and functional for nonliving things—it follows that category-specific deficits will be associated with disproportionate difficulties for a specific subtype of knowledge. In other words, the SFT predicts that patients with selective impairment for living things should show greater difficulties for visual knowledge of objects; patients with selective impairment for nonliving things should show greater difficulties with the functional attributes of objects. The theory is also necessarily committed to the reverse prediction: namely, selective damage to either the visual or the functional semantic subsystem should result in disproportionate difficulties for living or nonliving things, respectively. In short, what distinguishes the SFT from other accounts of category-specific deficits is its commitment to an association between deficits for modalities and for categories of knowledge.

Early reports of the relationship between category-specific deficits for living things and the ability to process their visual attributes were consistent with predictions from the SFT. Several studies reported that patients with disproportionate difficulties for living things were also disproportionately impaired in processing their visual relative to their functional attributes (for example, Basso, Capitani, and Laiacona, 1988; Silveri and Gainotti, 1988; Farah, et al., 1989). However, these studies have been criticized on methodological grounds (see Caramazza and Shelton, 1998). More recent, tightly controlled studies of patients with category-specific deficits for living things have found that they are equally impaired with visual and functional attributes of living things, and equally unimpaired with both attribute types of nonliving things (for example, Laiacona, Barbarotto, and Capitani, 1993; Laiacona, Capitani, and Barbarotto, 1997; Caramazza and Shelton, 1998; Lambon Ralph et al., 1998; Moss et al., 1998; Samson, Pillon, and De Wilde, 1998). A summary of the relevant results from several of these studies is shown in Table 7.3. Also problematic for the SFT are the results of two recent studies that have found that patients with disproportionate difficulties with visual attributes are *not* also disproportionately impaired in processing living things (Coltheart et al., 1998; Lambon Ralph et al., 1998). Thus, the central predictions of the SFT have not been confirmed.[6]

We don't have to assume a modality-based organization of conceptual knowledge in the brain in order for category-specific effects to "emerge" from a noncategorically organized system. If we were to assume that strongly correlated properties are represented in adjacent neural tissue and that members of natural-kind categories (for example, animals) share many properties in common, then we would expect that the semantic properties of natural-kind objects would be more likely to be found near one another and, consequently, more likely to be damaged together. The Organized Unitary Content Hypothesis (OUCH) is one instantiation of these principles (Caramazza

Table 7.3 Performance of patients with semantic category-specific deficits in property-judgment tasks with visual and functional/associative properties

	Living		Nonliving	
	Visual	Functional	Visual	Functional
EW (Caramazza and Sheridan, 1998)	0.67	0.74	0.96	0.99
GR (Laiacona et al., 1993)	0.55	0.57	0.91	0.84
GR (Laiacona et al., 1993)	0.73	0.69	0.95	0.95
JEN (Samson et al., 1998)	0.42	0.51	0.75	0.83

et al., 1990; Hillis, Rapp, and Caramazza, 1995). The core assumption in this model is that conceptual space is "lumpy," in the sense that semantic properties are not distributed uniformly across categories but tend to cluster together, independent of their modality. For example, objects that are made of certain kinds of stuff (texture, color, substance) have particular shapes, have certain kinds of odors, are likely to be capable of certain kinds of motion, and are also likely to be found in certain types of environments (for example, think of a horse); and objects that are shaped like a table and are made of certain kinds of stuff tend to be found in certain locations and are not likely to be capable of biological motion. In other words, the properties of members of semantic categories tend to cluster together and, therefore, tend to be damaged together, leading to category-like effects.

This model can account for the principal facts about category-specific deficits: it accounts for the fact that animate objects, fruits and vegetables, and artifacts can be damaged independently of one another, and for the fact that there is no interaction of modality by category in category-specific deficits. However, it fails to exclude the existence of unattested patterns of category-specific deficits. For example, there is nothing in the theory as currently formulated that would exclude the existence of a category-specific deficit restricted to just mammals or just vegetables or just vehicles. In fact, the theory fails to explain both why very narrow category-specific deficits (for example, birds but not fish) do not occur and why the boundaries of category-specific deficits are as have been observed.

The "computational" accounts of category-specific deficits share with OUCH the assumption that semantic categories differ in the degree of correlations and types of associations among the properties that characterize their members. However, the computational theories rely on assumptions about the manner in which properties interact in concept processing to explain the occurrence of category-specific deficits. For example, Devlin, Gonnerman, Andersen, and Seidenberg (1998) assume that living things share many more highly correlated properties than do nonliving things. They further assume that the activation state of any one property is a function of the activation state of its correlated properties. A consequence of this assumption in their computational model is that mild, diffuse damage to the conceptual system will result in a slight advantage for living things, while extensive, diffuse damage will result in disproportionate difficulties for living things. Durrant-Peatfield, Moss, and Tyler (1998; see also Moss et al., 1998) propose a similar theory but place greater emphasis on the *kinds* of properties that are correlated. They note that living things have many correlated properties, including perceptual and biological functions, whereas nonliving things have few shared properties but individual items have highly specific form-function correlations.

These computational models face two major difficulties. One difficulty is that it is not obvious how they can account for the dissociation between animals and plant life (fruits and vegetables) without making additional ad hoc assumptions. Greater difficulties are posed by the existence of cases of severe deficit to the category of nonliving things in the context of largely spared ability to process animate objects. For example, patient JJ (Hillis and Caramazza, 1991) performed very poorly with the category of inanimate objects despite nearly normal performance with animals. His performance in an object-naming task, at two points in the evolution of his illness, is shown in Table 7.4, together with the performance of patient PS, who shows the reverse pattern of difficulties. PS performed very poorly with the category of living things but nearly normally with nonliving things. These

Table 7.4 JJ's and PS's naming performance at six and thirteen months post-stroke

	Six months post		Thirteen months post	
	Animals	Nonanimals	Animals	Nonanimals
JJ	81	12	100	69
PS	47	93	61	92

Source: Hillis and Caramazza, 1991.

results show that the occurrence of disproportionate difficulty for inanimate objects is not dependent on the overall level of severity of deficit as would be expected by the two computational accounts reviewed here. Indeed, the two patients show contrasting patterns of category-specific disorders at comparable levels of severity of the deficit.

This brief review of semantic category-specific deficits has shown that the principal facts of this disorder are not easily accommodated without appeal to considerable structure in the organization of conceptual knowledge in the brain. Reductionist accounts of semantic category-specific deficits encounter severe difficulties explaining *why* it is that the categories of the disorder are just those that have been reported: the categories of conspecifics (body parts and faces), animate objects, fruits and vegetables, and artifacts. Furthermore, specific reductionist theories encounter additional difficulties with one or another aspect of the disorder. For example, the SFT incorrectly predicts that category-specific deficits should also be modality-specific deficits; and the computational (correlational) theories reviewed here incorrectly predict that disproportionate difficulty with inanimate objects should only be found in the context of moderately to severely impaired performance for animate objects. By contrast, the domain-specific hypothesis of conceptual organization provides a natural account for the facts of category-specific disorders. It correctly predicts that the categories of category-specific deficits should be just those that could plausibly have emerged through evolutionary pressures (but see Lambon Ralph et al., 1998; Moss et al., 1998). Reasonable candidates include the categories of conspecifics, animate objects, and plant life (and perhaps artifacts)—just the categories that have *reliably* been shown to be selectively damaged or spared in brain-damaged subjects and for which there are ontogenetic arguments that can be given for their functional autonomy (see, for example, papers in Hirschfeld and Gelman, 1994; and see Caramazza and Shelton, 1998, for further discussion of the parallels between category-specific deficits and the acquisition of the animate-inanimate distinction). It is not implausible to conclude, then, that the human mind is a collection of special-purpose devices, each dedicated to a narrowly defined function of which one set might be mechanisms for the classification and storage of distinct conceptual domains.

Notes

This chapter is adapted from Caramazza (1998). The writing of this paper was supported in part by NIH grant NS-22201. I thank Kathryn Link for her comments on an earlier version.

1. Although these cases are usually cited as examples of a category-specific deficit for living things, they are in fact much more complex. The two most thoroughly studied cases, those of JBR and SBY, were also impaired in processing the category of foods (and, in the case of JBR, the categories of musical instruments, precious stones, cloths, and metals—all inanimate objects).
2. This scheme captures most accounts of category-specific deficits. Some do not fit, however. For example, a recent proposal by Damasio and collaborators (Damasio et al., 1996) proposes that category-specific deficits result from damage to categorically organized "lexical" as opposed to conceptual representations. However, this account fails to explain the semantic character of the impairments in the detailed reports of patients with category-specific deficits. Furthermore, the evidence and arguments presented by Damasio et al. in favor of the claim that the lexical as opposed to the semantic system is organized categorically have been challenged on methodological grounds (see Caramazza and Shelton, 1998, n29).
3. Note that there is an important asymmetry here. Although the modularity theory of mind (for example, Fodor, 1983) does not entail that all cognitive processes be modular, the reductionist theory excludes the possibility that any cognitive process is modular.
4. However, Warrington (1981) and Laiacona, Capitani, and Barbarotto (1997) may have come close to proposing a taxonomic organization of conceptual knowledge.

5. It is important to emphasize that the domain-specific hypothesis of conceptual organization does not preclude there being other levels of organization within the conceptual system. This hypothesis only addresses the issue of between-domain organization. There is the further question of how conceptual knowledge is organized *within* domains. Depending on the assumptions one is willing to make about the organization of conceptual knowledge within domains, further expectations can be derived for the types of deficits that would be expected to follow from selective damage to specific brain areas. For example, if we were to assume that objects that share many properties tend to be represented in spatially adjacent areas (see OUCH below), then it might be possible to find finer-grained dissociations than domain-based categories.
6. For a detailed critique of the computational variant of the SFT (Farah and McClelland, 1991) see Caramazza and Shelton (1998).

References

Basso, A., Capitani, E., and Laiacona, M. 1988. Progressive language impairment without dementia: A case with isolated category specific semantic defect. *Journal of Neurology, Neurosurgery, and Psychiatry, 51,* 1201–1207.

Bruce, V., and Humphreys, G. W. 1994. Recognizing objects and faces. *Visual Cognition, 1,* 141–180.

Caramazza, A. 1997. How many levels of processing are there in lexical access? *Cognitive Neuropsychology, 14,* 177–208.

——— 1998. The interpretation of semantic category-specific deficits: What do they reveal about the organization of conceptual knowledge in the brain? *NeuroCase, 4,* 265–272.

Caramazza, A., Hillis, A. E., Rapp, B. C., and Romani, C. 1990. The multiple semantics hypothesis: Multiple confusions? *Cognitive Neuropsychology, 7,* 161–189.

Caramazza, A., and Shelton, J. R. 1998. Domain-specific knowledge systems in the brain: The animate-inanimate distinction. *Journal of Cognitive Neuroscience, 10,* 1–34.

Coltheart, M. 1985. Cognitive neuropsychology and the study of reading. In *Attention and Performance XI,* ed. M. I. Posner and O. S. M. Marin. Hillsdale, N.J.: Erlbaum.

Coltheart, M., Inglis, L., Cupples, L., Michie, P., Bates, A., and Budd, B. 1998. A semantic subsystem specific to the storage of information about the visual attributes of animate and inanimate objects. *NeuroCase, 4,* 353–370.

Damasio, H., Grabowski, T. J., Tranel, D., Hichwa, R. D., and Damasio, A. R. 1996. A neural basis for lexical retrieval. *Nature, 380,* 499–505.

De Renzi, E., and Lucchelli, F. 1994. Are semantic systems separately represented in the brain? The case of living category impairment. *Cortex, 30,* 3–25.

Devlin, J. T., Gonnerman, L. M., Andersen, E. S., and Seidenberg, M. S. 1998. Category-specific semantic deficits in focal and widespread brain damage: A computational account. *Journal of Cognitive Neuroscience, 10,* 77–94.

Durrant-Peatfield, M., Moss, H. E., and Tyler, L. K. 1998. The emergence of categories in a damaged PDP system. Paper presented to the meeting of the Cognitive Neuroscience Society, San Francisco, April.

Farah, M. J., and McClelland, J. L. 1991. A computational model of semantic memory impairment: Modality specificity and emergent category specificity. *Journal of Experimental Psychology: General, 120,* 339–357.

Farah, M. J., Hammond, K. M., Mehta, Z., and Ratcliff, G. 1989. Category-specificity and modality-specificity in semantic memory. *Neuropsychologia, 27,* 193–200.

Farah, M. J., and Wallace, M. A. 1992. Semantically-bounded anomia: Implications for the neural implementation of naming. *Neuropsychologia, 30,* 609–621.

Fodor, J. 1983. *The Modularity of Mind.* Cambridge: MIT Press.

Funnell, E., and Sheridan, J. S. 1992. Categories of knowledge? Unfamiliar aspects of living and non-living things. *Cognitive Neuropsychology, 9,* 135–153.

Gaffan, D., and Heywood, C. A. 1993. A spurious category-specific visual agnosia for living things in normal humans and nonhuman primates. *Journal of Cognitive Neurosciences, 5,* 118–128.

Gainotti, G., and Silveri, M. C. 1996. Cognitive and anatomical locus of lesion in a patient with a category-specific semantic impairment for living beings. *Cognitive Neuropsychology, 13,* 357–389.

Gainotti, G., Silveri, M. C., Daniele, A., and Giustolisi, L. 1995. Neuroanatomical correlates of category-specific semantic disorders: A critical survey. In R. A. McCarthy, ed., *Semantic Knowledge and Semantic Representations. Memory, 3,* nos. 3–4, 247–264. Hove, England: Erlbaum, Taylor and Francis.

Gelman, R. 1990. First principles organize attention to and learning about relevant data: Number and the animate-inanimate distinction as examples. *Cognitive Science, 14,* 79–106.

Hart, J., Berndt, R. S., and Caramazza, A. 1985. Category-specific naming deficit following cerebral infarction. *Nature, 316,* 439–440.

Hart, J., and Gordon, B. 1992. Neural subsystems for object knowledge. *Nature, 359,* 60–64.

Hillis, A. E., and Caramazza, A. 1991. Category-specific naming and comprehension impairment: A double dissociation. *Brain, 114,* 2081–2094.

Hillis, A. E., Rapp, B., and Caramazza, A. 1995. Constraining claims about theories of semantic memory: More on unitary versus multiple semantics. *Cognitive Neuropsychology, 12,* 175–186.

Hirschfeld, L. A., and Gelman, S. A, eds. 1994. *Mapping the mind: Domain specificity in cognition and culture.* New York: Cambridge University Press.

Laiacona, M., Barbarotto, R., and Capitani, E. 1993. Perceptual and associative knowledge in category specific impairment of semantic memory: A study of two cases. *Cortex, 29,* 727–740.

Laiacona, M., Capitani, E., and Barbarotto, R. 1997. Semantic category dissociations: A longitudinal study of two cases. *Cortex, 33,* 441–461.

Lambon Ralph, M. A., Howard, D., Nightingale, G., and Ellis, A. W. 1998. Are living and non-living category-specific deficits causally linked to impaired perceptual or associative knowledge? Evidence from a category-specific double dissociation. *NeuroCase, 4,* 311–338.

Moss, H. E., Tyler, L. K., Durrant-Peatfield, M., and Bunn, E. M. 1998. "Two eyes of a see-through": Impaired and intact semantic knowledge in a case of selective deficit for living things. *NeuroCase, 4,* 291–310.

Moscovitch, M., Winocur, G., and Behrmann, M. 1997. What is special about face recognition? Nineteen experiments on a person with a visual object agnosia and dyslexia but normal face recognition. *Journal of Cognitive Neuroscience, 9,* 555–604.

Plaut, D. C., McClelland, J. L., Seidenberg, M. S., and Patterson, K. 1996. Understanding normal and impaired word reading: Computational principles in quasi-regular domains. *Psychological Review, 103,* 56–115.

Premack, D. 1990. The infant's theory of self-propelled motion. *Cognition, 36,* 1–16.

Sacchett, C., and Humphreys, G. W. 1992. Calling a squirrel a squirrel but a canoe a wigwam: A category-specific deficit for artefactual objects and body parts. *Cognitive Neuropsychology, 9,* 73–86.

Samson, D., Pillon, A., and De Wilde, V. 1998. Impaired knowledge of visual and non-visual attributes in a patient with a semantic impairment for living entities: A case of a true category-specific deficit. *NeuroCase, 4,* 273–290.

Shallice, T. 1979. Case study approach in neuropsychological research. *Journal of Clinical Neuropsychology, 1,* 183–211.

Shelton, J. R., Fouch, E., and Caramazza, A. 1998. The selective sparing of body part knowledge: A case study. *NeuroCase, 4,* 339–351.

Silveri, M. C., and Gainotti, G. 1988. Interaction between vision and language in category-specific impairment. *Cognitive Neuropsychology, 5,* 677–709.

Stewart, F., Parkin, A. J., and Hunkin, N. M. 1992. Naming impairments following recovery from Herpes Simplex Encephalitis: Category-specific? *Quarterly Journal of Experimental Psychology, 44A,* 261–284.

Warrington, E. K. 1981. Neuropsychological studies of verbal semantic systems. *Philosophical Transactions of the Royal Society of London, Series B, 295,* 411–423.

Warrington, E. K., and McCarthy, R. 1983. Category specific access dysphasia. *Brain, 106,* 859–878.

——— 1987. Categories of knowledge: Further fractionations and an attempted integration. *Brain, 110,* 1273–1296.

Warrington, E. K., and Shallice, T. 1984. Category specific semantic impairments. *Brain, 107,* 829–854.

Discourse Structure, Intentions, and Intonation

8

Barbara J. Grosz

This chapter addresses language structure at the discourse level, describing investigations into the representations needed to support language processing at this level. The discussion that follows reviews research seeking to uncover the ways in which the sentences we speak group together into larger units, or discourse segments, and the ways in which segment groupings, and relationships between segments, influence discourse processing. The research has three complementary facets. One attempts to model the intentions of dialogue participants and to understand the ways in which these intentions determine discourse structure. Another seeks to understand intonational variation and the ways it indicates discourse structure. The third examines the ways in which choice of referring expression affects processing at the discourse level. The investigated structures and representations are rooted in computational models; they raise challenges for empirical investigations of human processing of dialogue.

Discourse Structure

Discourse is the fundamental unit of language use. Conversations, presentations, texts, and almost all other uses of language are multiple utterances in length. Language use is activity; it is one way to manipulate the environment. Manipulation of the environment is, however, typically a complex activity. It usually takes more than a single action to change the physical world—for example, in traveling, more than one motion is needed to move from one area of a city to another, and in cooking, more than a single chopping action or a single sautéing action is required to make a cassoulet. Likewise, it takes more than one sentence of language to "manipulate the environment" in a meaningful way. The multiple utterances that constitute a coherent discourse are not unstructured sequences, but structured entities constructed over time. Language use also occurs in context, not in a vacuum. Ultimately, to understand language and language processing requires that we understand the structure of discourses, the roles of context, and the representations to which discourse structure and context give rise. Furthermore, as described below, languages provide means of conveying information about discourse structure and context. Thus while understanding linguistic behavior requires representations of discourse structures, language itself provides a means of representing certain information about discourse structures.

The text in Box 8.1 and the dialogue in Box 8.2 are examples of discourses of the sort computational linguists and natural-language-processing researchers have studied in attempting to understand how language works at the discourse level. Each of these samples of language behavior comprises a number of discourse segments, and the structure of these segments—the relationships among segments—affects the meaning of individual phrases and sentences. For instance, the directions narrative of Box 8.1 includes a description of how to get from the Science Center to Harvard Yard, a method for recognizing Widener Library, and a description of where to get lunch. The phrase, "and then it's lunch time," indicates a shift of speaker purpose from providing information about getting to the library to providing information about getting lunch.

The dialogue in Box 8.2 illustrates a different facet of discourse structure. The italicized portion of it is a subdialogue. The overall dialogue relates to a joint task of a user and system to construct a hierarchical network of concepts. (The reader may consider this like the construction of a taxonomy; in this case, the taxonomy was to be used by an automated reasoning system.) The subdialogue concerns correcting a problem in the display of the network of concepts that is prohibiting the user from adding information to the network. Once

Box 8.1 Boston directions corpus sample narrative

"The first dormitory you see, will be Thayer. You want to go to the left of Thayer, and then you'll pass in between Thayer and Memorial Church, and that's the one with the steeple and the columns. So, if you go ar[-], proceed around Memorial Church to the front side of Memorial Church, and you look across Harvard Yard, it's called Tercentenary Theater, in that area, and there'll be a large building with, um, many columns, more than Memorial Church, and its says, quite clearly, along the facade, Harry [*sic*] Elkins Widener Memorial Library. So, that's Widener. You go up the steps, and do whatever you need to do there, and then it's lunch time. A good place to go, if you want sort of an uncomplicated lunch in a hurry, is One Potato Two Potato."

Box 8.2 Dialogue with correction subdialogue (Sidner, 1982)

USER: Show me the generic concept called "employee."
SYSTEM: OK. <System displays network>
USER: I can't fit a new individual concept below it. Can you move it up?
SYSTEM: Yes. <System revises display>
USER: OK, now make a new individual concept node.

the correction is made, the "OK, now" in the final utterance of the excerpt functions to move attention back to the main network construction task. Although this "correction subdialogue" is important for the overall accomplishment of the task, it is not something that could have been planned in advance. It arises spontaneously as the user and system carry out their task and is evidence of the dynamic nature of discourse structure.

We have shown that discourse structure is a complex that includes three interacting components: the linguistic structure, attentional state, and intentional structure (Grosz and Sidner, 1986). The linguistic structure comprises discourse segments and embedding relationships between them. For example, the italicized portion of Box 8.2 is a separate segment, one that is embedded in the larger segment that constitutes the full figure. A variety of different types of discourse have been examined in the computational linguistics literature and found to have this kind of structure, including arguments, task-subtask dialogues, information-seeking dialogues, descriptions, and narratives. Linguistic structure also includes certain features of utterances that convey discourse information, for example intonation in speech and paragraph markings in text.

The second component of discourse structure, attentional state, provides a dynamic record of the entities and attributes that are salient at a given point in the discourse, and as a result, it influences the processing of referring expressions. Attentional state reflects linguistic structure. Different entities are salient in different segments. An embedding of linguistic structure has a parallel in attentional state: the entities that are salient in the embedded segment are more highly focused than those in the embedding segment, though all are distinguished as being in the focus of attention of the discourse participants. These differences in salience allow the same expression to be used to refer to different entities at different times. For example, in the dialogue of Box 8.2, "the concept" could be used to refer to the generic "employee" concept in the outer, embedding segment, but would refer to the new individual concept in the embedded segment that is italicized in the box.

Both linguistic structure and attentional state rest ultimately on a structure of purposes or intentions of speakers or writers (Grosz and Sidner, 1990; Lochbaum, Grosz, and Sidner, 2000). The third component of discourse structure, intentional structure, represents these intentions and the relationships among them. We refer to these as "discourse segment purposes," or DSPs. The embeddings in linguistic structure reflect dominance relationships among DSPs, where one DSP is dominated by another if it in some way contributes to the satisfaction of the dominating DSP. For instance, the intention to describe a room is dominated by the intention to describe a house, because the room description contributes to the house description. Two DSPs are important in the dialogue fragment of Box 8.2: an intention to add information to the network (DSP_1) and an intention to fix the display (DSP_2). Fixing the display and satisfying DSP_2 contributes to DSP_1, and as a result, DSP_1 dominates DSP_2.

The next section provides a brief overview of intentional structure. We then examine evidence from analyses of the speech signal that language represents information about linguistic (discourse segment) structure, and subsequently turn to evidence of the relationship between attentional state and choice of referring expression.

Intentional Structure

Most instances of language behavior involve two or more participants: at least one speaker or writer, and one hearer or reader. In modeling the intentional structure of discourse, the different mental states of the various participants must be taken into account. The purposes, plans, and intentions that matter for discourse belong to more than one individual. We have shown that the intentional structure of dialogue requires a model of collaborative plans, not merely a model of individual plans (Grosz and Sidner, 1990), and have developed a model of collaborative planning, SharedPlans (Grosz and Kraus, 1996, 1999), which provides a foundation for modeling the intentional structure of dialogue (Grosz and Sidner, 1990; Lochbaum, 1995, 1998).

It may seem odd to claim that collaboration underlies all dialogue. For instance, arguments and formal debates, it might be argued, are examples of dialogues in which the participants clearly are not working together. However, even arguments are collaborative at some level; the participants in an argument collaborate at least in speaking a language they both can understand. Formal debates encompass even greater collaboration: debate participants agree to abide a set of rules; although they may disagree on the facts, they collaborate with respect to these rules.

Box 8.3 provides an English description of the basic components of the formal definition of SharedPlans. Each of the separate clauses in

Box 8.3 Informal definition of SharedPlan

Partial SharedPlan for GROUP to do action a in context C_a:

1. Forall G_1 in GROUP: G_1 intends-that GROUP do a
2. GROUP has a [partial] recipe for a
3. For each constituent act β in the recipe,
   a. some individual or subgroup, G_2, has a [partial] plan to do β,
   b. G_2 believes it can do β,
   c. GROUP mutually believe (a) and (β),
   d. Forall G_1 in GROUP: G_1 intends-that G_2 able to do β in context $C_{a/\beta}$

this definition can give rise to subsidiary plans. For instance, Clause 1 may give rise to subdialogues concerning whether to engage in a group activity. Clause 2 may engender subdialogues in which the participants discuss how they are going to perform some action (physical or mental). This clause represents a certain kind of "knowledge precondition"; agents cannot do an action unless they know how to do it, that is, they have some "recipe" (Grosz and Kraus, 1996) for doing it. Clauses (3b) and (3c) represent a different kind of knowledge precondition, knowledge of one's own or another agent's or group's ability to act. Lochbaum (1995, 1998) discusses the treatment of knowledge precondition subdialogues.

The dialogue in Box 8.2 contains an example of a subdialogue arising from Clauses (3b) and (3c). The participants in this dialogue, a user and a system, have a partial SharedPlan (PSP) to add some data, say *D*, to the displayed network fragment below some specified node, say N_1. However, the two conditions specified by Clauses (3b) and (3c) of the definition are unsatisfied: the user is not able to put data *D* below N_1, and as a result, the user and system cannot mutually believe the user has this ability. These unsatisfied conditions lead to a subsidiary SharedPlan for the user and system to free up some space for *D* below N_1.

SharedPlans provide the basic building blocks for intentional structure in dialogue (Lochbaum, 1995, 1998). Each segment of a dialogue has a corresponding SharedPlan, and subsidiary relationships between plans gives rise to a dominance relationship between the corresponding DSPs. For example, for the excerpt in Box 8.2, the overall dialogue corresponds to a SharedPlan for constructing the concept network, and the subdialogue corresponds to a subsidiary plan to remedy the Clause (3b) and (3c) deficits. More generally, each discourse segment has a DSP representing one participant's intention that the participants together construct (and hence execute) a SharedPlan. Intentions-that, denoted as "Int.Th(agent, proposition)," represent an agent's commitment to a proposition holding; they are analogous to intentions to do actions, but with some significant differences (Grosz and Kraus, 1996, 1999). In the general case, if the partial plan of two agents, G_1 and G_2, to do an action α—represented as $PSP(\{G_1,G_2\}, \alpha)$—includes as a subsidiary plan their partial plan to do some action γ—that is, $PSP(\{G_1,G_2\},\gamma)$—then for the dialogue connected with these activities, the DSP $Int.Th(G_1,PSP(\{G_1,G_2\},\alpha))$ dominates the DSP $Int.Th(G_2,PSP(\{G_1,G_2\},\gamma))$. Lochbaum (1995, 1998) has shown that a variety of different types of subdialogue types can be handled with this one mechanism, including task-subtask dialogues, information-seeking dialogues, correction dialogues, and knowledge-precondition dialogues.

Intonation and Discourse Structure

Written language has orthographic cues such as section headings, paragraph boundaries, and punctuation which can assist in identifying discourse structure. In spoken language, intonational variation provides similar, essential information about discourse structure. For instance, it may be used to mark discourse segment boundaries; to distinguish between different interpretations of phrases that can function either as cue phrases that indicate discourse segment boundaries or sententially to convey domain information; or to convey information about the discourse status of entities referred to by definite noun phrases and pronouns. In the absence of such intonational cues, complex reasoning about domain or task knowledge or complex plan inference is required to determine discourse segment boundaries and changes in attentional state. In this section I briefly review two ways in which intonational variation may be used to represent discourse information and thus decrease the processing required for understanding spoken discourse: the use of intonational properties to mark cue phrases and the use of intonational variation to indicate discourse segment boundaries.

Cue phrases not only serve in themselves to indicate discourse structure, but also provide a clear example of a way in which intonation affects interpretation. For example, Hirschberg and Litman (1987) examined uses of the word "now" in both its deictic (indicating a specific time) and cue (marking a discourse boundary) uses. The three examples in Box 8.4 illustrate the importance of intonational information. In each case, the string of words without pause ("uh") or orthographic markings would allow both interpretations of "now."

In Example (1), the "now" means that the speaker is currently fifty-eight years old; the "uh" indicates a phrase break and the grouping of the "now" with the "fifty-eight." In Example (2), the comma separates the "now" from the preceding material and thus leaves it indicating a shift in the discourse. Neither pause nor orthographic information is provided in Example (3) to make the intended interpretation clear. The speaker could mean that she has to pay the tax at the current time (deictic) or only be acknowledging that she has to pay one

Box 8.4 Deictic and cue uses of "now"
(from Hirschberg and Litman, 1987)

1. (deictic) I'm 58 now (uh) they forced me off the job—
2. (cue phrase) My husband retired and (uh) this is the first year, now what's this about (uh) quarterly income tax—
3. (?) So in other words I will have to pay the full amount of the (of the uh) tax now what about PA state tax?

tax and moving on to a new DSP, one that asks about another tax. Intonation is crucial to getting the right interpretation.

Hirschberg and Litman (1987) found differences in phrasing and intonational prominence (accenting) between deictic and cue uses. Deictic uses were always part of a larger phrase (60 percent were last in the phrase) and were almost always accented with a high or complex accent. In contrast, cue uses were often separate phrases (40 percent), and when part of a larger intonational phrase, were always initial and either accented low or deaccented. An analysis of the speech of Example (3) shows that it follows this latter pattern: the "now" is a separate phrase and clearly, even to non-native speakers of English, marking a discourse boundary.

Two challenges face researchers attempting to discover the relationship between intonational features and the structure of spoken discourse. First, the collection of corpora of spontaneous speech requires the development of new experimental methodologies. Whereas it is straightforward to have the same text read by many speakers, it is much more difficult to obtain similar samples of spontaneous speech from multiple speakers. Second, techniques must be developed to obtain reliable segmentations and labelings of the corpora. A variety of studies have shown that certain aspects of local and global structure can be conveyed by and predicted from variation in prosodic and acoustic features. Among the features studied are pitch range, pausal duration, speaking rate, amplitude, and accent type. However, most such studies have not used any independent analysis of discourse structure. We have undertaken a series of studies that employ an independent analysis of discourse structure based on Grosz and Sidner's (1986) tripartite theory to determine whether variation of prosodic-acoustic features with discourse structure is a reliable phenomenon (Grosz and Hirschberg, 1992; Nakatani, Hirschberg, and Grosz, 1995; Hirschberg and Nakatani, 1996). I review briefly the most recent of these studies.

We collected a corpus of monologues of people giving directions around the Boston area, the Boston Directions Corpus (BDC). The BDC consists of elicited, unrestricted monologues (20 minutes, 5000 words) of people doing ten, progressively more difficult, tasks. Box 8.5 gives examples of one of the easier tasks (no. 2) and a portion of

Box 8.5 Sample BDC tasks

Task #2: You are at the Harvard Square T stop. How would you get to Copley Station on the T?

Task #8: [A prospective graduate student is coming to visit Harvard from California. This student . . . has never been to Boston before.] The student must visit Widener Library in the morning and the office of your academic department in the afternoon. She will eat lunch at a place you recommend in the Square. How can she accomplish all these activities, starting and ending at the front of the Science Center?

one of the more complex tasks (no. 8). (The extract in Box 8.1 is from one speaker's Task no. 8.)

In collecting this corpus, we wanted to obtain samples of language use that involved planning in a restricted domain and that varied in length and complexity. We were also concerned with fluency and repeatability. The construction of the direction-giving tasks and the experimental design overall aimed specifically at constraining speakers sufficiently so that they would produce fluent speech. More important, to address the challenge of having similar samples from multiple speakers, we designed tasks intended to elicit approximately the same descriptions from different speakers. This goal was met. We used sixteen nonprofessional speakers. Their spontaneously generated directions were transcribed and minimally edited (to remove disfluencies), and they were then asked to read the transcriptions. We thus have both spontaneous and read versions of approximately the same language for each speaker.

In an initial study, "expert" labelers—students well versed in the tripartite theory of discourse (Grosz and Sidner, 1986)—segmented one speaker's monologues. Both spontaneous and read versions were segmented. To obtain a larger number of segmentations, we then developed an annotation scheme that is based on the tripartite model of discourse structure, but does not require familiarity with that model

Box 8.6 Sample DSPs

Give directions for tour of Harvard Yard, lunch, visit to department

Describe how to get from Science Center entrance of Harvard Yard to Widener: ". . . says quite clearly . . ."
Tell what to do at Widener: "You go up the steps . . ."
Describe lunch plans: "and then it's lunch time . . ."
Suggest One Potato Two Potato: "A good place to go . . ."

to enable labeling by nonexpert or "naive" labelers (Nakatani et al., 1995). The monologues of the four most fluent speakers were segmented by the trained "naive" segmenters; each monologue was analyzed by three segmenters. Box 8.6 gives one segmenter's DSPs for the directions sample given in Box 8.1.

Hirschberg and Nakatani (1996) report the results of measuring agreement among expert segmenters. When using text and speech (so intonational information was available to aid in their reactions), segmenters agreed on 80 percent of the labelings for read speech and 81 percent for spontaneous speech. (When text alone was used, the agreements fell to 57 percent and 61 percent, respectively.)

To determine acoustic-phonetic markers of discourse boundaries, we labeled the speech form using ToBI transcriptions (Pitrelli, Beckman, and Hirschberg, 1994) that follow Pierrehumbert's (1980) approach to describing intonational variation. In particular, the speech was labeled for phrasing (intermediate and intonational phrases), pitch range (distance between highest point in fundamental frequency and baseline), and intonational contour or tune (the sequence of high or low tones in fundamental frequency). Several significant acoustic-phonetic correlates of segment beginnings and endings were found (Hirschberg and Nakatani, 1996). For example, segment beginnings had a higher pitch range, longer preceding pauses, and shorter subsequent pauses than midsegment utterances, whereas segment ending utterances had lower pitch range, shorter preceding pauses, and longer subsequent pauses. These results, which are similar to correlations found for the read speech of a professional speaker (Grosz and Hirschberg, 1992), are the first such results obtained for spontaneous speech.

Attentional State and Reference

The Attentional State Model of Grosz (1977) and Grosz and Sidner (1986) distinguishes local focusing mechanisms from global focusing mechanisms. Attention at the local level is modeled by a "backward-looking center," Cb, a set of "forward-looking centers," Cf, and rules relating centering status to form of expression. Attention at the global level is modeled by a push-down stack of focus spaces. Whereas local attentional state concerns the influence of immediate memory for the linguistic form of an utterance on the interpretation of a subsequent utterance, global attentional state is concerned with the overall discourse and situational context and its affect on interpretation (Grosz, 1977).

Centering theory (Grosz, Joshi, and Weinstein, 1983, 1995) is intended to model focus of attention at the local level. It stipulates a number of constraints, including the uniqueness of the Cb, the ranking of elements of the Cf, and the dependence of choice of form of referring expression on centering status. Its main claim is that to the extent a discourse adheres to these constraints, it will place a smaller inference load on the reader or hearer and thus appear more coherent. Global focusing (Grosz, 1977) concerns a more global coherence that is determined by hierarchical relationships among discourse segments and discourse segment purposes; it will be considered here only with respect to its interaction with the local level.

Experimental studies of comprehension have provided substantial insight into centering and manner of realization (that is, choice of referring expression). Gordon, Grosz, and Gillom (1993) identified a set of circumstances in which a sentence is read more slowly when it contains a repeated-name rather than a pronoun and found evidence that this "repeated-name penalty" marks the backward-looking center. Their studies (1) confirmed that there is a single backward-looking center (the Cb), but a ranked list of forward-looking centers (the Cf);

(2) determined that the Cb is preferentially realized by a pronoun rather than by a repeated name or definite description; (3) identified grammatical role as a key indicator of the Cb, and surface position as unimportant; and, (4) found that both grammatical role and surface position affect the ranking of the elements of the Cf. More particularly, these studies have shown that comprehension is impaired when a repeated name rather than a pronoun is used to realize a single entity in an utterance that is central to the discourse segment.

Gordon and Hendrick (1997) examined the extent to which centering provides a useful framework for analyzing intrasentential constraints on the interpretation of pronouns and names through a series of studies that systematically examined judgments of the acceptability of co-reference by native English speakers who were naive to contemporary linguistic theory. Their studies showed that notions of linguistic prominence, expressed by the construct of a set of forward-looking centers ordered in terms of accessibility, make an important contribution to understanding the patterns of acceptable co-reference within sentences. Additional studies have examined the effect of centering on the interpretation of ambiguous pronouns and of the interaction of passivization and pronominalization.

Nakatani (1997a,b) has examined interactions between attentional state and intonational prominence. In studying a twenty-minute narrative (Nakatani, 1997a), she noticed that a significant portion of the referring expressions did not follow the standardly accepted rules for accent. For instance, she found that 23 percent of the pronouns in subject position were accented and 45 percent of the full lexical forms in direct-object position were not accented. She recast traditional notions of given and new in terms of global and local attentional state and argued that accent serves as an inference cue, marking preservation of and changes in attentional status. The analysis of her corpus confirms that lexical form reflects level of attentional state, with pronominal forms adhering to local constraints and full forms adhering to global constraints. Grammatical position reflects salience at the local level. When grammatical and referential forms align (that is, pronominals in subject position or full forms in direct-object position), accent may be used to convey additional discourse information. Prominence or accent is a way in which language represents shift of attention to a new Cb or marks the global (re)introduction of a referent. Nonprominence indicates maintenance of the current attentional state. In Nakatani's corpus, the accented subject pronouns shifted attention to a new Cb, whereas the nonprominent full direct-objects referred to entities already highly salient globally. Nakatani (1997b) contains a more extensive analysis of the relationship between attentional state, prominence, and lexical form in the Boston Directions Corpus.

Conclusion

Work in computational linguistics demonstrates that language has a structure at the discourse level. Furthermore, it has been shown that discourse structure depends on intentional structure and that, in dialogue, intentional structure rests on collaborative plans. Perhaps most important for this volume, our research has shown that language represents information about changes in linguistic structure and about attentional state. Studies of intonation and cue phrases provide evidence of the former; studies of the differences in use and accenting of pronouns as compared with names or descriptions provides evidence of the latter.

References

The work reported in this paper was supported by grants IRI-90-09018, IRI 94-04756, IRI-93-08173, IRI 95-25915, and CDA-94-01024 from the National Science Foundation.

Gordon, Peter, Barbara Grosz, and Laura Gillom. 1993. Pronouns, names, and the centering of attention in discourse. *Cognitive Science, 3* (17), 311–347.

Gordon, P. C., and R. Hendrick. 1997. Intuitive knowledge of linguistic coreference. *Cognition, 62,* 325–370.

Grosz, Barbara. 1977. The representation and use of focus in a system for understanding dialogs. *Proceedings of the Fifth International Joint Conference on Artificial Intelligence.* Cambridge, Mass.

Grosz, Barbara, and Julia Hirschberg. 1992. Some intonational characteristics of discourse structure. *Proceedings of the 1992 International Conference on Spoken Language Processing* (ICSLP-92).

Grosz, Barbara, Aravind Joshi, and Scott Weinstein. 1983. Providing a unified account of definite noun phrases in discourse. *Proceedings of the 21st Annual Meeting of the ACL,* 44–50.

——— 1995. Centering: A framework for modeling the local coherence of discourse. *Computational Linguistics, 21* (2), 203–225.

Grosz, Barbara, and Sarit Kraus. 1996. Collaborative plans for complex group action. *Artificial Intelligence, 86* (2), 269–357.

Grosz, Barbara, and Sarit Kraus. 1999. The evolution of SharedPlans. In *Foundations of Rational Agency,* ed. M. Wooldridge and A. Rao, 227–262. Netherlands: Kluwer Academic Press.

Grosz, Barbara, Martha Pollack, and Candace Sidner. 1989. Discourse. In *Foundations of Cognitive Science,* ed. M. Posner. Cambridge: MIT Press.

Grosz, Barbara, and Candace Sidner. 1986. Attention, intentions, and the structure of discourse. *Computational Linguistics, 12* (3), 175–204.

——— 1990. Plans for discourse. In *Intentions in Communication,* ed. P. Cohen, J. Morgan, and M. Pollack, 417–444. Cambridge: Bradford Books/MIT Press.

Hirschberg, Julia, and Diane Litman. 1987. Now let's talk about now: Identifying cue phrases intonationally. *Proceedings of the 25th Annual Meeting of the Association for Computational Linguistics,* Stanford, Calif.

Hirschberg, Julia, and Christine Nakatani. 1996. A prosodic analysis of discourse segments in direction-giving monologues. *Proceedings of the Annual Meeting of the Association for Computational Linguistics,* Santa Cruz, Calif.

Lochbaum, Karen E. 1995. The use of knowledge preconditions in language processing. *Proceedings of the International Joint Conference on Artificial Intelligence* (IJCAI-95), ed. Chris S. Mellish, 1260–1266. San Mateo, Calif.: Morgan Kaufmann Publishers.

——— 1998. A collaborative planning model of intentional structure. *Computational Linguistics, 34* (4), 525–572.

Lochbaum, Karen E., Grosz, Barbara J., Sidner, Candace. 2000. Discourse structure and intention recognition. *A handbook of natural language processing: Techniques and applications for the processing of language as text,* ed. R. Dale, H. Moisl, and H. Somers, 123–146. New York: Marcel Dekker.

Nakatani, Christine H. 1997a. Discourse structural constraints on accent in narrative. In *Progress in speech synthesis,* ed. J. van Santen, R. Sproat, J. Olive, and J. Hirschberg, 139–158. New York: Springer-Verlag.

——— 1997b. The computational processing of intonational prominence: A functional prosody perspective. Ph.D. dissertation, Harvard University.

Nakatani, Christine H., Barbara J. Grosz, David D. Ahn, and Julia Hirschberg. 1995. Instructions for annotating discourse. Harvard University, *TR-21–95.*

Nakatani, Christine H., Julia Hirschberg, and Barbara J. Grosz. 1995. Discourse structure in spoken language: Studies on speech corpora. *Proceedings of the AAAI Spring Symposium on Empirical Methods in Discourse Interpretation and Generation.* Palo Alto, Calif.: AAAI.

Pierrehumbert, Janet B. 1980. The Phonology and phonetics of English intonation. Ph.D. dissertation, Massachusetts Institute of Technology. Distributed by the Indiana University Linguistics Club.

Pitrelli, John, Mary Beckman, and Julia Hirschberg. 1994. Evaluation of prosodic transcription labeling reliability in the ToBI framework. *Proceedings of the 3rd International Conference on Spoken Language Processing,* 2, 123–126. Yokohama.

Sidner, Candace L. 1982. Protocols of users manipulation of visually presented information with natural language. BBN Labs, Report 5128, Cambridge, Mass.

Discussion: Section 2

FROM THE FLOOR: Thank you [François Recanati] for giving me this terminology for these concepts. But I am not quite sure I understand: indexical concepts are clearly related to a fairly short list of words or verbal expressions. And deferential concepts, if I am understanding them correctly, must refer to everything else. Right?

If you think about children acquiring language, they are acquiring ten words a day or something like that. Most of those words are not acquired in ostensive contexts; most of those words are acquired deferentially. And most of what we know about most things is acquired deferentially.

It seems if you're suggesting that a sort of a binary analysis—the doctor knows what arthritis is, and the woman does not—whereas, for most concepts as most of us use them, sort of an analog model would be better. The doctor knows more about arthritis than the woman, but he does not really know all that much about it either. If he did, he could cure it.

So, what I am asking is whether you're thinking of this as something that is limited in the way that indexical concepts are limited? Or whether this is in fact an explanation for everything that we know that is represented verbally?

FRANÇOIS RECANATI: Thanks for the question. Actually, first, indexical concepts are not so limited; I have described this unlimited character here by using an operator that can apply to anything. So of course that can be multiplied, as it were. But you have the same with indexicality in some concepts like demonstrative concepts: this thing, this man, this house, and so on. So there is also "this title" as well.

But you're quite right about the pervasiveness of the deferentiality, especially in acquisition. So that is really a problem of another character. It seems that there are two distinct phenomena. In a sense deference is everywhere, and if we want to capture it, we have to use some sort of analog notion. You're quite right.

However, there must be a threshold somewhere. At a certain point it seems that we can talk of mastery of the concept, right, quite right, that it is sort of graded. But still we must be able to make a difference. For example, I can hear a language, I do not know the language at all. I can hear a sentence in the language, I can repeat that sentence. Would you say there is a continuum with that, on one hand, and the full mastery of a field or domain that you know, on the other? It seems that there must be some point somewhere. But in any case, that is a problem which I—I mean, I realize there is a problem here, and I am sort of working at it, but I have no answer to provide.

FROM THE FLOOR: Is looking at the location of the brain lesions helpful for distinguishing between the different models of categorical knowledge?

ALFONSO CARAMAZZA: The patients that have been reported are very heterogeneous in their lesion localization. However, patients who show category-specific deficits for living things tend to have damage that involves the temporal and parietal lobes. Patients who show deficits for nonliving things also tend to have damage involving the temporal and parietal areas. That is, you cannot on the basis of the evidence that has been presented show dissociations. Now, of course, it could be that brain damage as reported is just too gross a level of analysis, and, in fact, that is what I think.

If you're asking me to comment on the neuroimaging data, I think these, too, are ambiguous. People have shown involvement of the inferior temporal lobe for animate things but also for inanimate things. Others have shown involvement of posterior areas for animals as well as for inanimate things. So I could not say that either the analysis of brain lesions or neuroimaging data are sufficient to make the distinction.

FROM THE FLOOR: Do you get the sense that there exists at present a topography of semantic knowledge in the brain?

CARAMAZZA: No, I do not think so.

FROM THE FLOOR: Is this simply because the lesions and imaging data have not been analyzed correctly?

CARAMAZZA: Yes, I believe that is right. I think this does have to do with the poverty of the observations themselves. We do not have the techniques at this time to demonstrate the desired dissociations. Now, a prediction of the hypothesis I presented is precisely that there should be considerable separation in terms of neural structures for the different categories. But exactly where to look for them, and what they are, we do not—I certainly do not—have the foggiest idea.

FROM THE FLOOR: At one point early in your talk you said that the tree is constructed as you go along. Do you not have to know where you're going?

BARBARA GROSZ: Many of us, especially when we are not giving a formal presentation, start talking before we know completely what we are going to say. I fact, this is especially true if one is carrying on a dialogue, because one does not know ahead of time what the other person will say. In my early work I would draw complete trees and people would complain that they applied for some types of discourse, but not to free discourse. Let me draw an analogy for you. Think about two people working together to build a tower of blocks. Let us say, for the sake of argument, that one of them has red blocks and the other has blue blocks, but they may not have drawn out the full architectural plan detailing what parts will be blue and what parts red. Then, one of them puts down a block, the other one puts down a few blocks, and so on, as they work together interactively to construct this tower. It is the same thing with language, in particular with dialogue. An important point here is that I may start a discourse saying that what I want to do is to convince you that a certain thesis is correct, and I have some idea about what I am going to cite as the main points. But I do not know exactly what sentences I am going to utter. I do not know ahead of time the 39th sentence in my paragraph, before I begin.

One does not have to have a mental model of the complete discourse.

STEPHEN KOSSLYN: I was just wondering whether your theory would address a related phenomenon. Because I have been struggling to learn French. I notice that this phenomenon of not knowing exactly what I am going to say occurs at the level not only of the sentence but of the phrase itself. Sometimes I get stuck—the blocks fall down. So, I am wondering whether there is something, working memory, for instance, that might explain how the same sorts of phenomena might operate at a more micro level.

GROSZ: I have not looked at that at the subutterance level, but I think it will show the same kind of phenomenon. Let me see whether I can find the definition of shared plans here among my slides, because this is actually an important part of what I am trying to show in my talk. Notice that the slide says "partial shared plan." The part that addresses what you have said is that which says that the group has a partial recipe. That is, the speakers know in part how they are going to go about doing what they want to do. They set about doing it, and if something happens, they go back and they may correct the recipe and change it.

The speaker has a plan for the utterance, he starts executing it, it falls apart, so he starts building the tower again.

FROM THE FLOOR: How does the process of going back affect syntactic structure?

CARAMAZZA: Allow me to respond to that question. Katherine Bock has shown that in the production of a sentence, if you come to a point where there is a word of very low frequency, which you can not retrieve, then you will retrieve a higher-frequency word and be forced to change the syntactic structure as a consequence. So yes, there are those problems that affect syntactic structure.

Section 3
Verbal Variants

It is fair to say that, as a rule, an aphasic patient is aphasic in all the languages he or she knows. It is also true, however, that in some cases one of the languages seems much more affected than the other ones. This is true also for recovery, whereby one of the languages, usually the one being spoken in the rehabilitation environment, recovers better than the others. This discovery should not be too surprising. We have noted that illiterate subjects (notably those who are illiterate not because of some mental deficiency, but because of lack of socioeconomic opportunity—an important distinction) have more difficulties naming objects presented in front of them after right hemisphere lesions than literate controls. This indicates that the way one learns about the objects of the world determines, in part, the areas that will participate in the content representations. The term "content representations" is chosen here, rather than the processes used to access and otherwise manipulate the representations, because illiterate subjects do not become more or less agrammatic from lesions causing Broca's aphasia, and they do not get Broca's aphasia more commonly from right hemisphere lesions. It is worth remembering, in this light, that Broca's first patient, Leborgne, was most likely illiterate, as were most people from his socioeconomic level at that time in Europe and elsewhere. It is probably safe to hypothesize that there is more variability in verbal language mechanisms where it concerns content than where it concerns process, and to the extent to which culture influences the way an individual learns about the objects in his/her environment (more than just literacy versus illiteracy), one should expect differences in the brain's organization for different languages.

It is known that linguistic similarity or dissimilarity matches more closely than any other cultural phenotype the genetic proximity between two ethnic-racial groups. This raises the question of whether the language of a particular group was selected for by natural selection forces, as were other phenotypes, and the corollary question of whether a particular group is best adapted to comprehend and speak a particular language. As ludicrous as this proposal seems, and the enormous success of some people who have migrated across two drastically different cultural and linguistic environments speaks to this ludicrousness, it might be tempered by findings in very young French babies of preference for their native language over a foreign language. Clearly other explanations may be brought to bear here, whereby a baby may have indeed captured the emotional prosody and even some phonetic qualities in its native language while still in the womb. Or, it may be something about French? (Russian babies also prefer French!)

There are complications in thinking about multilingualism, because, in addition to the cultural issues and differences in the surface structure of languages, they are often learned at different ages, so that the same brain is not used to learn each one. Plasticity changes with age, and it is safe to propose that the learning of one language changes the brain for learning another language. This effect, it appears, can be seen almost at birth, leading Jacques Mehler to doubt the existence of perfect bilingualism (see Chapter 10). Catherine Snow, in Chapter 9, tackles the question of whether children learn a second language better, more efficiently, and faster than do adults. This is a highly contested topic—Snow's conclusions are not mainstream—but she does raise interesting issues that are ultimately amenable to scientific discovery.

In Chapter 10 Franck Ramus and Mehler hail the scientific method for discovering the structure and function of the human mind, an approach illustrated by the workings of cognitive psychology and its allies evolutionary psychology, cognitive neuroscience, and cognitive modeling. Then they cite interesting experimental approaches in newborn infants that have produced data pertaining to the question of what these infants pay attention to when they are able to distinguish a change from one language to another. As another illustration of the strength of the methods, they provide information on the question of what factors play a role in the differential representation of two languages in the brain in bilinguals. Finally the question is raised as to what cognitive psychology is actually studying, when it studies mental processes. Relative to the topic of this section, where does the variability in verbal language lie? In other words, are there levels where the variability can be demonstrated (because it is there where it exists) and levels where it cannot (because there is no variability). This type of questioning implies that there is some central processing module that equalizes all knowledge and does not distinguish among languages, which instead are phenomena of more peripheral mental function. Moreover, the workings of the central module cannot be discovered. There is a parallel conflict in neuroscience, as areas farther away from sensory input channels are more difficult to study. At this stage of our knowledge, however, it is difficult to escape the conclusion that the central module lives in the frontal lobe.

Chapter 11, which is the final verbal-language chapter and which closes this section, represents a transition to nonverbal languages. Here Stanislas Dehaene presents work he has done, some in collaboration with Laurent Cohen, on the representation of numbers in the brain. Arithmetic knowledge involves on the one hand a symbolic representation and processing system and on the other a sense of quantity, which would belong not to a verbal process but rather to some other form of knowledge representation and manipulation. These two systems have to meld in some way: hence the transition between verbal and nonverbal languages. Interesting results are emerging from functional imaging studies that implicate widely varied systems in the brain for the different forms of representations of numbers. Some are shared with verbal processes, others are not; but they are activated together only when numbers are processed under certain conditions that open a window to the interaction between verbal and nonverbal language systems.

Second Language Learners and Understanding the Brain

9

Catherine E. Snow

In 1967 the appearance of Eric Lenneberg's book *Biological Foundations of Language* reorganized thinking about the relationship between the brain and languages and introduced a notion—of a critical period for language learning—which subsequently became so powerful that it lives on in folk psychology and in policy debates despite increasing doubts about its correctness.[1] This chapter reexamines the critical period hypothesis from the perspective of data about second language learning. One of the strengths of Lenneberg's formulation of the hypothesis was precisely that he built an argument for it on the basis of several different kinds of behavioral data—that is, the predictable timing of milestones of normal first language acquisition and the difficulties of first language acquisition when it is slowed or delayed by brain injury, mental retardation, or social deprivation. Declines in second language learning ability with age formed only a tiny part of Lenneberg's argument, though it is the aspect of his thinking that has attracted the most subsequent attention. Addressing Lenneberg's various arguments in their entirety is impossible here, but it should be pointed out that all have been challenged (see Snow, 1987; Harley and Wang, 1997; Birdsong, 1999; Marinova-Todd, Marshall, and Snow, 2000).

Crucial to Lenneberg's argument was the claim of a correlation between the time course of the decline of language acquisition ability and the time course of brain growth and organization, which he described as ending at puberty. Advances during the last thirty years in brain imaging techniques, in our understanding of dendritic pruning and cell death as features of early brain development, and in our capacity to measure functional and metabolic activity in the brain have greatly reorganized the picture Lenneberg masterfully pieced together from the very partial data available to him. Limitations of length and knowledge prevent me from addressing claims about irreversible changes in the brain that would be a crucial component of a comprehensive discussion of the critical period hypothesis, since it posits permanent changes in learning ability *associated with* changes in the brain. Suffice it to note that assessing behavioral claims derived from the critical period hypothesis is made much more difficult by the ambiguity concerning which change in the brain might be posited as the crucial one that limits further learning. The period of biological grace was originally assumed to be associated with incomplete brain lateralization, and subsequently has been variously identified in the literature with the ongoing processes of myelinization, of localization, of dendritic pruning, and of establishing well-reinforced neural networks, and with high levels of glucose uptake. Lenneberg's own proposal, that the accomplishment of lateralization set the limit, has been demonstrated to be incorrect, but many alternate hypotheses remain on the table and account for suggestions that the critical period might end as early as age five or as late as age twelve.

Age Differences in Speed of Second Language Acquisition

Most nonspecialists are of the opinion that the critical period reveals itself in the speed with which young children acquire second languages. This belief is held strongly, for example, by Ron Unz, who has made it the basis of his political movement to ban bilingual education programs in favor of one-year kindergarten immersion programs for English-language learners in California and elsewhere. Unz and many of his supporters state explicitly that older arrivals in the United States may need a few years to learn English well enough to function in school, but ridicule the notion that five-year-olds are unable to master English in a year.

In fact, hard data about the actual accomplishments of second language learners of different ages leaves little doubt that the five-year-olds, at the end of one year of immersion, will have learned considerably less than older children or adolescents with the same exposure, and even that adults will learn more than older children if they are provided with equivalent learning conditions. This pattern of correlation between age of initial exposure to a second language and speed of acquisition during the first year or so of exposure holds true over an age range from three to sixty at least for English speakers learning Dutch in naturalistic settings (Snow and Hoefnagel-Höhle, 1977), immigrants of various language backgrounds to Sweden (Ekstrand, 1976) and to the United States (Fathman, 1975), English speakers learning Russian in formal settings where the Total Physical Response method was used (Asher and Price, 1967), English speakers in French immersion programs (Genesee, 1983; Harley, 1986), and in every study where roughly comparable learning conditions were available to older and younger learners. These studies diverge from "common sense" in using actual assessments of second language skill: vocabulary size; control over grammar as revealed in correctness of spontaneous speech or writing; performance on imitation, translation, or grammaticality judgment tasks; fluency; pronunciation; and auditory discrimination of phonemic contrasts. Interestingly, the common-sense view that younger children are faster learners derives primarily from informal assessments of conversational ability, in contexts where young children can choose what to say, can use a high proportion of routinized or semi-analyzed speech, and can often participate effectively with relatively little linguistic competence. Young learners do manage social interaction at that level relatively well, but they do not develop a deeper knowledge of the language nearly as quickly as older learners.

Age Differences in Ultimate Second Language Attainment

The ability of young second language learners to pass as native speakers is perhaps the strongest argument in support of the critical period hypothesis. Ultimate attainment levels in the second language generally show an advantage for younger learners, who are much more likely to end up indistinguishable from native speakers than older learners. It is clear, though, that decline with age in average attainment is associated with an increase in variability—that some percentage even of the oldest group of learners achieves nativelike competence. Methodological problems with ultimate attainment studies abound:

1. As Birdsong (1992) has convincingly argued, only adult learners who have had a reasonable chance to become proficient ought to be included in these studies, which in fact often incorporate casual and short-term learners, particularly in the older groups.
2. These studies have often compared childhood learners who are shifting from first language (L1) to second language (L2) dominance, and who essentially abandon L1 (a very high likelihood outcome for young, especially for preliterate, L2 learners) with adult learners who maintain L2 while acquiring L1. The task of speaking a second language well while maintaining a first language is obviously more difficult. Furthermore, first language maintenance implies commitment of time to L1 (whether to speaking it, or to reading and writing it), a disruptive factor younger L2 learners are typically not confronted with.
3. These studies often compare adult L2 learners who are receiving or have received formal instruction (sometimes counterproductive instruction, often from nonnative speakers of the target language who speak with and teach non-native phonological systems) to child learners in naturalistic learning environments.
4. These studies have often ignored the role of literacy in L1 and in L2 in influencing the course of L2 acquisition. Almost inevitably older learners will have more consolidated first language literacy skills and will seek to represent their knowledge of L2 using writing. Indeed, older learners given a choice of learning methods typically choose more formal, grammar-translation methods in which written presentation of material is frequent and starts very early in the learning process. The average literate adult speaker of English has in her lifetime encountered billions of occurrences in print of, for example, the letter "p," and has automatically decoded that grapheme by producing a phonological representation of the aspirated, relatively long voice-onset time (VOT) version of "p" which is typical of spoken English almost

all of those times. When this adult starts to learn Spanish, in which the letter "p" represents a nonaspirated, short VOT bilabial stop, the overwhelming strength of the association of written "p" with English /p/ may flood out the knowledge that Spanish "p" is pronounced differently. Thus one might actually expect better pronunciation from adults who learn a language without reading it, or who learn a language with an unfamiliar orthography (and an orthography in which the tendency to link new graphemes to old ones is avoidable). Systematic analysis of pronunciation correctness under varying conditions of second language orthographic knowledge has not been undertaken.

5. Many studies of ultimate attainment of second language skill have failed to note the degree of variability among native speakers on the phenomena being studied. Evidence that second language speakers are ranked by native-speaking judges as, for example, 4.2 on a 5-point scale could be seen as proof of nonnative attainment, but in fact some native speakers might be ranked that low as well. Particularly in the domain of minor, highly conditioned phonological and grammatical rules, levels of performance of native speakers might well deviate considerably from the presumed norm, so native speaker controls are needed as much as different age groups.

Work carried out by Birdsong has been, perhaps, the most sophisticated in demonstrating the capacity of adult second language learners to achieve nativelike levels of performance. Birdsong (1989) has pointed out that native speakers are neither consistently normative, nor stable, in their performance on grammatical tasks. Studying twenty English speakers who had been resident in Paris for more than three years (initial exposure after puberty in all cases), and who were selected to be very proficient speakers of French, Birdsong (1992) found that fifteen fell within the range established by twenty demographically equivalent native French speakers on grammaticality judgment tasks. Birdsong argues explicitly that many studies of ultimate attainment in adult second language learners have included learners who had had insufficient opportunity to acquire the second language to a high level, and that the relevant data have to do with the range of attainment, not the mean. Strikingly, even in the data reported by Johnson and Newport (1989), the study most repetitively cited in support of a critical period for second language acquisition, some of the adult learners scored above the level achieved by some of the younger learners.

Case studies of other adult learners support the possibility of nativelike proficiency. Ioup, Boustagui, Tigi, and Moselle (1994) report on two native speakers of English who functioned in ways indistinguishable from native speakers in Arabic, after living in Egypt for a few years. Both were judged to be native speakers by most judges: one of the two performed in a way indistinguishable from that of native speakers on grammaticality judgments, while the other made a few deviant (overinclusion) judgments. Notably, both these women were married to Egyptian Arabic speakers and spent most of their time functioning in Arabic—Birdsong similarly noted that the subjects in his study who were most likely to achieve native levels of performance were those who spent all their time (during some period) communicating in French.

The presumed impossibility of adult attainment of nativelike performance in the domain of accent has been challenged as well by the work of Bongaerts and his colleagues (Bongaerts, 1999; Bongaerts, Planken, and Schils, 1995; Bongaerts et al. 1997), studying native speakers of Dutch who had learned English or French. This work, like Birdsong's, was careful to select subjects who had a real chance to become nativelike, and found that half the Dutch speakers scored as high or higher than native English speakers.

Markham (1997) carried out an interesting variant of ultimate attainment studies, asking native speakers of various languages to judge imitations of utterances in those languages produced by Swedish first language speakers who had not had any particular phonetic training but were self-judged good language learners. Markham instructed the judges that the speakers were native speakers who had lived outside their native countries for some time—thus in effect biasing the judgments toward seeking dialectical or individual variation rather than foreign language influences. Most of the imitators' productions were judged nativelike most of the time.

In short, while an average adult learner's ultimate attainment in an L2 is likely to be lower than that of a younger learner, in fact adults under optimal circumstances can achieve nativelike performance in domains that include minor grammatical rules and pronunciation of unfamiliar sounds as well as in the more commonly mastered domains of vocabulary, pragmatics, and regular grammatical rules. Adults who do become nativelike in an L2 are typically those who immerse themselves full time in the L2 for some period, and they still may achieve nativelike levels only after two to three years. This level of attainment for adults typically does not involve drastic diminution of proficiency in the first language—whereas younger children may well lose much or all of their first language skill in a similar time period, and thus may end up with the easier task of displaying nativelike proficiency in the second-learned language without ongoing interference from a need to process the first language regularly or alternatively. Particularly in the domain of pronunciation, but also for rapid syntactic processing, proficient bilinguals, particularly those who live in bilingual communities and code switch frequently, often show a merged or midpoint pattern of performance that may be heard as not quite nativelike in either language. These merged systems can even be adopted by monolinguals as standard regional varieties—for example, the southwestern English spoken by many monolinguals has the reduced vowel repertoire of Spanish.

Age Differences in Process of Second Language Acquisition

Assessing the process of second language learning is a complex task. Enormous individual differences exist within groups of any age. Some simple facts are clear. Older and younger learners are all capable of naturalistic, untutored second language learning, although older learners may express a preference for formal teaching support. Older learners may be more inclined to use literacy, memory aids, and expressly formulated rules than younger learners; indeed, this tendency may account for their more rapid initial progress. However, quite young second language learners engage in metalinguistic and metacognitive activities such as asking for translations and formulating explicit rules, so the age differences may well be more quantitative than qualitative.

Explicit analyses of types of errors committed by younger and older learners have found no age differences (see Harley and Wang, 1997, and Snow and Hoefnagel-Höhle, 1977 for reviews). Snow, Smith, and Hoefnagel-Höhle (1980), for example, compared performance on a nonsense-word-based elicitation of morphologically inflected forms among English-speaking learners of Dutch and found similar errors, similar sequences of approach to nativelike performance, and similar (incorrect) rules or generalizations across the age groups. Thus while Lenneberg's hypothesis posits a much more natural process for younger than for older language learners, the reflexes of that greater naturalism in approaches to the task or in stages on the way to high proficiency are hard to find.

Age Differences in Brain Localization of Early versus Late Learned Languages

Discussions of the critical period hypothesis were reinitiated in 1997 with the appearance of a widely publicized study that used functional magnetic resonance imaging to show that aspects of later learned second languages were localized in cortical areas distinct from those of primary or early learned second languages (Kim et al., 1997). This study constituted a pioneering use of newly available technologies to confirm conclusions that others had drawn using much older methods. Cross-case analyses of polyglot aphasics have typically identified a small but significant number of cases where patterns of damage and/or recovery differ sharply across the patient's various languages, suggesting differential localization (Paradis, 1977; Albert and Obler, 1978). Techniques involving brain stimulation during surgery reveal that somewhat differently localized sites control similar processes (such as naming) in the two languages of bilinguals (Ojemann, 1983). Although early hypotheses about the localization of later learned languages suggested a greater likelihood of bilateral representation (for example, Gordon, 1980; Sussman, Franklin, and Simon, 1982), it is striking that Kim et al.'s findings identified divergent *within hemisphere* localization.

The real question about the finding of age-of-learning differences in brain localization is whether it implies anything about behavior or about critical periods. Even the Kim et al. finding does not imply that the later learned language is more poorly learned—simply that it is localized differently. Furthermore, the age cutoff for new localization indicated by this study was age eight—well before the age when nativelike attainment becomes unlikely. It is, in fact, not surprising that later acquired capacities have somewhat different brain localizations than early ones, nor would it be surprising if it emerged that bilingual brains are organized somewhat differently from monolingual brains. Such facts, even if proved, will not impel any particular conclusion concerning the existence of a critical period for language learning.

Age Differences in Nonbiological Factors Related to Second Language Learning

Age differences in second language outcomes can be taken as evidence in support of a critical period only if those age differences can be somehow specifically linked to differences in brain parameters. As noted above, that link has not been proved. At the same time, there are many differences in the context of second language learning that might well relate to outcomes, and that would have to be excluded as accounting for age differences in order to isolate brain factors as the cause.

Bilingualism

A very powerful difference between early and late second language learners concerns the likelihood that such learners will end up bilingual. Young children, when placed in a situation where learning a second language becomes crucial, often respond by ceasing to acquire their first language and ultimately, in many cases, by losing the first language. Thus early second language learning is unlikely to produce good bilinguals, unless special steps are taken to protect, maintain, and support continued development in the first language.

Literacy as Route to Learning

The availability of literacy as a form of representation of language is much more likely to affect older than younger learners. Markham (1997) has argued that neutralizations of phonetic or phonemic contrasts in the orthographic system may well have a negative influence on older learners, for whom much learning may come through reading, but leave younger learners relatively unscathed.

Mute Period

Children often are allowed a silent period, whereas adults in formal learning settings are encouraged to speak in the L2 early on, and in informal learning settings often need to communicate in the L2 at early stages of acquisition. A period of intense, auditory exposure to the second language before attempting to produce it may be helpful in enabling the learner to hear (and thus produce) subtly different phonetic features, new phoneme distinctions, and unfamiliar sequences or stress patterns. Neufeld (1977, 1980) has had considerable success in facilitating the nativelike production of a foreign language by adults who listen for several hours before being allowed to speak. This artificially induced mute period may protect the learner from using first language phonological categories to represent the second language system, thus enabling higher levels of production performance.

The frequent occurrence of a mute period among child learners also suggests that the reported ease of second language acquisition in young children may reflect more the inability of adults to acknowledge young children's efforts (and their suffering) than any real age difference in the difficulty of the task. The subjectively experienced challenge of second language acquisition is something adults can report on, but that for young children is perceptible only through their experiences of social withdrawal, depression, and their retreat into a silent period during first exposure to the second language. Just as we perform surgery on infants without anaesthetic in the belief their pain is less serious than adults' pain, we use a belief in the critical period to shield us from the recognition that young children find second language learning no less traumatic than adults find it.

Affective/Personal Identification with Second Language Group

Interestingly, a second domain for which a critical period ending about puberty has been proposed is the domain of cultural membership. Minoura (1992) has argued that it is impossible to fully acquire the rules of a second culture and thus to feel like a native member of that culture after about age ten. Although the correctness of the cultural critical period has been widely questioned, it is clear that the organization of social roles and the existence of a structure of social rules is somewhat transparent to young children, who simply learn to function in their various environments, but that such roles and structure can become an object of reflection and thus of potential conflict for older children. Precisely because conforming to peer-established norms is such an important aspect of successful adolescence, adolescents may well suffer more conflict about the adaptations needed in a new environment. This conflict can lead to negative affect directed toward the new group and/or to decisions to retain a distinct personal identity.

Scovel (1988) has made a closely related argument concerning age differences across the entire span from childhood into adulthood, suggesting that affective factors vary considerably more than biological capacities across this age range. The stronger emotional ties of older learners to a first language, a first culture, and the associated group may explain their disinclination to lose the first language, thus accounting for the greater incidence of bilingualism among older learners and for the persistence of identifying accents, which serve as external markers of partial rather than full membership in the new group. This hypothesis is also consistent with the suggestion in the ultimate attainment studies that learners who marry or cohabit with native speakers, in other words those who have the most intimate and positive emotional association with the second language group, are most likely to attain nativelike proficiency.

Intensity of Exposure

Children typically acquire a second language in school—in situations where everyone speaks it and where its acquisition is a prerequisite to their functioning in all realms. In many second language settings, adults may continue to perform many of their functions in the first language—for instance, leisure reading, writing, work-related talk, maintenance of contacts with friends and relatives. The importance of intensity of exposure to the second language may help explain a fairly robust finding that is quite puzzling to the critical period adherents, namely that the correlation between mean levels of attainment in the second language and age does not diminish in adulthood (Hakuta, Bialystok, and Wiley, submitted). In other words, just as eight-year-old arrivals are more likely to become nativelike than fifteen-year-old arrivals, twenty-eight-year-olds are more likely to become nativelike than thirty-five-year-olds. These age differences in adulthood probably reflect the conditions of life in adulthood and associated differences in motivation and intensity of exposure.

Conclusion

The notion of a critical period for language learning is highly appealing for many reasons: it absolves us adults of our failures in language learning, it justifies educational policies that lead to rapid assimilation and promote English monolingualism for new immigrants, while at the same time it supports investment in enrichment language-teaching programs for middle-class, mainstream schoolchildren. Nonetheless, the behavioral data are inconsistent with the existence of a critical period, and the correlation between changes in the brain and changes in behavioral capacities that would be needed to support the critical period hypothesis is absent. Adults learn second languages relatively quickly and can learn them extremely well under the right conditions—which are exactly the same conditions under which younger learners succeed. There are many likely explanations for the difference in rate of success of younger and older learners, ranging from intensity of exposure to necessity of success to affective emotional processes differentiating their situations. These explanations impel us to seek age differences in the domains of the social and the emotional—not the biological.

Note

1. The genius of Lenneberg's book was to coordinate data from across varying fields of endeavor to build the argument for the critical period hypothesis. Since 1967, each of his claims has in fact been challenged, and most have been convincingly rejected. On the brain development side, current views of the changes in brain organization that occur during childhood are fundamentally different from Lenneberg's view of developmental lateral-

ization, and emphasize much more the role of experience in organizing the brain than the structure of the brain in organizing experience. None of the processes hypothesized to account for the critical period show any particular culmination or cessation at puberty. If behavioral changes in language acquisition possibilities indeed cluster around puberty—and some of them seem to—then that suggests precisely that biological explanations for those changes are particularly unconvincing ones.

References

Albert, M., and Obler, L. 1978. *The bilingual brain: Neuropsychological and neurolinguistic aspects of bilingualism.* New York: Academic Press.

Asher, J., and Price, B. 1967. The learning strategy of the total physical response: Some age differences. *Child Development, 38,* 1219–1227.

Birdsong, D. 1989. *Metalinguistic performance and interlinguistic competence.* Berlin: Springer-Verlag.

——— 1992. Ultimate attainment in second language acquisition. *Language, 68,* 706–755.

Birdsong, D., ed. 1999. *The critical period hypothesis and second language acquisition.* Mahwah, N.J.: Erlbaum.

Bongaerts, T. 1999. Ultimate attainment in foreign language pronunciation: The case of very advanced late foreign language learners. In *The critical period hypothesis and second language acquisition,* ed. D. Birdsong. Mahwah, N.J.: Erlbaum.

Bongaerts, T., Planken, B., and Schils, E. 1995. Can late starters attain a native accent in a foreign language? A test of the critical period hypothesis. In *The age factor in second language acquisition,* ed. D. Singleton and Z. Lengyel, 30–50. Briston, Pa.: Multilingual Matters.

Bongaerts, T., van Summeren, C., Planken, B., and Schils, E. 1997. Age and ultimate attainment in the pronunciation of a foreign language. *SSLA, 19,* 447–465.

Ekstrand, L. 1976. Age and length of residence as variables related to the adjustment of migrant children, with special reference to second language learning. In *Proceedings of the Fourth International Congress of Applied Psycholinguistics,* vol. 3, ed. G. Nickel. Stuttgart: Hochschulverlag.

Fathman, A. 1975. The relationship between age and second language learning productive ability. *Language Learning, 25,* 245–253.

Flege, J., Frieda, E., and Randazza, L. 1998. Lexical factors and segmental accuracy in second language speech production. *SSLA, 20,* 155–187.

Genesee, F. 1983. The bilingual education of majority language children: The immersion experiments in review. *Applied Psycholinguistics, 4,* 1–46.

Gordon, H. 1980. Cerebral organization in bilinguals: 1. Lateralization. *Brain and language, 9,* 225–268.

Hakuta, K., Bialystok, E., and Wiley, E. Submitted. Critical evidence: A test of the critical periods hypothesis for second language acquisition. Available on www.stanford.edu/~hakuta/docs.

Harley, B. 1986. *Age in second language acquisition.* Clevedon, U.K.: Multilingual Matters.

Harley, B., and Wang, W. 1997. The critical period hypothesis: Where are we now? In *Tutorials in bilingualism: Psycholinguistic perspectives,* ed. A. de Groot and J. Kroll. Mahwah, N.J.: Lawrence Erlbaum Associates.

Ioup, G., Boustagui, E., Tigi, M., and Moselle, M. 1994. Reexamining the critical period hypothesis: A case of successful adult SLA in a naturalistic environment. *Studies in Second Language Acquisition, 16,* 73–98.

Johnson, J., and Newport, E. 1989. Critical period effects in second language learning: The influence of maturational state on the acquisition of English as a second language. *Cognitive Psychology, 21,* 60–99.

Kim, K. H., Relkin, N. P., Lee, K. M., and Hirsch, J. 1997. Distinct cortical areas associated with native and second languages. Letter to *Nature, 388,* 171.

Lenneberg, E. 1967. *Biological foundations of language.* New York: Wiley.

Marinova-Todd, S., Marshall, D. B., and Snow, C. E. 2000. Three misconceptions about age and second language learning. *TESOL Quarterly, 34,* 9–34.

Markham, D. 1997. *Phonetic imitation, accent, and the learner.* Travaux de l'Institut de linguistique de Lund 33. Lund: University of Lund Press.

Minoura, Y. 1992. Sensitive period for the incorporation of a cultural meaning system: A study of Japanese children growing up in the United States. *Ethos, 20,* 304–339.

Neufeld, G. 1977. Language learning ability in adults: A study on the acquisition of prosodic and articulatory features. *Working Papers in Bilingualism, 12,* 45–60.

——— 1980. On the adult's ability to acquire phonology. *TESOL Quarterly, 14,* 285–298.

Ojemann, G. 1983. Brain organization for language from the perspective of electrical stimulation mapping. *Behavioral and Brain Sciences, 6,* 261–285.

Paradis, M. 1977. Bilingualism and aphasia. In *Studies in Neurolinguistics,* vol. 3, ed. H. A. Whitaker and H. Whitaker. New York: Academic Press.

Scovel, T. 1988. *A time to speak: A psycholinguistic inquiry into the critical period for human speech.* New York: Harper and Row.

Snow, C. E. 1987. Relevance of the notion of a critical period to language acquisition. In *Sensitive periods in development: Interdisciplinary perspectives,* ed. M. H. Bornstein, 183–209. Hillsdale, N.J.: Erlbaum.

Snow, C. E., and Hoefnagel-Höhle, M. 1977. Age differences in the pronunciation of foreign sounds. *Language and Speech, 20,* 357–365.

Snow, C. E., Smith, N. S. H., and Hoefnagel-Höhle, M. 1980. The acquisition of some Dutch morphological rules. *Journal of Child Language, 7,* 539–553.

Sussman, H., Franklin, P., and Simon, T. 1982. Bilingual speech: Bilateral control? *Brain and Language, 15,* 125–142.

In Praise of Functional Psychology 10

Franck Ramus and Jacques Mehler

In this chapter we defend a view of cognitive science that asserts the important role that linguistics, philosophy of mind, and computer science play in the effort to discover how the mind works. Moreover, this *functional approach* acknowledges that the study of information processing implemented by experimental psychology gives unity to cognitive science and makes it possible to link formal discoveries with biology.

We will first argue that there is little hope of reaching an understanding of how the mind works if experimental psychology is bypassed. Second, we will argue that psychological measurements are more telling when they are broken down into finer-grained components using the methods of neuroscience. Next, we will argue that neuroscience provides the conceptual basis to understand how mental abilities develop. In sum, although the functional approach has not yet been successful with the study of the central faculties of the mind—thinking, problem solving, and conceptual representations—there is no reason to be skeptical. The scientific method has aided our understanding of many other areas of the physical and biological world, and should be helpful here as well.

Studying the Mind

Humans have the drive to think, speak, and learn. Humans, moreover, are unique in their ability to reason about the functioning of the mind. Humans experience color and pitch, smell and texture, feelings and emotions, which gives them the ability to link their states of mind to exogenous or endogenous stimuli. This, in turn, allows them to do research linking their subjective experience to counterpoint measures made with physical equipment. This simple truth reminds us of the importance of psychology in science. Similarly, there is no way in which we can study natural categories, beliefs, and desires without taking mental states seriously.

As soon as humans began constructing a culture, they started exploring the mind (Mithen, 1996). Naive or folk theories of psychology may have begun many thousands of years ago, and basically they are still with us. Philosophers explored the mind more systematically, and Greek philosophers attained the most advanced understanding of how the human mind works given the nonexperimental means available to them. In the late nineteenth century Wundt became the first to use experimental methods to study the mind. He nevertheless believed that thought, concepts, and the other higher mental processes, with the exception of memory and language, could not be studied experimentally. Wundt became a model for many psychologists who began the systematic exploration of the mind in the different laboratories that sprang up at the start of the twentieth century. Perception, attention, memory, learning, and language became the objects of systematic studies.

Psychology, having discovered how the human operator encodes the visual and auditory stimuli, has devised methods to link these findings to the physiology of vision and audition. Similarly, students of memory have developed an understanding of how humans store and recall sequences of words, digits, pictures, and other stimuli. They have further identified separate subsystems, one for storing events and another for storing skills and rule-governed procedures. These psychological discoveries have made it possible to expand the study of memory by exploring its neurological substrates.

The study of language illustrates the most prolific and successful use of the methods drawn from experimental psychology. The examples of acoustic phonetics, phonology, lexical access, and parsing will suffice to illustrate the success that empirical science has attained in the psycholinguistic domain. Although we are far from understanding how concepts are represented and how sentences are understood, the methods that have solved many of the difficult problems of biology and physics will, when used to explore the mind, lead to new insights. Cognitive psychology, for example, has made progress by adopting the functional approach.

In Praise of Cognitive Psychology and Its Methodology

Cognitive psychology explores how knowledge is acquired, represented, and used. It is complemented by a number of disciplines. For instance, in cognitive development one explores how the infant acquires knowledge; in cognitive neuropsychology one attempts to discover what parts of the cognitive apparatus have ceased to function after trauma. More recently, evolutionary psychology, cognitive neuroscience, and cognitive modeling have emerged.

Cognitive psychology has paid special attention to how types of information are processed. The hope is to segregate subdomains, each of them having specialized learning routines to adapt to the environment. Theorists postulate specialized information-processing structures, or modules, for such subdomains and try to state the specific learning that is required for a particular module to gain knowledge. For instance, psycholinguists postulate a series of modules to explain how humans learn to speak. Theoreticians usually assume that modules are sensitive to specific signals and that the module responds with a coded output whenever a given signal is detected. Thus phonological structures receive inputs from the acoustic-phonetic structures and generate an output that is fed into the lexical access structures. Likewise, syntactic structures respond to information delivered by the mental lexicon, and so forth.

In our laboratory we have sought to understand how infants learn language from the acoustic signals in their surrounds. This endeavor requires the collaboration of linguists, acoustic-phoneticians, and computer scientists, as well as the cooperation of colleagues who act as informants on many different languages. These efforts led us to reformulate a thesis that has been scrutinized by linguists, namely, that languages can be arranged into a limited number of rhythmic classes.

As we will argue below, our explorations led to results that can be used to formulate neurological predictions.

Language Classes

Developmental psycholinguists have explored the dispositions allowing infants to learn the language in their surrounds, thus uncovering many specific dispositions and capacities. We still have to clarify which inputs the child may consider as potentially capable of conveying linguistic information. For instance, it appears that utterances from signed and from spoken language are scanned with special interest by infants. More research is needed on this question, however. A further question is how infants raised in a multilingual milieu segregate inputs from the different languages, thus avoiding the confusion that would otherwise arise.

To investigate this second issue, we decided to examine the infant's ability to discriminate utterances from different languages. Mehler et al. (1988) explored how neonates and two-month-olds react to a language change after they are habituated to utterances in one language and tested with utterances in another. It was discovered that neonates were able to discriminate between two languages and, moreover, that their ability to discriminate was preserved even when the utterances were low-pass filtered.[1] In contrast, when speech was played backward no discrimination was observed, suggesting that there are sequential constraints that have to be maintained in order for infants to judge them as a linguistic input.

Comparing the behavior of neonates with that of two-month-olds resulted in a surprising finding. While the former were capable of distinguishing any pair of languages, the latter reacted only when they were asked to contrast the maternal language with another language (Mehler et al., 1988; Christophe and Morton, 1998). We asked ourselves what cues infants were using to perform this task. In our quest we were helped by Nazzi, Bertoncini, and Mehler's (1998) finding that French-born infants have no difficulty discriminating English from Japanese though they failed to discriminate Dutch from English. Nazzi and his collaborators conjectured that languages fall into rhythm classes. Pike (1945), Abercombie (1967), and others had the intuition that Romance languages have a syllabic rhythm; Germanic languages, a stress-timed rhythm; and languages like Japanese, a mora-timed rhythm. These different rhythmic percepts were thought to arise because different languages, having units of different sizes that are used as primitive speech acts, would have isochrony over these units. In other words, Romance languages would have syllable isochrony, Germanic languages, feet isochrony and Japanese, mora isochrony.

Isochrony is not a simple notion and it deserves close scrutiny. Researchers who attempted to validate it using acoustic-phonetic measures failed (see Dauer, 1983). Yet Nazzi et al.'s research supports the notion that languages fall into rhythmic categories. They reported that infants who were able to discriminate a mix of Spanish and Italian utterances from a mix of English and Dutch utterances failed to discriminate a mix of Spanish and Dutch sentences from one of Italian and English utterances. They speculated that it is easy for infants to discriminate syllable-timed utterances from stress-timed utterances even when the utterances of each class come from several languages. In contrast, they cannot discriminate a mix of utterances from languages in two different classes, for example, Spanish and English, from another such mix, for example, Italian and Dutch. Although this result per se is not sufficient to render the rhythmic class hypothesis credible, there are other results in the literature that correspond well with the hypothesis.

Mehler et al. (1993) found that when one listens to compressed sentences (sentences speeded up with speech-editing software that changes duration without altering other spectral properties), comprehension is difficult but improves with practice. There is no awareness that one is making subtle changes in the processing algorithms, yet the perceptual scores improve. Dupoux and Green (1997) showed that the improvement resists a speaker change, and Mehler et al. (1993) showed that understanding was not required, since adaptation could transfer to an unfamiliar language. Pallier et al. (1997) showed that Spanish subjects become better at processing compressed Spanish test sentences after listening to compressed Italian or Greek even though they were incapable of understanding either Greek or Italian. Furthermore, they did not benefit from prior exposure to compressed Japanese or English. This pattern of results suggests that one's language-processing algorithm becomes tuned to the rhythmic properties of the habituation sentences, regardless of understanding. If habituation and test sentences are in languages of the same rhythmic class, perception of the test sentences improves as compared with the control condition. Subjects can experience interference when they listen to the test sentences in a language of a different rhythmic class than the habituation language. Thus these results also suggest that there is some psychological reality to the notion of rhythmic class, even though the measures of acoustic phonetics have not established its validity.

Nazzi (1997) asked people to rate filtered utterances of foreign languages as a function of the perceived proximity to their native tongue. The experiment is reminiscent of what one feels when entering a noisy, crowded room in which many conversations are being held at the same time. In such a situation, one may suddenly notice that one's attention is attracted toward an acoustic signal. It often turns out that the signal is a sentence in our maternal language. However, there are times when we think that we are listening to a conversation in our maternal language, but we are mistaken. As one pays more attention, one realizes the mistake. In such cases, will one confuse, say, English, with any other language with the same likelihood? Using low-pass filtered speech, Nazzi showed that this was not the case. Indeed, some foreign languages are rated as more similar to the maternal language than others. Since the filtered utterances were not understandable, Nazzi reasoned that the distance of languages must be determined by their acoustic-phonetic properties.

It then became evident that if low-pass filtering is a procedure to neutralize the influence of meaning in sentence processing, it also has many drawbacks. We thus devised and used a more flexible system to explore speech processing (Ramus and Mehler, 1999). Using a speech synthesizer and real sentences in several languages, we made utterances without meaning but with total control over their acoustic-phonetic and prosodic properties. Basically, every phoneme was systematically replaced by another phoneme. In one manipulation we replaced all phonemes of a natural class (stops, nasals, and so on) to just one phone of that class, for example, all stops by /t/, all nasals by /n/, and so forth. This transformation removes meaning, leaving the phonotactics, rhythm, and intonation unchanged. In a more radical transformation we replaced all consonants by /s/ and all vowels by /a/ and optionally flattened the fundamental frequency. Proceeding in this way we were able to remove selectively intonation cues or rhythmic cues. When only rhythmic cues were preserved the task was feasible, provided the source languages were sufficiently different, but not otherwise. In a series of studies, we included English, Polish, Spanish, and Japanese. Discrimination results from experiments carried out with French adult subjects were consistent with the notion that natural languages fall into rhythmic groups or classes (Ramus et al., submitted).

In another study, Ramus, Nespor, and Mehler (1999) extensively measured the proportion of time that is taken up by vowels and by consonants in utterances drawn from eight languages and several native speakers per language. They used these measurements to provide a phonetic account of the rhythm classes and to simulate language discrimination experiments previously made on infants and adults. They were able to show great consistency between the rhythmic class hypothesis, the subjects' behaviors, and acoustic-phonetic measurements in the speech signal.

This work allows us to unify into a single major conjecture a great deal of psycholinguistic work that has been carried out in our laboratory. It allows us to try to project experiments with infants, asking such questions as: Which acoustic cues is the infant most sensitive to when s/he is reacting to a change of language? Are the same cues used all throughout development when making this kind of discrimination? How specific are these abilities to the human language module? In a study we conducted in collaboration with Marc Hauser, we have shown that the acoustic properties humans use to represent utterances may also be used by tamarin monkeys. Indeed, like infants, monkeys distinguish a language change and fail to distinguish the contrast when the utterances are played backward. This result, though preliminary, is compatible with the view that the language endowment has inherited some of its properties from the ape's acoustic system. (Ramus et al., 2000).

The above illustration of the functional cognitive approach at work is partial, because it leaves out the important role that the neurosciences are beginning to play in cognitive science. It is desirable to correct this oversight for at least two reasons: first, the tools to explain development are to be found within the neurosciences; second, the neurosciences have provided us with methods to explore brain activity in healthy volunteers. Now experiments similar to those in experimental psychology can be run, adding measures of brain activity to the behavioral measures.

Psycholinguists have often been fascinated by the apparent difficulty people have when they are learning a language late in life. Some psycholinguists argue that there is a critical period in which to learn a first language, although most of the observations bear on the late learning of a second language (see Chapter 9). Foreign accent is but one of the many features that are generally associated with late second language (L2) acquisition. This has been a traditional area of research, but little has been learned and there are many controversies among specialists about the source and reality of such difficulties. Last, the aphasiological study of bilinguals who have suffered stroke is disconcerting. Indeed, neuropsychology has not set down clear principles to understand how first and second languages are preserved or lost in bilingual patients who have suffered a cerebrovascular accident.

The advent of brain-imaging and the improved quality of the functional explorations of bilingual processing have instilled new life into this domain. Positron emission tomography (PET) and functional magnetic resonance imaging (fMRI) now encourage novel explorations into how the brain represents first and second languages in healthy bilinguals, as a function of age of L2 acquisition, proficiency attained with L2, and distance between L1 and L2. (For details of all the results that have been gathered, see Perani et al., 1996, 1998; Dehaene et al., 1997.) It appears that the age of L2 acquisition has a lesser weight than attained L2 proficiency to predict the cortical representation of L2. Results make it clear why cortical lesions in the bilingual may have such different consequences compared with the effects of similar lesions in monolinguals. We still do not know why the older one gets, the more difficult it becomes to learn a second language. This question is currently being addressed with new tools and concepts. Notions such as plasticity, remapping of cortical structures, and many other neuroscience concepts are providing an explanatory framework that psychology did not have before. It is hoped that the new entente of psychology and neuroscience will bring progress to both disciplines.

Challenges to the Approach

Despite its success, cognitive psychology has often been the target of criticism or skepticism from colleagues. These critics are often assumed to be the social psychologists, the personality experts, or the researchers of the emotional side of cognition whose agenda is different from that of standard cognitive psychologists. Most of the time, however, the skeptics are found among the most central players of the young discipline of cognitive psychology itself. We will discuss here only two types of reservations, which seem to us quite important. One comes from some philosophers of mind and perhaps a few linguists, who argue that cognitive psychology, even when it is good, deals only with the most marginal aspects of the mind. The other comes from neuroscientists who argue that or behave as if they believe that by studying molecules, neural receptors, neurons and neural nets, the properties of the mind will become, one by one, crystal clear.

Colleagues like Fodor, among others, have argued that cognitive science neglects the truly important properties of the mind, and for this reason it (and cognitive psychology) is and may well remain in a rather primitive state. Fodor (1983) proposed that the mind is organized in terms of vertical modules that provide information to the central or horizontal module about the state of the surrounds (internal or external). Vertical modules respond rigidly, with great speed and efficiency, to specific stimuli. It is those peripheral modules that Fodor claims are the ones cognitive science is targeting for study. In contrast, the central system has generally been neglected or has resisted scrutiny. What is even worse, Fodor claims, is that cognitive scientists have no idea how to correct this state of affairs.

Of course, it is difficult to disagree with the assertion that the central system is the most important component we need to crack to understand how the human mind works. Indeed, the central system mediates the rational capacities, that is, thinking, solving hitherto unsolved problems, and elaborating knowledge and culture. The central system, Fodor argues, cannot function using only specific kinds of information. Rather, the central system almost by definition has to be capable of handling all kinds of information. Thanks to the central system, scientific theories are elaborated. Still, to elaborate scientific theories it is necessary to pay attention and to think about data that one cannot determine a priori. Who would have predicted that looking at vestigial organs would inform biologists of what many consider central issues to the understanding natural history? Or that neglecting friction would help formulate a first-order theory of physics? Fodor argues that it is precisely the indeterminate nature of the information that is efficiently handled by the central system that puts the current models and theories in cognitive science in crisis. Cognitive science has successfully used computational models to explain many kinds of processes. Those models work because all the work is being done by the syntactic properties of the model. However, if the problem to be solved requires the efficient use of isotropic information, Fodor argues, syntactic devices may turn out to be unsuitable. Thus Fodor, like Wundt one hundred years earlier, reaches the conclusion that the truly interesting higher mental processes cannot be studied scientifically or that we do not have the faintest clue how to go about it.

Fodor's argument seems airtight. We cannot offer a convincing counterargument, even though we are not persuaded that his position, compelling as it sounds, is justified. We trust that the discovery of new and unforeseen facts and theories will little by little erode the protective walls that make the horizontal module so resistant to scientific scrutiny. Fodor has raised an important point that we can no longer ignore. Even so, cognitive psychology is quickly making tremendous progress. We prefer to pursue our explorations of peripheral properties of the human mind in the hope that progressively there will remain less and less of the central core to explain. The worst that could happen is that Fodor will turn out to have been right. If so, then nobody will have helped solve the mystery of how the central module works. In that case, cognitive scientists will acknowledge Fodor's insights.

Cognitive science is also often challenged by neuroscience. Neuroscience is a discipline that has grown enormously and encountered great success in its exploration of how the nervous system works. Cognitive neuroscience is helping us to understand how the brain operates and how some cognitive modules are neurally actualized. The success of the neurosciences has often led some practitioners to think that the study of neural processes in vitro, so to speak, will generate cognitive insights that will render branches like cognitive psychology almost obsolete.

This view is wrong. Essentially, to understand how the mind works, the theories and models of cognitive processing must be linked with the underlying neural mechanisms. This requirement arises for the sake of completeness and because it is always necessary to link a function to its organ. We believe that this is gradually what will happen, and for the most part there need be no clash between disciplines. Neuroscience, however, needs to accept the fact that the methods that have allowed psychologists to understand learning, memory, language, and many other abilities are not only useful but also essential. Cognitive neuroscience, of course, is offering us new methods that make it possible, and relatively easy, to observe brain activity in awake and performing subjects. This development, rather than challenging the validity of cognitive psychology, has made it even more evident that to study brain structures we need to link them to the behaviors and functions that the structures sustain. This view is gaining support, and neuroscientists and cognitive scientists are now working in better concert.

Conclusion

The functional approach that we favor makes use of all the disciplines that cognitive science draws on. It is an approach that highlights the importance of studying the formal properties of the faculties of the human mind and asks how it is that each one of them comes to be mastered and how each one is represented by the brain. This perspective allows us to have a biological perspective on the functioning of the mind without losing sight of the fact that it is the mind that creates culture and that this in turn may influence the way in which we behave and interact with other social beings.

Note

1. That is, only the part of the spectrum below 400 Hz was played.

References

Abercrombie, D. 1967. *Elements of general phonetics.* Chicago: Aldine.

Christophe, A., and Morton, J. 1998. Is Dutch native English? Linguistic analysis by 2-month-olds. *Developmental Science, 1,* 215–219.

Dauer, R. M. 1983. Stress-timing and syllable-timing reanalyzed. *Journal of Phonetics, 11,* 51–62.

Dehaene, S., Dupoux, E., Mehler, J., Cohen, L., Paulesu, E., Perani, D., van de Moortele, P.-F., Lehéricy, S., and Le Bihan, D. 1997. Anatomical variability in the cortical representation of first and second languages. *NeuroReport, 8,* 3809–3815.

Dupoux, E., and Green, K. 1997. Perceptual adjustment to highly compressed speech: Effects of talker and rate changes. *Journal of Experimental Psychology: Human Perception and Performance, 23,* 914–927.

Fodor, J. A. 1983. *Modularity of mind.* Cambridge: MIT Press.

Mehler, J., Jusczyk, P., Lambertz, G., Halsted, N., Bertoncini, J., and Amiel-Tison, C. 1988. A precursor of language acquisition in young infants. *Cognition, 29,* 143–178.

Mehler, J., Sebastian, N., Altmann, G., Dupoux, E., Christophe, A., and Pallier, C. 1993. Understanding compressed sentences: The role of rhythm and meaning. *Annals of the New York Academy of Science, 682,* 272–282.

Mithen, S. 1996. *The prehistory of the mind.* London: Thames and Hudson.

Nazzi, T. 1997. Du rythme dans l'acquisition et le traitement de la parole. Ph.D. dissertation, Ecole des Hautes Etudes en Sciences Sociales, Paris.

Nazzi, T., Bertoncini, J., and Mehler, J. 1998. Language discrimination by newborns: Towards an understanding of the role of rhythm. *Journal of Experimental Psychology: Human Perception and Performance, 24* (3), 1–11.

Pallier, C., Sebastian-Gallés, N., Dupoux, E., Christophe, A., and Mehler, J. 1997. Perceptual adjustment to time-compressed speech: A cross-linguistic study. *Memory and Cognition, 26,* 844–851.

Perani, D., Dehaene, S., Grassi, F., Cohen, L., Cappa, S., Dupoux, E., Fazzio, F., and Mehler, J. 1996. Brain processing of native and foreign languages. *NeuroReport, 7,* 2439–2444.

Perani, D., Paulesu, E., Galles, N. S., Dupoux, E., Dehaene, S., Bettinardi, V., Cappa, S., Mehler, J., and Fazio, F. 1998. The bilingual brain: Proficiency and age of acquisition of the second language. *Brain, 121,* 1841–1852.

Pike, K. L. 1945. *The intonation of American English.* Ann Arbor: University of Michigan Press.

Ramus, F., Dupoux, E., Zangl, R., and Mehler, J. Submitted. An empirical study of the perception of language rhythm.

Ramus, F., Hauser, M., Miller, C., Morris, D., and Mehler, J. 2000. Language discrimination by human newborns and by cotton-top tamarin monkeys. *Science, 288,* 349–351.

Ramus, F., and Mehler, J. 1999. Language identification with suprasegmental cues: A study based on speech resynthesis. *Journal of the Acoustical Society of America, 105,* 512–521.

Ramus, F., Nespor, M., and Mehler, J. 1999. Correlates of linguistic rhythm in the speech signal. *Cognition, 73,* 265–292.

Verbal and Nonverbal Representations of Numbers in the Human Brain

11

Stanislas Dehaene

There is a domain of language in which we are all, in some sense, bilinguals: the domain of numbers. Like any other category of words, numbers can be spoken (/four/, /forty/) or spelled out (FOUR, FORTY). However, we are all familiar with a third symbolic notation, Arabic numerals (4, 40). Furthermore, numbers can also be conveyed in nonsymbolic ways such as sets of dots (::).

The human brain must contain mental representations and processes for recognizing, understanding, and producing these various notations of numbers and for translating between them. Hence the number domain provides a manageably restricted area within which to study the representation of symbolic information in the human brain and the interplay between verbal and nonverbal formats of representation. The lessons that numbers can teach us about the organization of symbol systems in the human brain may also turn out to be generalizable to other linguistic domains.

The Quantity Representation

Moyer and Landauer's (1967) seminal study of number comparison provided the first strong evidence for a quantity representation of numbers in human adults. Measuring the time that it takes to select the larger of two digits, they found a *distance effect:* number comparison becomes systematically slower as the distance between the two numbers decreases. It is easier to decide, say, that 9 is larger than 5 than to decide that 9 is larger than 8. The effect was later extended to two-digit numerals (Dehaene, Dupoux, and Mehler, 1990). The reaction time curve for deciding whether a two-digit number is larger or smaller than 65 is remarkably smooth and shows no significant discontinuities at decade boundaries. Reaction times are influenced by the ones digit, even though the tens digit is sufficient to respond: subjects respond "smaller" more slowly to 59 than to 51, although the 5 in the decades position readily indicates that both of these numbers are smaller than 65.

These results suggest that subjects do not compare numbers digit by digit. Rather, they appear to mentally convert the target Arabic numeral into a continuous quantity, which they then compare to the reference quantity using a psychophysical procedure similar to the one used for comparing line lengths, weights, or other physical quantities. Several models of number comparison suppose that the human brain incorporates an *analogical representation of numerical quantities* that may be likened to a number line. In this representation, numbers are represented not by discrete symbols such as digits or words, but by distributions of activation whose overlap indicates how similar the quantities are. Experiments with normal subjects confirm that the conversion from digits or number words to the corresponding quantities is fast and automatic and even occurs unbeknownst to the subject (review in Dehaene and Akhavein, 1995).

The Triple-code Model

The triple-code model was introduced by Dehaene (1992; Dehaene and Cohen, 1995) in an effort to provide testable hypotheses about the relationship between the various codes for numbers and their implementation in the human brain. The model postulates three main representations of numbers:

- A visual Arabic code, localized to the left and right inferior ventral occipito-temporal areas, and in which numbers are represented as identified strings of digits. This representation, which we call the visual Arabic number form by analogy with Shallice's

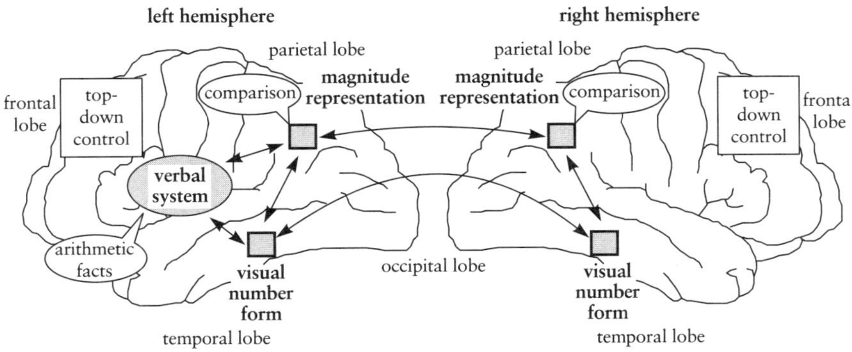

Figure 11.1. Schematic anatomical and functional architecture of Dehaene and Cohen's (1995) triple-code model. The three cardinal representations of number (two of them distributed bilaterally) are shown in light gray.

visual word form, is used during multidigit operations and parity judgments (for example, knowing that 12 is even because the ones digit is a 2).

- An analogical quantity or magnitude code, subserved by the left and right inferior parietal areas, and in which numbers are represented as points on an oriented number line. This representation underlies our semantic knowledge about numerical quantities, including proximity (for example, 9 close to 10) and larger-smaller relations (9 smaller than 10).
- A verbal code, subserved by left-hemispheric perisylvian language areas, in which numbers are represented as a parsed sequence of words. This representation is the primary code for accessing a rote verbal memory of arithmetic facts (for example, "nine times nine, eighty-one").

Figure 11.1 shows the patterns of interconnections that are postulated in the model. In the left hemisphere, all three cardinal representations (Arabic, verbal, and quantity) are interconnected by bidirectional translation routes, including a direct asemantic route for transcoding between the Arabic and verbal representations. In the right hemisphere, there are similar routes for translating back and forth between Arabic and quantity representations, but there is no verbal representation of numbers. Finally, it is assumed that the homologous Arabic and quantity representations in the two hemispheres are interconnected by direct transcallosal pathways. The system operates under the top-down control of frontal lobe and anterior cingulate, where the goals of the calculation and the information-processing pathways appropriate to implement them are specified.

Number Processing in Split-brains

A strength of the triple-code model is that it specifies cerebral localizations, however coarse, for the various representations of numbers. As a result, the model can predict the effect of specific anatomical lesions on number processing. A case in point is the "split-brain" syndrome. When the corpus callosum is severed, the model predicts that the left hemisphere should remain able to perform all sorts of calculations, because it contains the three cardinal representations of numbers (Arabic, verbal, and quantity). The right hemisphere, however, should be able to recognize Arabic numerals, to retrieve the quantity that they represent, but not to read aloud or to perform calculations dependent on the verbal code. This predicted pattern of results is exactly what is found, both in the classical literature on split-brains (Gazzaniga and Hillyard, 1971; Gazzaniga and Smylie, 1984; Seymour, Reuter-Lorenz, and Gazzaniga, 1994) and in a recent single-case study of number processing following an infarct of the posterior half of the corpus callosum (Cohen and Dehaene, 1996). When digits 5 and 6 are flashed in the left hemifield, the patients' right hemisphere can decide that 5 is smaller than 6, but it cannot read the digits aloud or calculate 5 + 6. Similar results suggesting a right hemispheric ability restricted to quantitative processing have been obtained in patients with extended left hemispheric lesions (Dehaene and Cohen, 1991; Grafman et al., 1989). Patient NAU, for instance, could not tell whether 2 + 2 was 3, 4, or 5—but he knew that it had to be smaller than 9.

Number Processing in Pure Alexia

Similar dissociations between impaired linguistic processing of numbers and preserved manipulation of numerical quantities are found in pure alexia (Cohen and Dehaene, 1995). Patients GOD and SMA suffered from highly similar infarcts of the left ventral occipito-temporal area, a region involved in high-level visual identification. Both were totally unable to read words. Arabic numerals were slightly better preserved: multidigit numerals were misread on 60–80 percent of trials and single digits on 8–18 percent of trials. Calculation on written operands was also impaired. For instance, when presented with 2 + 3, the patients might say *seven*. That these calculation errors were due to a misidentification of the digits was shown by (a) the patients' perfect ability to perform the same calculation with spoken operands, and (b) the patients' reading errors in calculation: for instance, 2 × 3 might be read *two times five* and then solved as *ten*, indicating that the patients correctly computed the sum of the operands that they had misread.

So far, this deficit might be understood as a selective impairment of the Arabic number identification module. Contradicting this hypothesis, however, but in agreement with the triple-code model's hypothesis of a right-hemispheric digit identification and quantity processing system, both patients GOD and SMA compared Arabic numerals with remarkable accuracy. For instance, when presented with 44 pairs of two-digit numerals, neither of them made any errors in pointing to the larger number, while they made respectively 89 percent and 91 percent errors in reading the very same pairs aloud. Some of the reading errors inverted the order of the numbers. For instance 78 76 was read as *seventy eight, seventy nine*—yet the patient correctly pointed to 78 as the larger number. These two pure alexia cases thus suggest that access to number semantics can be fully preserved, even when number identification for the purpose of reading is severely compromised. These observations have been replicated (Miozzo and Caramazza, 1998) and extended to show that even elementary calculations such as subtractions can remain preserved (for example, a pure alexic patient might read 3 – 1 incorrectly as *nine minus one*, but then go on to say the correct result, *two*) (Cohen and Dehaene, 2000).

In detail, how does the triple-code model account for these pure alexia cases? In those cases, the lesion affected the left ventral occipito-temporal area and therefore predictably impaired the left visual word and number identification system. Hence left-hemispheric verbal areas could not be directly informed about the identity of the visual word or digit, resulting in a severe impairment in reading aloud. Since the memory retrieval of rote arithmetic facts is assumed to depend on the verbal format, this reading deficit entailed a calculation deficit—the patients could not turn 3 × 3 into the verbal format *three times three*, which was necessary for them to retrieve the result *nine*. Yet the verbal circuit itself was intact and connected to auditory input/output circuits; it was only deprived of visual inputs. Hence the patients could still calculate when an arithmetic problem was read aloud to them. And finally, their right hemisphere was fully intact, including its visual identification and magnitude representation areas. According to the triple-code model, these preserved right-hemispheric circuits (and connections to the left-hemispheric quantity representation) were the basis for the patients' ability to compare the magnitudes of Arabic numerals that they failed to read aloud (Cohen and Dehaene, 1995).

A New Classification of Acalculias

The triple-code model also accounts for some of the types of acalculias and their anatomical correlates. According to the model, there are two basic routes through which a simple single-digit arithmetic problem such as 4 + 2 can be solved. In the first, direct route, which works only for overlearned addition and multiplication problems, the operands 4 and 2 are transcoded into a verbal representation of the problem ("four plus two") which is then used to trigger completion of this word sequence using rote verbal memory ("four plus two, six"). This process is assumed to involve a left cortico-subcortical loop through the basal ganglia and thalamus. In the second, indirect semantic route, the operands are encoded into quantity representations held in the left and right inferior parietal areas. Semantically meaningful manipulations are then performed on these internal quantities, and the resulting quantity is then transmitted from the left inferior parietal cortex to the left-hemispheric perisylvian language network for naming. The model assumes that this indirect semantic route is used whenever rote verbal knowledge of the operation result is lacking, most typically for subtraction problems.

The two types of acalculic patients predicted by these two routes for calculation have now been identified (Dehaene and Cohen, 1997). There are several published cases of acalculia following a left subcortical infarct (Whitaker, Habiger, and Ivers, 1985; Corbett, McCusker, and Davidson, 1988; Hittmair-Delazer, Semenza, and Denes, 1994). In a recent case of a left lenticular infarct, Dehaene and Cohen (1997) showed that, as predicted by the model, only rote verbal arithmetic facts such as 3 × 3 were impaired (together with rote verbal knowledge of the alphabet, nursery rhymes, and prayers). Quantitative knowledge of numbers was fully preserved, as shown by the patient's intact number comparison, proximity judgment, and simple addition and subtraction abilities. Hittmair-Delazer, Semenza, and Denes (1994) likewise observed a preservation of conceptual, quantitative, and algebraic manipulations of numbers in their severely acalculic patient with a left subcortical lesion.

Conversely, the model predicts that lesions of the left inferior parietal area, typically resulting in Gerstmann's syndrome, affect calculation because they destroy quantitative knowledge while preserving rote verbal abilities. Indeed, Dehaene and Cohen (1997) observed a case of Gerstmann's syndrome who could still read aloud numbers and write them down to dictation, still knew rote addition and multiplication facts such as 2 + 2 and 3 × 3, and yet failed even in the simplest of quantitative tasks. He made 16 percent errors in larger-smaller comparison, 75 percent errors in simple subtractions (including gross errors such as 3 – 1 = 3 or 6 – 3 = 7), and 78 percent errors in number bisection (stating, for instance, that 3 falls in the middle of 4 and 8). The deficit was highly specific to the category of numbers, since the patient performed quite well in finding the middle of two letters, two days of week, two months, or two notes of the musical scale. We have now observed several such cases of severe number bisection deficits following lesion of the inferior parietal area. These cases support the triple-code model's hypothesis that this area is critical for representing and manipulating number as quantities.

Imaging the Parietal Representation of Quantities

Brain-imaging techniques now allow for the visualization of the cerebral circuits involved in number processing in normal subjects, without resorting to the study of pathological lesion cases. Imaging studies have confirmed that the inferior parietal lobe, in both hemispheres, is critically involved in the internal manipulation of numerical quantities. In an early study Roland and Friberg (1985), with a primitive PET (positron emission tomography) technique, reported bilateral frontal and inferior parietal activity during a repeated subtraction task, a result that has been confirmed in more recent fMRI (functional magnetic resonance imaging) studies (Burbaud et al., 1995; Rueckert et al., 1996). Most recently, we have found bilateral parietal activity during much simpler calculation tasks. In PET, intraparietal activation was found during multiplication of two single digits (Dehaene et al., 1996). In fMRI, similar activation is found when a single digit is flashed and subjects must compare it with 5, multiply it by 3, or subtract it from 11 (see Figure 11.2; see also Chochon et al., 1999). The accuracy of fMRI images obtained from single subjects allowed for a much tighter localization of the activated tissue, which is confined to the banks of the middle portion of the intraparietal sulcus, extending anteriorily into the depth of the postcentral sulcus. Activity is left-lateralized during multiplication, right-lateralized during comparison, and bilateral during subtraction, in agreement with previous studies using event-related potentials (Dehaene, 1996; Kiefer and Dehaene, 1997). Most interestingly, little or no parietal activation is found when subjects simply have to name a single Arabic digit. Hence, in agreement with the triple-code model, parietal activity is not found when subjects merely have to process numerical symbols (such as recognizing a digit or producing a number name), but only when they have to mentally represent and manipulate the corresponding quantity.

The triple-code model makes specific predictions concerning the nature of the parameters that should or should not affect parietal lobe activity during number processing. A first prediction is that the quantity representation should be more active during tasks that draw upon an approximate sense of numbers than during tasks that require exact arithmetic fact retrieval, which can be mediated at least in part by rote verbal memory processes. This prediction was recently confirmed with fMRI (Dehaene et al., 1999). Second, notational changes, such as presenting numbers in Arabic or in verbal form, should affect activity in visual and verbal areas, but not within the parietal system, which is supposed to encode numerical quantities in a notation-independent quantity code. The parietal system should, however, be affected by changes in the size of the numerical quantities involved, and in the dis-

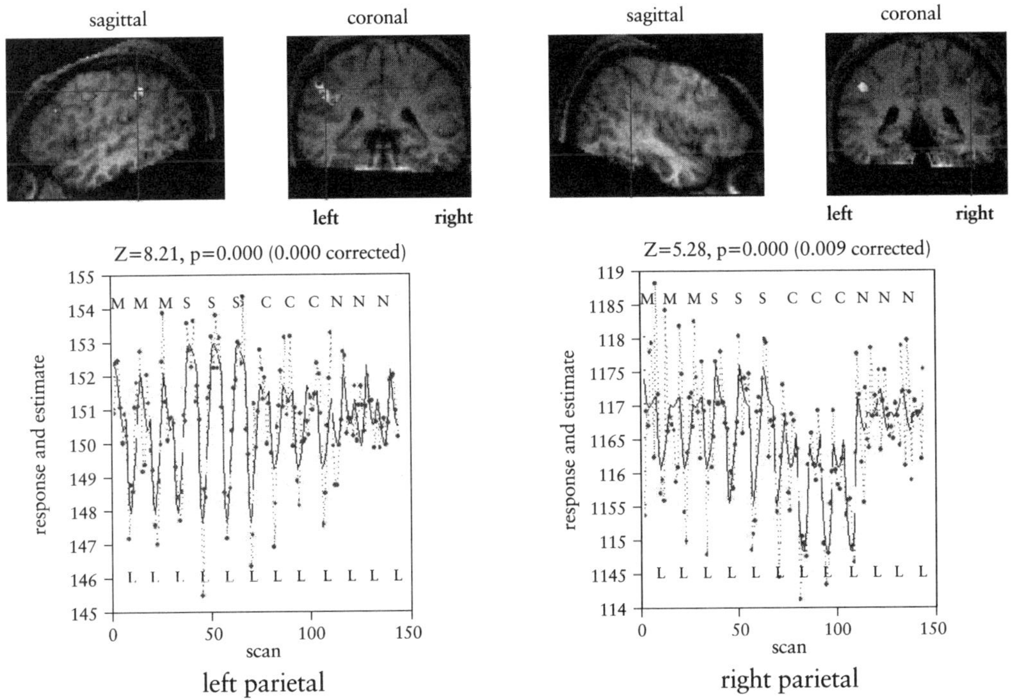

Figure 11.2. The banks of the intraparietal sulcus are active in both hemispheres during number-processing tasks (data from Chochon et al., 1999). Plots indicate activation as a function of time as the subject alternated blocks of comparison (C), multiplication (M), subtraction (S), and number-naming tasks (N) with blocks of letter-naming (L). Areas conjointly activated in the three calculation tasks (C, M, S) were determined with SPM96 software in an individual subject (voxelwise $p < 0.001$, corrected to $p < 0.05$). These areas are postulated to participate in the cerebral substrates of quantity knowledge.

tances between them. This prediction has been confirmed using event-related potentials. In a multiplication task, late event-related potentials recorded over left parietal electrodes were affected by the size of the operands (for example, 2×3 versus 7×9), but not by the auditory or visual modality in which they were presented (Kiefer and Dehaene, 1997). And likewise, in a number comparison task, electrical activity over left and especially right parietal electrodes was affected by the distance between the numbers to be compared (for example, 1 and 5 versus 4 and 5), but not by whether the numbers were presented visually as words or as digits (Dehaene, 1995). The latter variable only affected early visual ERPs: as predicted by the triple-code model, visual activity was bilateral for digits and left-lateralized for number words.

Conclusion

Neuropsychological and brain-imaging studies suggest that multiple brain areas are involved in representing numbers mentally. Each area contributes a different code for numbers, and different mental operations are preferentially executed using specific codes. The rich variety of arithmetical operations that can be executed by humans is presumably based on a constant interplay between symbolic and semantic representations for numbers. The human brain possesses both notation-specific cortices where specific number notations are recognized and/or produced, and notation-independent cortices, within the intraparietal sulcus, where numbers are represented in a nonsymbolic semantic quantity code. I speculate that other categories of knowledge, whether for persons, animals, actions, or colors, will be found to rest on a similar organization, with distributed cortical representations for the various input and output symbolic codes in which these concepts can be conveyed, as well as nonverbal category-specific cortical representations of their semantic dimension.

References

This chapter is based on an updated and abbreviated version of a chapter entitled "Levels of Representation in Number Processing," by S. Dehaene and

L. Cohen, which appeared in 1997 in *The Handbook of Neurolinguistics*, edited by Brigitte Stemmer and Harry A. Whitaker (New York: Academic Press). Neuropsychological cases were studied in tight collaboration with L. Cohen. F. Chochon, P. F. van de Moortele and D. Le Bihan provided invaluable help with the fMRI. My research on number processing is sponsored by a centennial fellowship from the McDonnell Foundation.

Burbaud, P., Degreze, P., Lafon, P., Franconi, J.-M., Bouligand, B., Bioulac, B., Caille, J.-M., and Allard, M. 1995. Lateralization of prefrontal activation during internal mental calculation: A functional magnetic resonance imaging study. *Journal of Neurophysiology, 74,* 2194–2200.

Chochon, F., Cohen, L., van de Moortele, P. F., and Dehaene, S. 1999. Differential contributions of the left and right inferior parietal lobules to number processing. *Journal of Cognitive Neuroscience, 11,* 617–630.

Cohen, L., and Dehaene, S. 1995. Number processing in pure alexia: The effect of hemispheric asymmetries and task demands. *NeuroCase, 1,* 121–137.

——— 1996. Cerebral networks for number processing: Evidence from a case of posterior callosal lesion. *NeuroCase, 2,* 155–174.

——— 2000. Calculating without reading: Unsuspected residual abilities in pure alexia. *Cognitive Neuropsychology, 17(6),* 563–583

Corbett, A. J., McCusker, E. A., and Davidson, O. R. 1988. Acalculia following a dominant-hemisphere subcortical infarct. *Archives of Neurology, 43,* 964–966.

Dehaene, S. 1992. Varieties of numerical abilities. *Cognition, 44,* 1–42.

——— 1995. Electrophysiological evidence for category-specific word processing in the normal human brain. *NeuroReport, 6,* 2153–2157.

——— 1996. The organization of brain activations in number comparison: Event-related potentials and the additive-factors methods. *Journal of Cognitive Neuroscience, 8,* 47–68.

Dehaene, S., and Akhavein, R. 1995. Attention, automaticity, and levels of representation in number processing. *Journal of Experimental Psychology: Learning, Memory and Cognition, 21,* 314–326.

Dehaene, S., and Cohen, L. 1991. Two mental calculation systems: A case study of severe acalculia with preserved approximation. *Neuropsychologia, 29,* 1045–1074.

——— 1995. Towards an anatomical and functional model of number processing. *Mathematical Cognition, 1,* 83–120.

——— 1997. Cerebral pathways for calculation: Double dissociation between rote verbal and quantitative knowledge of arithmetic. *Cortex, 33,* 219–250.

Dehaene, S., Dupoux, E., and Mehler, J. 1990. Is numerical comparison digital: Analogical and symbolic effects in two-digit number comparison.

Journal of Experimental Psychology: Human Perception and Performance, 16, 626–641.

Dehaene, S., Tzourio, N., Frak, V., Raynaud, L., Cohen, L., Mehler, J., and Mazoyer, B. 1996. Cerebral activations during number multiplication and comparison: A PET study. *Neuropsychologia, 34,* 1097–1106.

Dehaene, S., Spelke, E., Stanescu, R., Pinel, P., and Tsivkin, S. 1999. Sources of mathematical thinking: Behavioral and brain-imaging evidence. *Science, 284,* 970–974.

Gazzaniga, M. S., and Hillyard, S. A. 1971. Language and speech capacity of the right hemisphere. *Neuropsychologia, 9,* 273–280.

Gazzaniga, M. S., and Smylie, C. E. 1984. Dissociation of language and cognition: A psychological profile of two disconnected right hemispheres. *Brain, 107,* 145–153.

Grafman, J., Kampen, D., Rosenberg, J., Salazar, A., and Boller, F. 1989. Calculation abilities in a patient with a virtual left hemispherectomy. *Behavioural Neurology, 2,* 183–194.

Hittmair-Delazer, M., Sailer, U., and Benke, T. 1995. Impaired arithmetic facts but intact conceptual knowledge—a single case study of dyscalculia. *Cortex, 31,* 139–147.

Hittmair-Delazer, M., Semenza, C., and Denes, G. 1994. Concepts and facts in calculation. *Brain, 117,* 715–728.

Kiefer, M., and Dehaene, S. 1997. The time course of parietal activation in single-digit multiplication: Evidence from event-related potentials. *Mathematical Cognition, 3,* 1–30.

Miozzo, M., and Caramazza, A. 1998. Varieties of pure alexia: The case of failure to access graphemic representations. *Cognitive Neuropsychology, 15,* 203–238.

Moyer, R. S., and Landauer, T. K. 1967. Time required for judgements of numerical inequality. *Nature, 215,* 1519–1520.

Roland, P. E., and Friberg, L. 1985. Localization of cortical areas activated by thinking. *Journal of Neurophysiology, 53,* 1219–1243.

Rueckert, L., Lange, N., Partiot, A., Appollonio, I., Litvar, I., Le Bihan, D., and Grafman, J. 1996. Visualizing cortical activation during mental calculation with functional MRI. *NeuroImage, 3,* 97–103.

Seymour, S. E., Reuter-Lorenz, P. A., and Gazzaniga, M. S. 1994. The disconnection syndrome: Basic findings reaffirmed. *Brain,* 117, 105–115.

Whitaker, H., Habiger, J., and Ivers, R. 1985. Acalculia from a lenticular-caudate lesion. *Neurology, 35* (suppl. 1), 161.

Discussion: Section 3

Language Processing and Linguistic Diversity

CATHERINE SNOW: We've seen some very interesting data from Pat Kuhl that show that in the first year of life babies already have language-specific patterns of perception. Then there are the data from Jim Flege, which show differentiation among different phonemes in the first language with respect to approach to the second language as a function of age. How do you reconcile those two? I mean, the native language perceptual system is set, Kuhl and Werker and other people would suggest, by a year. And yet with respect to acquiring a second language age differences continue to emerge in a gradual sort of way over the first several years.

JACQUES MEHLER: It does not seem to me that the picture that has emerged from the work of Kuhl and Werker allows one to say that it is a case of all or none. I think that the language acquisition faculty is complex, and that there are some settings that are established very early. There must be more than one way to achieve near perfection in the second language. For instance, Chinese linguists speaking English may perform very well by using a cognitive, isotropic approach. This does not mean that they have the ability to speak fast in the way in which native speakers do. All of us know that, for instance, you take two scotches in the evening and, if you are a bilingual, you might not suffer equally in the two languages. The point here is that in one of the languages you may need more cognitive involvement. I think, therefore, that the formula is complex, and the fact that we can almost simulate perfection does not mean that the representations are the same.

STEPHEN KOSSLYN: I would like to hear, if possible, a resolution to Jacques Mehler's and Catherine Snow's talks. On the one hand, I was very enthusiastic about Catherine's cheery words about learning language, a second language, as an adult. On the other hand, Jacques gave us the news that one gets configured as a baby, and that this is it for life. Can you talk to each other, and see whether we can work this out?

MEHLER: The evidence suggests that when one looks in a systematic way at the performance of people who are very high proficiency learners of a second language—the way Helen Neville, Flege, and some people in my lab have done—one finds extremely important, measurable differences. This does not say that one cannot attain high levels of performance such that the layperson will be fooled. We hear foreign speakers with charitable receptive equipment. Why are we charitable? I believe it is because we have to cope with a large variety of dialects, accents, and so on. Now, take somebody who has lived in Paris for forty years and sounds French. Now you ask a trained phonologist whether he can distinguish that person from a native speaker. I think that they will be able to tell them apart easily. The data I have presented here supports this claim.

SNOW: On the other hand, the data I presented from Bohart's lab, for example, showed a total overlap in the judgments of trained phonologists and English teachers when comparing native English speakers to native Dutch speakers.

MEHLER: Well enough, but there is another issue, which I did not introduce into this discussion, and which seems important to me. It has to do with the distance between L1 and L2. Okay. It seems to me that if you rated me as a foreign speaker of Greek, according to my model, I could attain (I have not done it) a very high level of performance. I could cheat anybody in Greek, because Greek has phonological and rhythmical properties very similar to Argentine Spanish. On the other hand, if I went from Japanese to Dutch, or from Mandarin to English, then I bet you that you would easily find differences.

SNOW: That is an empirical question. Here is another issue to put on the table with regard to the Flege data that you showed. One of the major differences between child second language learners and adult second language learners is the degree to which they maintain their native language. One of the factors that we do not take into account at all when comparing degree of variability in ultimate attainment among child learners, and among adolescent and adult learners, is the psycholinguistic cost of maintaining separate phonological systems, separate phonetics systems, separate auditory discrimination systems simultaneously inside the same head. Flege's three-year-old learners—Italian learners of English—by the time he tested them, were monolingual English speakers, not Italian-English bilinguals.

GALABURDA: To what extent does learning English as the second language make a difference in this discussion, since there is so much background English around the world through cable TV, movies, and so on? This presumably could serve to expose even infants to the sounds of English and in that way prevent their atrophy?

MEHLER: If you have traveled for even one day inside Japan, you will realize that all the exposure to English has not helped much.

ALFONSO CARAMAZZA: I would like pursue this a little bit further. I am not sure I understand what the difference between the two positions is. What is the claim that you are making, Catherine? Are you saying that there is nothing special about language acquisition? That one acquires language the way one acquires chess, backgammon, and so on? If that is the claim, then, how do you account for the evidence that has been brought forward about first language acquisition? I mean, a second language to me is a very difficult thing. I am bilingual, but I know that my judgments in English stink. I look at English sentences I write and they seem to be fine. This is because they look Italian. Then people point out to me that they are not English. And what about first language acquisition? How does your story square with the fact that we learn language when we are very young, but we do not learn calculus? Perhaps we could, if we trained. Perhaps, if babies were shown calculus, they would learn it very quickly. I would rather doubt it.

SNOW: Basically, the claim that I would want to make about first language acquisition is that people have attributed to very young children much of the structure of language, which in fact emerges (I would add remarkably and miraculously), but not until considerably later. I am also claiming that syntactic knowledge is a product of language acquisition, not a precondition to language acquisition. So, from this point of view, I would argue that, in fact, second language acquisition and first language acquisition are quite different in terms of cognitive challenge, because one goes into second language acquisition armed with previous knowledge of phonetic, phonological, lexical, semantic, and syntactic systems. These can operate negatively on the process of acquiring the second language, but also positively.

The major claim I would make is that acquiring a language involves acquiring a communicative system first and a formal system second, the latter a byproduct of the communicative system. Also, the major difference between second language learning and first language learning is that the formal system interferes with the communicative system. I think that if once could re-create for second language acquisition affective and social conditions that support first language acquisition, one would end up with something much closer to native-like attainment. In other words, my position is that it is the conditions of acquisition that differentiate the two, not the state of the brain.

Verbal and Nonverbal Representations of Numbers in the Human Brain

CARAMAZZA: Stanislas [Dehaene], might you want to make a distinction between number sense and quantity sense? If you ask the right hemisphere to answer the question about which difference is larger, 9/8 or 99/8, can the right hemisphere do it? And, does the right hemisphere need number sense to be able to answer that question, which may be different from a quantity sense?

DEHAENE: This is a very good question. The answer is no, it does not need number sense. It is quite possible that the right hemispheric system is more limited than the left, and we can envision all sorts of hypotheses, including the idea that Stephen Kosslyn has proposed for order of domains. This is that the right hemisphere has a continuous representation for numbers whereas the left has a categorical representation through the use of verbal labels for quantities.

However, for the moment, there are really no hard data to prove this.

FROM THE FLOOR: What do you think are the boundaries of this natural conceptual system? Does it apply to fractions? Does it apply to negative numbers? Also, do you think that there are any interactions with the form of notation? So, for instance, if you ask someone to say which is bigger, 5.9×10^{17} or 1.9×10^{18}, are you going to find a magnitude effect totally independent of notation?

DEHAENE: The last task you mentioned would not be done by an animal, and clearly requires a symbolic system. In that case, it is probably not going to be performed by the parietal system. There is evidence indicating that if you have to compare two six-digit numbers, you do it serially and do not show the "holistic" effect I showed you. So again, there is an interplay between the two systems, which we have to disentangle.

We do not know the limits of the system, but we have at least a good model for how it could work. This is the so-called accumulator model, which has been derived from the animal and infant literature, and which supposes that all you have is the ability to accumulate quantity. Some kind of water-and-bucket model of arithmetic, whereby if you have some different amounts accumulated in your head, you can add two amounts and get an approximate result. This could be the limits of the system.

With regard to fractions, David Premack showed some interesting data in chimpanzees that seem to suggest that they can work with notations of one half and one quarter, which are also concepts for which we have words in natural languages. So maybe there is some innate ability for fractions.

CARAMAZZA: Stan, you have raised a really important point. The issue now is how to connect this symbolic system with this continuous system. How do you go from something that is continuous to something that has all of the qualities that we attribute to numbers, which you mentioned? What is the link?

DEHAENE: You are quick to point out a missing link. There are several missing links. We did propose, with Jean-Pierre Changeux, a neural network model that organizes to detect numbers in the outside world and could be connected to arbitrary output systems that could be likened to naming the different numbers. That was one concrete model aimed at performing this link. It was not a complete model for how the child does it, certainly not. There are lots of transition points as a child acquires the language of numbers, which are extremely subtle. I think that what is happening is that as the child acquires a language for numbers, there is a simultaneous modification of the semantic system. I do not think that, initially, animals have representations of numbers that are sufficiently accurate to discriminate 19 from 18. This is because they are subject to the distance effect and to the increasing inaccuracy typical of larger numbers. Somehow, however, as the child acquires a vocabulary for numbers, she becomes able to attribute separate meanings to each item.

CARAMAZZA: Yes, but there is a supposition in your story that there is merely a quantitative difference between what a chimp, a rat, or a pigeon can do, and what a human can do. You have not convinced me that, in fact, there is not a qualitative jump, in terms of what humans do when they use numbers.

You insist, and I think correctly, that there are similarities between humans and nonhuman animals, but the differences are equally striking. It is the case that a pigeon cannot do 2 + 2 = 4. Perhaps a rephrasing of Hereford's position might be reasonable, and it is that the ability to have number sense is tied up directly with language.

DEHAENE: So, I think, you are actually redefining number. Maybe the solution is somewhere in between. But, certainly it is not the case that, as Piaget among others proposed, nonverbal organisms are devoid of genuine number abilities or that infants are devoid of genuine numerical abilities. I really want to call these abilities genuine number representations. They are obviously not identical to the ones that we have as adults, and I agree that the transition from the infant to the adult system needs to be worked out. That I view as a very important missing link.

ELIZABETH SPELKE: May I just say one thing on this point? Stan already mentioned that there is plenty of evidence for number representations in infants. But there is also something curious, which

Karen Wynn's early studies of counting bring out when children start learning number words. This is that it seems to be extremely difficult for children to figure out what words like "two" and "three" mean at a time when figuring out what words like "tree" and "cow" mean seems to be going very, very rapidly. I think that this finding supports the idea that there is some nontrivial mapping that has to be made here, perhaps reflecting the notion that the preverbal number representations of number do not perfectly correspond to the verbal representations.

DAVID CAPLAN: Do we have imaging data on where the symbolic numerical manipulations are?

DEHAENE: We have both imaging and lesion data. First, the lesion data. We find a double dissociation in the patients I showed you. With a left lesion in the language system—we reported a patient with a left subcortical lesion—the patient was not able to do verbal arithmetic but had a perfect number sense. The converse was seen in our Gerstmann patient, with a parietal lesion missing the language system.

With neuroimaging the demonstration of the dissociation is more difficult, but we do find striking differences in different tasks. For instance, when one does mental multiplication, activation is confined to the left hemisphere, although it does include the left parietal system. There is no reason why one should not use the parietal system, which is available even though it may not be necessary. The important point is that the activity is completely left lateralized. Conversely, activation is bilateral if one does subtraction. It may even be right lateralized, something that I did not show in my talk.

GALABURDA: If you do the same experiments but use equivalent percentage changes rather than equivalent number changes, do you still get the same effect?

So, for instance, a change from 4 to 2 represents a greater percentage change than a change from 35 to 33.

DEHAENE: Yes, you still get the same effect. But you're absolutely right. The effect depends more—something I did not say—on the ratio of the two numbers than on the actual difference. It is more difficult to decide that 9 is larger than 8, than to decide that 2 is larger than 1.

KOSSLYN: Just one last point on Stan's work. As you know, you get exactly the same results with names of animals. So, for instance, if I ask you which is bigger, a hamster or mouse, it takes you more time than which is bigger, a hamster or an elephant. What makes you think that what you find is specific to numbers per se, as opposed to something much more general?

DEHAENE: I suppose that there are commonalities, which suggests that maybe size is represented also in a similarly analog way. But noncommonalities are also found. For example, I compared letter processing as opposed to number processing, and even though there was a similar temporal order in both cases, there also were striking dissociations.

KOSSLYN: The reason I bring it up is that there are fairly well worked out models for how the brain coordinates the continuous kinds of representation with the discrete kinds, in the case of the animal, which maybe could apply more broadly to include numbers and quantities.

Nonverbal Representation

II

Although it is clear that language is used to express thoughts, it is also clear that it cannot be *the* "language of thought": if we actually thought in terms of language, why would we ever have difficulty putting a thought into words? Moreover, words are ambiguous, but thoughts are not. For example, the statement "The student found the solution" may have a different meaning in a chemistry class (where liquid was found) than in a math class (where the answer was found). But one's thoughts are never ambiguous in this way; one is never uncertain what sort of solution one has in mind. Language is a tool, one way in which information is represented and processed by the brain.

Given that there are at least two ways of representing information, language and something more conceptual (which is unambiguous and must be mapped into language), the door is open—why just two? Why not multiple forms? Many kinds of representations may be involved in thinking. One candidate, which was the central focus of the British Associationists (such as John Locke), is mental images. Indeed, these philosophers felt that thought consisted of sequences of images. But this idea also falls short. Just as words are ambiguous, so are images: for example, an image of a rectangle could be a rectangle or part of a box seen from the side. Moreover, images are notoriously limited when it comes to specifying classes or abstractions. What, for example, is the image for "beauty"? An image of the goddess Venus? But how then could we represent Venus per se?

Nevertheless, there is ample evidence that imagery does play a role in mental life, if only as a tool for expressing thoughts. Thus it is not surprising that imagery figures in many of the chapters to follow. However, imagery is itself not a single type of representation, and it draws on numerous specific brain systems. In fact, as we shall see, the representations that underlie our ability to move also play roles in imagistic thought. Rather than a single language of thought, we have many, and these different forms work together.

This part of the volume has three sections. The first is "Perception and Language," which is a bridge from the previous material. Looking at the most mental of the perceptual processes, imagery, we seek connections with perception and language. Some of these chapters focus on the role of the first cortical visual area (known as area 17 or V1) in imagery. This issue is important because if imagery can activate the first cortical areas that process vision, it can affect our perception. In this case, thought and perception may not be distinct, but instead may be intimately connected in both directions—perceptions affect our thoughts, but our thoughts color our perceptions.

We then turn to "Visual and Motor Representations." The key idea is that both the input *and* the output systems provide basic representations that can be used in broader contexts. Imagery is often conceived solely in terms of stored perceptual representations that are activated in the absence of the immediate appropriate sensory input, but motor representations can also be used in imagery. For example, consider what happens when you decide whether your right elbow would rest on your left leg if, when seated, you cupped your left knee in your right hand. Most people report that to make the decision, they imagine making the required movement. Moreover, such imagery is often multimodal, involving both perceptual and motoric representations and processes (did you "see" your arm during the previous exercise, as well as feel it?).

The third and final section, "Representations in the World," takes us into even higher-level representations. Here we look at applications of visual and motoric nonverbal representations. By considering these applications, we learn not only about representations in the head but also about the extent to which we are social creatures who use the world in some sense as an extension of our own minds, a prosthetic device, as it were. Other people extend our capabilities—and vice versa. Throughout, we see how different sorts of representations contribute to thought and how each plays a role as a language of the brain.

Section 4
Perception and Language

In this section we consider the relationship between perceptual, imagistic, and verbal representations. Imagery arises when stored perceptual information is activated, creating a percept-like representation in short-term memory. Imagery and language are often treated as diametrically opposed, but in fact they have several key features in common. Both rely to greater or lesser extents on the perceptual system, albeit spoken language relies on audition and most imagery on other modalities. Moreover, both operate within strict systems of rules, although grammatical rules govern the ways that discrete sounds can be arranged and interpreted in spoken language, whereas perceptual principles and learned regularities about the behavior of objects govern imagery (even if the "learned regularities" include gross errors in how objects actually behave, as occurs when one visualizes many physical changes). In addition, imagery and language must interact, in both directions. For example, we can visualize a novel arrangement of furniture in a room upon hearing a description, and once having formed such an image we then can describe it.

The final chapter in this section is not on imagery, but rather on the development of perceptual and conceptual knowledge. This knowledge clearly underlies imagery, but also makes contact with the material in the section's first three chapters in another way. Although the literature on imagery and on what Alan Baddeley has called "working memory" rarely reference each other, they are in fact intimately related. Working memory is the system that allows one to use stored information when reasoning. Thus imagery is in fact an aspect of working memory. According to Baddeley, working memory includes three components: a "central executive," a "visual-spatial sketchpad," and an "articulatory loop." The latter two are considered forms of short-term memory, and can be used in tandem. Notice that the former is crucial for holding at least some types of visual images in mind, and the latter for storing the sounds of words. It is likely that the two forms of representation, visual-spatial and articulatory, often work together, and are "managed" by at least some of the same set of processes. However, imagery is more than the kinds of spatial representations Baddeley considered; images also serve to depict shapes and other visual properties.

Indeed, all of the chapters in this section can be regarded as fleshing out specific aspects of the working-memory system. In Chapter 12 Bernard Mazoyer and his colleagues use functional neuroimaging to examine which brain systems are engaged when one builds images based upon descriptions; they find evidence that imagery and language are intimately interconnected, but nevertheless are distinct. Both draw on working memory, but do so in different ways. Michel Denis, in Chapter 13, shows that images that are formed on the basis of descriptions have properties very much like images formed on the basis of perceptual information. Thus the operations that occur in working memory can translate one form of representation to the other. Next, Denis Le Bihan and his colleagues focus in Chapter 14 on the nature of the representations that underlie imagery per se and provide evidence that even the earliest visual structures are sometimes recruited during imagery. The parts of the brain used in imagery appear to depend in part on precisely that which one is visualizing, including the sorts of linguistic characters one visualizes. These authors show fascinating differences in neural activation depending on the form of Japanese writing that their subjects visualize. This finding suggests that the "visual spatial sketchpad" is too coarsely characterized; the normally purely visual parts of the brain (in the occipital lobe) are a different system from the more general spatial parts (in the parietal lobes), and each apparently can be activated separately. Finally, in Chapter 15 Elizabeth Spelke presents developmental work that indicates that Baddeley's view is an even greater oversimplification. She argues that there are many "modules" that are task specific, not part of a general system. Moreover, she argues that perceptual representations are used in special ways by humans, probably because of the interplay between nonverbal representations and language. This interplay changes over the course of development, however; in fact, in some ways children's cognitive structures are more similar to those of lower animals than to those of adult humans.

Visual and Language Area Interactions during Mental Imagery

12

Bernard Mazoyer, Emmanuel Mellet,
and Nathalie Tzourio

The human brain relies on two main systems for mental representation: language and visual mental imagery. Language conveys symbolic representations that allow human communication; mental imagery operates on internal representations and as such is a major component of human thought. The neural bases of both systems have been extensively studied over the past several years, using either positron emission tomography (PET) or functional magnetic resonance imaging (fMRI), and appear to be quite segregated: while language is supported by a leftward asymmetrical temporal and inferior frontal cortical network (Mazoyer et al., 1993), visuo-spatial mental imagery appears to rely on a bilateral occipito-parieto-frontal network, as shown by studies in which subjects first memorized visual percepts and later generated a mental image based on the reactivation of their representations in long-term memory (Mellet et al., 1995).

Strong interactions exist, however, between the two language and imagery systems and permit an easy transfer from one representation mode to the other: one can indeed easily build a mental image from a verbal description (Denis and Cocude, 1992) or conversely give an oral description of a mental image. Moreover, mental images of an object or a scene generated on the sole basis of a verbal description exhibit properties similar to those of images based on perceptual experience. In particular, cognitive operations, such as mental scanning or distance comparison, show chronometrical patterns similar to those executed on an image that reactivates stored visual information (Denis, Gonçalves, and Memmi, 1995; De Vega et al., 1996).

These findings raise the following question: do operations on mental visual images, that arise not from a visual experience but from a linguistic one, recruit visual areas? Previous work has indeed shown that brain regions involved during auditory language may be interacting in a complex manner with those involved in visual tasks: for example, deactivations of the superior temporal cortex and of the left inferior frontal cortex were reported during a visual exploration task (Mellet et al., 1995), while the occipito-parietal cortex appears to be deactivated by some auditory language tasks (Shulman et al., 1997). In this chapter, we report on two brain activation PET experiments that were designed to drive visual mental imagery by language stimuli of increasing linguistic content.

Creating Visual Mental Images from Verbal Descriptions

In a first study (Mellet et al., 1996), subjects had to construct mental objects, made of assembled cubes, that they had never seen. Adding cubes to the construction was done upon auditory spatial instructions (left, right, up, down, back or front) (Figure 12.1). This operation, performed in total darkness, implied on-line translation of the semantic content of the verbal stimuli into picture-like representations. This task was contrasted both to a silent resting condition and to listening to a series of phonetically matched words having low imagery content. After the completion of the mental imagery task, it was controlled by asking the subject to visually identify, from a choice of four, the objects he had just constructed. The major finding of this study was a co-activation of visual and language areas, namely activations of the bilateral superior temporal cortex and of the bilateral occipito-parietal cortex (the so-called dorsal visual pathway) and of the right inferior temporal cortex (Figure 12.1). This result supports the hypothesis that temporal language areas can convey the information directly to the associative visual areas, both structures being necessary and sufficient for changing the nature of the information. Note that there was no activation of the early visual areas during the mental construction task, indicating that top-bottom visual processes were

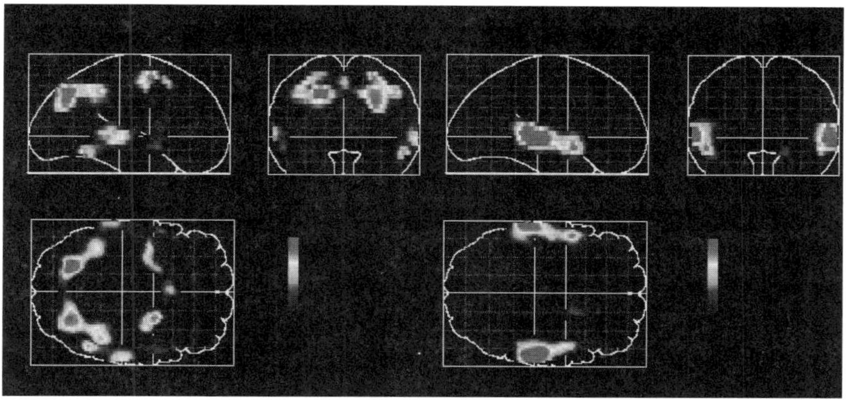

Figure 12.1. Statistical parametric maps resulting from the comparison of (1) mental construction of 3D cube assemblies according to verbally delivered directional words, and (2) passive listening of words without any visual imagery activity. Note the bilateral activation of occipito-parietal regions (the dorsal route) as well as the prefrontal activity, which is likely to reflect the working memory activity. Also note the right inferior temporal gyrus activation, which may translate the object-processing component of the task (adapted from Mellet et al., 1996).

not necessary. It was of particular interest as well that the left inferior frontal cortex was not activated during the mental imagery task, in contrast with its activation during word listening.

This first study was followed by several other ones that reported conflicting results. Mental evocation of memories, a task likely to be accompanied by visual images, was claimed to evoke deactivation in inferior occipital and parietal areas (Fink et al., 1996b). Similarly, rCBF (regional cerebral blood flow) decreases were found during visual imagery of previously learned objects, as compared with rest, in superior and inferior occipital, in superior and inferior parietal, and in inferior temporal cortices (Buckner et al., 1996). The authors of this last study claimed that this fact could be explained by a cross-modal inhibition, given the auditory directed attention paid to the stimuli. In contrast, recent studies have reported visual area activation during imagery tasks cued from words (Kosslyn et al., 1995; D'Esposito et al., 1997; Ghaem et al., 1997). One must note, however, that in all these studies, the language stimuli were restricted to single words or simple verbal instructions, making them quite different from usual speech. In addition, these studies were designed in such a way that listening to the language stimulus and generating the mental image were subsequent to each other rather than simultaneous.

In a second PET activation study, we investigated the cerebral areas involved in a task that closely intermingled language and visual mental imagery (Mellet et al., 1998). In this protocol, the subjects, while listening to concrete words and their definition, had to generate a mental image of the corresponding object or animal and adjust this image to the definition. This condition was again compared both with "rest" and with a condition during which concrete word definitions were replaced by abstract ones. Task execution was a posteriori, controlled by having the subjects recall as many words that they heard during the PET scan as possible, showing the classical facilitation effect for concrete words. When compared with rest, the concrete word definition condition elicited bilateral activations in the superior temporal sulcus, related to the language comprehension, together with bilateral activations in the fusiform and inferior temporal gyri, reflecting, as suggested earlier, the involvement of the ventral route during the mental imagery of objects (Figure 12.2). This study confirms that high-order visual areas can be activated when an imagery task and a language comprehension task are performed simultaneously. Interestingly, when compared with the conditions of either rest or abstract word definitions, additional activations were found in two areas of the prefrontal cortex, very likely reflecting both the visuo-spatial and the object working-memory components of the task (Courtney et al., 1996). In contrast, activations during the abstract definition condition were restricted to the superior and middle temporal cortex, being more intense in the right temporal cortex during this condition than during the concrete definition task. As such, these results demonstrate that, although verbal representation and visual mental images are distinct cognitive entities (Paivio, 1986), the so-called cross-modal inhibition does not prevent a coactivation of visual and language areas, even under intense linguistic processing of the stimuli. Within this framework, the larger activation of right temporal language areas in the abstract definition than in the concrete definition tasks suggests that language areas can be solicited to address a representation more when language is the only source of information than when imagery and language are used in conjunction.

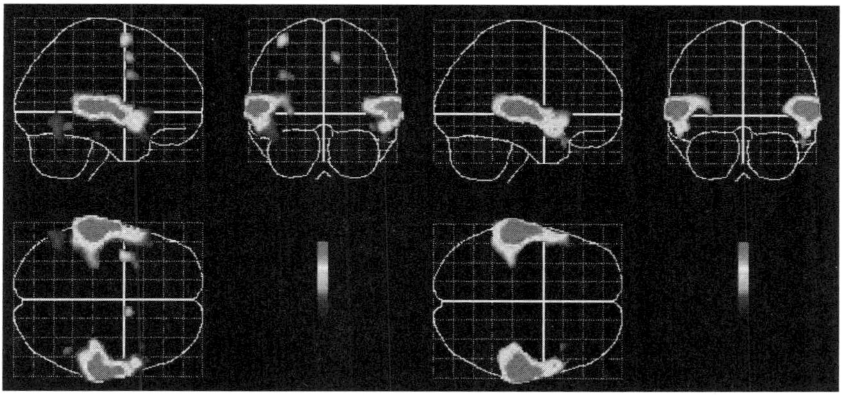

Figure 12.2. Statistical parametric maps resulting from the comparison of (1) listening to concrete words and their definition that elicited, in addition to language processing, a visual imagery activity and (2) listening to abstract words and their definition that resulted in language processing only. Note the bilateral activation of the inferior temporal/fusiform gyri (the ventral route), specific to the mental imagery activity, as well as the prefrontal activity that may reflect the involvement of working memory (adapted from Mellet et al., 1998).

Hemispheric Lateralization of Mental Imagery

Although the left hemisphere functional dominance for language is well established in right-handers (Mazoyer et al., 1993), such a functional hemispheric asymmetry for mental imagery remains under debate. In this regard, a recent fMRI study has reported left-lateralized activations of the inferior temporal and fusiform gyri during mental image generation of an object or animal upon listening to its name, the control task being to listen to an abstract word (D'Esposito et al., 1997). According to the authors, this finding reflects the specific role of the left hemisphere in mental image generation, in disagreement with the bilateral ventral areas activations, reported in the previous section, during concrete word mental image generation while listening to its dictionary definition (Mellet et al., 1998). Note that bilateral (Kosslyn et al., 1993) or right-lateralized (Mellet et al., 1996) activations of the same areas during mental image generation of letters or complex forms, respectively, had been previously reported.

It thus seems difficult to conclude that there is exclusive participation by either one of the hemispheres in mental image generation.

Rather, a bilateral participation that does not imply that the two hemispheres play identical roles appears more likely. Similar to what has been described in the perceptive domain (Fink et al., 1996a), the right hemisphere could be specialized in the processing of the global attributes of a mental image, whereas the left hemisphere could process the local ones. There are, however, few evidences of such a dichotomy in the literature. Another factor that might play a role in functional lateralization is the complexity of the image. In the visual perception domain, activations of the right inferior temporal and fusiform gyri have been reported during complex form discrimination (Faillenot et al., 1997; Schacter et al., 1995). Similar findings have been observed during the mental imagery of letters (Kosslyn et al., 1993) or schematic objects (Mellet et al., 1996). A right ventral activation has also been found during mental imagery of concrete words upon listening to their definition: in this latter study, the definitions contained a detailed description of the object/animal, allowing the generation of a complex mental image (Mellet et al., 1998). Accordingly, the absence of a right ventral activation in the study of D'Esposito et al. (1997) could be due to the high frequency at which the subjects had to generate mental images (1 Hz), which limited their complexity.

Concerning the left hemisphere, the inferior temporal and nearby fusiform gyri seem to be recruited by the perception of forms that can be named, that is, for which a lexical entry exists (Kosslyn et al., 1994). The same finding seems to be valid in the visual mental imagery domain: these left ventral areas were activated when subjects were asked to generate mental images of objects (Mellet et al., 1996; D'Esposito et al., 1997; Ghaëm et al., 1997; Mellet et al., 1998), or even of letters (Kosslyn et al., 1993) and in the transcription of phonemes in visualized graphemes (Démonet et al., 1994). Functional lateralization during mental imagery may thus depend on two different characteristics of the mental images to be generated: complexity, which would modulate the degree of involvement of the right hemisphere ventral route, and "lexicality," which would drive the left hemisphere participation. Within this framework, the finding of bilateral activations in several studies could reflect the simultaneous contribution of both components in the proposed tasks (Kosslyn et al., 1993; Mellet et al., 1998).

References

The authors are deeply indebted to Michel Denis (CNRS-LIMSI, Orsay) for an invaluable and long-standing collaboration.

Buckner, R. L., Raichle, M. E., Miezin, F. M., and Petersen, S. E. 1996. Functional anatomic studies of memory retrieval for auditory words and visual pictures. *J. Neurosci., 16* (19), 6219–6235.

Courtney, S. M., Ungerleider, L. G., Keil, K., and Haxby, J. V. 1996. Object and spatial visual working memory activate separate neural systems in human cortex. *Cereb. Cortex, 6,* 39–49.

Démonet, J.-F., Price, C., Wise, R., and Frackowiak, R. S. J. 1994. A PET study of cognitive strategies in normal subjects during language tasks: Influence of phonetic ambiguity and sequence processing on phoneme monitoring. *Brain, 117,* 671–682.

Denis, M., and Cocude, M. 1992. Structural properties of visual images constructed from poorly or well-structured verbal descriptions. *Mem. Cogn., 20,* 497–506.

Denis, M., Gonçalves, M. R., and Memmi, D. 1995. Mental scanning of visual images generated from verbal descriptions: Towards a model of image accuracy. *Neuropsychologia, 33,* 1511–1530.

D'Esposito, M., Detre, J. A., Aguirre, G. K., Stallcup, M., Alsop, D. C., Tipett, L. J., and Farah, M. J. 1997. A functional MRI study of mental image generation. *Neuropsychologia, 35,* 725–730.

De Vega, M., Intons-Peterson, M. J., Johnson-Laird, P. N., Denis, M., and Marschark, M. 1996. *Models of visuospatial cognition.* New York: Oxford University Press.

Faillenot, I., Sakata, H., Costes, N., Decety, J., and Jeannerod, M. 1997. Visual working memory for shape and 3D-orientation: A PET Study. *Neuroreport, 8,* 859–862.

Fink, G. R., Markowitsch, H. J., Reinkemeier, M., Bruckbauer, T., Kessler, J., and Heiss W.-D. 1996a. Cerebral representation of one's own past: Neural networks involved in autobiographical memory. *J. Neurol. Sci., 16* (13), 4275–4282.

Fink, G. R., Halligan, P. W., Marshall, J. C., Frith, C. D., Frackowiak, R. S. J., and Dolan, R. J. 1996b. Where in the brain does visual attention select the forest and the trees? *Nature, 382,* 626–628.

Ghaëm, O., Mellet, E., Crivello, F., Tzourio, N., Mazoyer, B., Berthoz, A., and Denis, M. 1997. Mental navigation along memorized routes activates the hippocampus, precuneus, and insula. *Neuroreport, 8,* 739–744.

Kosslyn, S. M, Alpert, N. M., Thompson, W. L., Chabris, C. F., Rauch, S. L., and Anderson, A. K. 1994. Identifying objects seen from different viewpoints: A PET investigation. *Brain, 117,* 1055–1071.

Kosslyn, S. M., Alpert, N. M., Thompson, W. L., Maljkovic, V., Weise, S. B., Chabris, C. F., Hamilton, S. E., Rauch, S. L., and Buoanno, F. S. 1993. Visual mental imagery activates topographically organized visual cortex: PET investigations. *Journal of Cognitive Neurosicence, 5,* 263–287.

Kosslyn, S., Thompson, W. L., Kim, I. J., and Alpert, N. M. 1995. Topographical representations of mental images in primary visual cortex. *Nature, 378,* 496–498.

Mazoyer, B. M., Dehaene, S., Tzourio, N., Frak, G., Murayama, N., Cohen, L., Salamon, G., Syrota, A., and Mehler, J. 1993. The cortical representation of speech. *Journal of Cognitive Neuroscience, 5,* 467–479.

Mellet, E., Tzourio, N., Crivello, F., Joliot, M., Denis, M., and Mazoyer, B. 1996. Functional anatomy of spatial mental imagery generated from verbal instructions. *J. Neurosci., 16,* 6504–6512.

Mellet, E., Tzourio, N., Denis, M., and Mazoyer, B. 1995. A positron emission tomography study of visual and mental spatial exploration. *Journal of Cognitive Neuroscience, 7,* 433–445.

Mellet, E., Tzourio, N., Denis, M., and Mazoyer, B. 1998. Cortical anatomy of mental imagery of concrete nouns based on their dictionary definition. *Neuroreport, 9,* 803–808.

Paivio, A. 1986. *Mental representations: A dual coding approach.* New York: Oxford University Press.

Schacter, D. L., Reiman, E., Uecker, A., Polster, M. R., Yun, L. S., and Cooper, L. A. 1995. Brain regions associated with retrieval of structurally coherent visual information. *Nature, 376,* 587–590.

Shulman, G. L., Fiez, J. A., Corbetta, M., Buckner, R. L., Miezin, F. M., Raichle, M. E., and Petersen, S. E. 1997. Common blood flow changes across visual tasks: II. decreases in cerebral cortex. *Journal of Cognitive Neuroscience, 9,* 648–663.

Can the Human Brain Construct Visual Mental Images from Linguistic Inputs?

13

Michel Denis

Language and visuo-spatial cognition, two key components of the human cognitive system, interact in a variety of communicative situations. This is particularly true when people generate verbal messages with the intention of having other people construct visual images of spatial configurations. These situations typically involve two people. One person (A) has knowledge of a certain configuration; the other (B) does not, but for some reason needs information contained in it. If A is a cooperative person and is ready to share information with B, A may attempt to convey this information to B. But consider the case where the only means available to A is the spoken language. This kind of interaction is driven by the speaker's objective of having his or her listener construct a surrogate representation as similar as possible to the representation the addressee would have built from direct perception of the configuration. By "*similar,*" I mean "*carrying the same information*" (similar in content), but also "*displaying information in a similarly nonlinguistic format*" (structurally isomorphic), and consequently "*likely to support the same kind of processing.*"

The situations considered here illustrate a basic theoretical problem encountered by the human cognitive system when it has to make two representational subsystems cooperate in spite of their different structural and functional properties. Such cooperation sometimes results in friendly communication, but many cases illustrate its difficulty or cost for at least one of the partners involved. The research program developed in our laboratory is twofold. In one part of the program, we investigate the speaker's cognitive processes, and in the other, those of the listener. I will only briefly refer to our studies on the speaker's processes in this chapter. Discourse production studies have shown that one of the main problems in describing spatial configurations is the "linearization problem" (Levelt, 1989). This problem arises because the outputs of the linguistic system are inherently linear, so that describing any multidimensional entity forces the speaker to make choices about the order in which the component parts of the entity are introduced. Following Levelt's pioneering work, we showed that certain descriptive strategies are more spontaneously used than others, in particular those strategies that place less demand on working memory during the description, for both speakers and listeners. For instance, people required to start their description of a spatial network from a specific point are more likely to describe first the branches that will minimize the number of elements to be stored in working memory during the description, or the duration of such storage. Interestingly, although this strategy was repeatedly shown to be readily available, people who use it do not seem to have any intuition that this is because it lowers the memory load of their addressees. A wide variety of descriptive strategies are also used in unconstrained conditions, but only a subset of them is easy for the listener to process (Denis, 1996; Taylor and Tversky, 1996).

This chapter focuses on the listener's side, that is, on the person who has to convert a spoken input into an internal, presumably visuospatial, representation. We can begin to understand this person's cognitive situation by considering the differences between the representations elicited by the inspection of visual configurations and those resulting from the processing of descriptions. First, it is common to stress the differences between the *structure of information* in visuospatial configurations and in verbal descriptions. Although configurations make information simultaneously available (even though visual inspection is a sequential process), verbal information has an inherently sequential structure. This results from the fact that two statements cannot be made simultaneously, but must be sequential. A second contrasting feature is that visual configurations clearly display their content, while descriptions require the encoding of objects and their transformation into chains of arbitrary symbols. Third, a configuration displays its content in such a way that all the relations among its parts are visible. Not only does an observer see the objects that make up the configuration, but he or she cannot avoid noticing their spatial relationships. A verbal description, by contrast, typically indicates a limited number of such relations, leaving room for the generation of inferences. Some of these inferences may be well founded; others can be no more than "best guesses," because some relationships are not completely described. For instance, in a spatial configuration, if a triangle is *"to the right"* of a square (from the observer's perspective), one speaker may consider it useful to state this relational information explicitly. Another describer may produce less determinate discourse by simply stating that the triangle is *"beside"* the square. Underspecification of a spatial relationship does not invalidate the description, but it lowers its informational value, which may have important consequences in some situations. Last, while a configuration shows itself just as it is, verbal descriptions may emphasize certain objects or relations by using special rhetorical devices.

Let us now turn to *processing*. One important distinction between configurations and descriptions is due to the differential amount of constraint that is placed on processing. The processing of configurations typically involves relatively few constraints. For instance, there is a quasi-infinity of sequences in which the visual exploration of a scene may be accomplished by an observer. In contrast, the structure of information in descriptions greatly constrains processing. A listener has no other choice than to adopt the sequence that has been selected by the speaker, which may have serious consequences if the sequence does not fit in with the listener's expectations. Another important contrast is in the nature of the representations obtained by the processing of configurations or descriptions. The result of processing a configuration is a representation of that configuration (whatever its form), whereas a verbal description is believed to result in a dual representation, consisting of both a representation of the description itself (including surface features, such as the specific sentences used) and a representation of the configuration. An important issue then is to determine whether the representation of visuo-spatial information has any distinct characteristics depending on the fact that a configuration or its description were originally processed. Last, what about the brain mechanisms involved in the processing of configurations and descriptions? There are well documented differences between the brain regions activated by perceptual (visual) and by verbal inputs. The specific point to consider here is whether the representations constructed from text processing involve the same or distinct cerebral regions as those used for reviving past visual experience.

In order to investigate these issues, we needed a task that made it possible to assess the internal structure of images derived from perception or language. We had to find a task that not only required subjects to generate images, but also allowed the experimenter to assess the similarity of the cognitive operations executed on these images. The task that seemed to meet these requirements best was the mental scanning task originally developed by Stephen Kosslyn in the early phase of his theory building (Kosslyn, Ball, and Reiser, 1978; Kosslyn, 1980). In this task, subjects first learned a visual configuration containing several objects, each at a specific location. In the island map that made the paradigm popular, seven geographical features were located in such a way that the distances between each pair of objects were different. Once the subjects had memorized the configuration and the precise location of landmarks, they were asked to scan mentally between each pair of objects, and the scanning times were recorded. The most notable finding from the experiments conducted by Kosslyn and his associates was that scanning times increased linearly with increasing distance between objects. When times were averaged over subjects, there was a significant positive correlation between time and distance. This finding was considered to be one of the most significant building blocks of the theory of visual mental imagery, by reflecting the structural isomorphism of the visual image to the configuration it represents. Since this finding, the distance effect in mental scanning has been interpreted as showing that visual images incorporate the metric information present in the original configuration (Denis and Kosslyn, 1999). The mechanisms that explore the visual image are assumed to operate on a cognitive entity that includes the spatial characteristics that were processed during perception.

The research program that Marguerite Cocude and I have been operating over the past years has consisted of creating situations in which subjects built an image of a spatial configuration without any perceptual cues, using only a verbal description, and then mentally scanned the newly constructed image. The rationale here was that analysis of the scanning processes should provide an indirect, but valid and reliable, indication of the structure of the visual images processed. Because the outline shape of the island used by Kosslyn was far too complex to be described verbally, we replaced it by a simpler circular shape; we also used a descriptive device that made it possible to locate each landmark precisely at the periphery of the island in clockwise order. We used the conventional directions of aerial navigation, stating for instance that a landmark was located "*at one o'clock*" or "*midway between two and three.*" Our first experiments thus compared two conditions. In the first condition, subjects studied the island map (following the same procedure as in Kosslyn's experiments). In the second condition, subjects learned the description and were instructed to construct a vivid, detailed visual image from the description. These subjects were presented with the description three times. The subjects in both groups were then tested in a standard mental scanning task. The results from subjects who learned the map replicated the finding that the time to scan between landmarks increased with the distance between the two landmarks. In the verbal learning condition, response times resulted in a similar distance effect, but the correlation coefficient was somewhat lower, and absolute scanning times were longer than in the map learning condition. These results suggested that the visuo-spatial representation constructed after three exposures to the verbal description did include some metric information, but reached less structural integration than did an image resulting from actually seeing the map. However, the question was whether this difference was due to the linguistic nature of the input or to the fact that the amount of learning involved in the description condition had simply been insufficient. We answered this question by repeating the description condition, but this time the subjects were presented with the description six times, that is, they were forced to invest more in the processing of their images. This learning condition resulted in a scanning performance that was very similar in pattern and chronometric values to the performance following visual learning. Thus, for a moderate rate of learning, an image constructed from a verbal description may not attain the structural coherence of an image derived from perception. Additional learning of the description may result in the image's reaching coherence and having veridical metric properties that make it cognitively similar to a perceptually based image (Denis and Cocude, 1989).

In subsequent studies, we showed that the structural qualities of images constructed from verbal descriptions were sensitive to variations likely to create more difficult conditions for processing information and building a coherent, integrated visual image. When subjects were exposed to descriptions providing information in a random order (instead of the highly expected clockwise order used up to now), subjects had much difficulty in scanning their images after three learning trials. The absence of a significant correlation between response times and distances indicated that the subjects' mental images had no internal structure at this phase of learning. Three more exposures to the description were needed for subjects to achieve scanning performance indicating that their images validly reflected the metrics of the described configuration (Denis and Cocude, 1992). When subjects were tested after every two learning trials, the gradual process of image elaboration and the progressive increase in image accuracy were still more evident (Denis, Gonçalves, and Memmi, 1995). These findings suggested that the capacity of images to reflect accurately the object they stand for is not an all-or-nothing property, but results from stepwise elaboration.

Mental scanning was used as a test of the structural coherence and metric value of images for investigating effects of the semantics of the descriptions. We wanted to determine whether the manipulation of some landmark descriptions could bias the mental representation and subsequently its scanning. One such attempt consisted of increasing the cognitive salience of some landmarks by providing a narrative containing many concrete, vivid details. The results, in fact, showed that there was no difference between the scanning times toward salient or nonsalient landmarks. This suggested that, on the one hand, the time-distance correlation in mental scanning is a robust phenomenon. On the other hand, very strong effects of the subjects' visuospatial capacities were found. Subjects with high scores on a visuospatial test (the Minnesota Paper Form Board) produced the pattern typical of mental scanning, whereas subjects with low scores produced responses whose chronometric characteristics indicated that their images had no consistent structural properties after the same amount of learning. These images probably contained a large amount of noise, which resulted from the difficulty experienced by the subjects in maintaining their mental representations at a sufficiently high level of activation when learning the descriptions, then scanning the resulting images (Denis and Cocude, 1997).

The results of these experiments document the structural similarities between images and the perceptual events from which they were formed, and the similarities between images reconstructed after perceptual experience and those newly constructed from verbal descriptions. In addition to behavioral evidence, an important question remains. Do the systems that control these cognitive events involve the same or different brain structures? Little information is available on the brain structures that are involved in visual imagery based on verbal inputs. But it seems at first sight reasonable to assume that the same neural substrate is activated whatever the origin of the image. Our first neuroimaging study conducted with Bernard Mazoyer and Nathalie Tzourio used single photon emission computerized tomography (SPECT). The subjects took part in two cognitive tasks. One task consisted of mentally conjugating abstract, irregular verbs, and the other consisted of performing mental scanning over the island that had been previously learned from a purely verbal description. When they were performing the verbal task, high visuo-spatial imagers showed a selective increase in blood flow in the left sensorimotor cortex over the resting state. When they imagined and mentally scanned the map, there was a significant increase in blood flow in the left temporo-occipital cortex. This result was compatible with the idea that visual representations constructed from visual experience and those constructed from descriptions involve the same cortical areas. However, no activation of the primary visual cortex was found (Charlot et al., 1992).

The issue of the involvement of the primary visual cortex in visual imagery remains open. Kosslyn, Le Bihan, and others have reported positron emission tomography (PET) and functional magnetic resonance imaging (fMRI) data indicating that early visual areas are activated in visual imagery, thus supporting the assumption that the visual areas subserving visual imagery are identical to those subserving visual perception (Kosslyn et al., 1993; Le Bihan et al., 1993; Kosslyn, 1994; Kosslyn et al., 1995). However, these areas are not activated during visual imagery in all subjects, and it is likely that they are activated only by tasks that require high-resolution images (Ogawa et al., 1993; D'Esposito et al., 1997). There is also some evidence suggesting that early visual areas are not always involved in visual imagery, but that the temporo-occipital and parieto-occipital areas represent objects and scenes in visual imagery. In an experiment that compared PET activations in perceptual and imagery conditions, Mellet collected data showing that visual scanning of a map and mental scanning of an image of the map involved a common network of cerebral structures, including a bilateral superior external occipital region and a left internal parietal region. A further critical finding was that bilateral activation of the primary visual areas occurred in the perceptual condition, while these areas were not activated during the processing of a visual image (Mellet et al. 1995).

The involvement of regions belonging to the dorsal route in the mental scanning of a previously learned visual configuration is in line with current assumptions about the role of the parieto-occipital cortex in the spatial processing of mental images. These findings suggest that mental imagery involves the same distinction as in the visual system between the dorsal route, which is in charge of processing the spatial attributes of visual stimuli, and the ventral route, which processes their figural attributes. A further attempt to investigate the capacity of the brain to generate images based on verbal descriptions was reported by Mellet. This research was intended to establish whether a network specialized for visuo-spatial processing can be activated by purely verbal inputs. The subjects were trained to construct visual images of objects they had never seen before from verbal instructions. These objects were three-dimensional cube assemblies. PET was used to monitor variations in regional cerebral blood flow while the subjects constructed the images. The results showed that the mental imagery task activated a bilateral occipito-parieto-frontal network, including the superior occipital cortex, the inferior parietal cortex, and the premotor cortex. The right inferior temporal cortex was also activated in this task, but there was no activation of the primary visual areas (Mellet et al., 1996; see also Mellet et al., 2000).

To conclude, these data first confirm that at least some mental imagery tasks may not involve any detectable participation of early visual areas. However, they do not exclude that these areas may be activated in specific circumstances. A recent review of the neuroimaging literature has established that whether high resolution is required in an imagery task predicts the activation of the primary visual areas during that task (Thompson and Kosslyn, 2000). Second, the data reported above provide evidence that the dorsal route can be recruited in the absence of any visual input. This is an important finding, since it indicates that the involvement of the dorsal route for spatial processing is not linked to the modality under which information was presented. This network can be activated by visual stimuli or verbal inputs, provided these inputs elicit the construction of visuo-spatial images. Thus while the brain has long been studied for its capacities to process language, visual information, and a number of other inputs, the newest insight from the studies summarized here is that not only can the brain process verbal information (which is obviously not a subject of debate), but, more important, it can translate it into nonverbal representations whose properties are similar to those of visual images derived from perception.

References

Charlot, V., Tzourio, N., Zilbovicius, M., Mazoyer, B., and Denis, M. 1992. Different mental imagery abilities result in different regional cerebral blood flow activation patterns during cognitive tasks. *Neuropsychologia, 30,* 565–580.

Denis, M. 1996. Imagery and the description of spatial configurations. In M. de Vega, M. J. Intons-Peterson, P. N. Johnson-Laird, M. Denis, and M. Marschark, *Models of visuospatial cognition,* 128–197. New York: Oxford University Press.

Denis, M., and Cocude, M. 1989. Scanning visual images generated from verbal descriptions. *European Journal of Cognitive Psychology, 1,* 293–307.

——— 1992. Structural properties of visual images constructed from poorly or well-structured verbal descriptions. *Memory and Cognition, 20,* 497–506.

——— 1997. On the metric properties of visual images generated from verbal descriptions: Evidence for the robustness of the mental scanning effect. *European Journal of Cognitive Psychology, 9,* 353–379.

Denis, M., Gonçalves, M.-R., and Memmi, D. 1995. Mental scanning of visual images generated from verbal descriptions: Towards a model of image accuracy. *Neuropsychologia, 33,* 1511–1530.

Denis, M., and Kosslyn, S. M. 1999. Scanning visual mental images: A window on the mind. *Current Psychology of Cognition, 18,* 409–465.

D'Esposito, M., Detre, J. A., Aguirre, G. K., Stallcup, M., Alsop, D. C., Tippett, L. J., and Farah, M. J. 1997. A functional MRI study of mental image generation. *Neuropsychologia, 35,* 725–730.

Kosslyn, S. M. 1980. *Image and mind.* Cambridge: Harvard University Press.

——— 1994. *Image and brain: The resolution of the imagery debate.* Cambridge: MIT Press.

Kosslyn, S. M., Alpert, N. M., Thompson, W. L., Maljkovic, V., Weise, S. B., Chabris, C. F., Hamilton, S. E., Rauch, S. L., and Buonanno, F. S. 1993. Visual mental imagery activates topographically organized visual cortex: PET investigations. *Journal of Cognitive Neuroscience, 5,* 263–287.

Kosslyn, S. M., Ball, T. M., and Reiser, B. J. 1978. Visual images preserve metric spatial information: Evidence from studies of image scanning. *Journal of Experimental Psychology: Human Perception and Performance, 4,* 47–60.

Kosslyn, S. M., Thompson, W. L., Kim, I. J., and Alpert, N. M. 1995. Topographical representations of mental images in primary visual cortex. *Nature, 378,* 496–498.

Le Bihan, D., Turner, R., Zeffiro, T. A., Cuénod, C. A., Jezzard, P., and Bonnerot, V. 1993. Activation of human primary visual cortex during visual recall: A magnetic resonance imaging study. *Proceedings of the National Academy of Sciences USA, 90,* 11802–11805.

Levelt, W. J. M. 1989. *Speaking: From intention to articulation.* Cambridge: MIT Press.

Mellet, E., Kosslyn, S. M., Mazoyer, N., Bricogne, S., Denis, M., and Mazoyer, B. 2000. Functional anatomy of high resolution mental imagery. *Journal of Cognitive Neuroscience, 12,* 98–109.

Mellet, E., Tzourio, N., Crivello, F., Joliot, M., Denis, M., and Mazoyer, B. 1996. Functional anatomy of spatial mental imagery generated from verbal instructions. *Journal of Neuroscience, 16,* 6504–6512.

Mellet, E., Tzourio, N., Denis, M., and Mazoyer, B. 1995. A positron emission tomography study of visual and mental spatial exploration. *Journal of Cognitive Neuroscience, 7,* 433–445.

Ogawa, S., Tank, D. W., Menon, R., Ellermann, J. M., Merkle, H., and Ugurbil, K. 1993. Functional brain MRI of cortical areas activated by visual mental imagery. *Society for Neuroscience Abstracts, 19,* 976.

Taylor, H. A., and Tversky, B. 1996. Perspective in spatial descriptions. *Journal of Memory and Language, 35,* 371–391.

Thompson, W. L., and Kosslyn, S. M. 2000. Neural systems activated during visual mental imagery: A review and meta-analyses. In *Brain mapping: The systems,* ed. J. C. Mazziotta and A. W. Toga, 535–560. San Diego: Academic Press.

Making Area V1 Glow in Visual Imagery

14

Denis Le Bihan, Isabelle Klein, and Michiko Dohi

Investigators have long debated the role of the cortical visual system in the processes underlying mental imagery. An issue of particular interest concerns the degree to which the processes that are operative in visual perception are the same processes involved in the generation of visual imagery and whether visual representations are shared between imagery and perceptual processes (Hebb, 1968; Kosslyn and Pomerantz, 1977; Farah, 1984b). The finding that brain activity in relation to mental imagery occurs in at least some of the same locations as those seen during perception would be strong evidence that these two mental experiences share common physiological mechanisms. Previous clinical and experimental studies provide support for the spatial co-localization of these processes (Farah, 1988; Kaufman et al., 1992). The clinical evidence is the finding that lesions to the occipital lobe in the human that result in disorders of visual perception can also result in visual imagery deficits (Farah, 1984a). The most compelling experimental evidence comes from functional neuroimaging studies demonstrating concordance between the neuroanatomical regions in occipital cortex activated by visual perception and imagery tasks in the same individual. Although the details of the results differ among experiments, all have found *extrastriate* visual areas that have been activated both when the stimulus is perceived and when it is recalled (Roland et al., 1987; Goldenberg et al., 1989; Charlot et al., 1992). In contrast, activation in *striate* cortex related to visual recall has been more difficult to demonstrate with apparent conflicting results in the literature.

Several factors may have contributed to this discrepancy. Differences in methodology may be responsible to some extent. For instance, a lack of sensitivity or a limited spatial and temporal resolution inherent in some techniques may prevent detection and localization of the activated regions. The one previous positron emission tomography (PET) study that investigated visual recall using tomographic measurements at higher resolution demonstrated small but statistically nonsignificant activation in the calcarine fissure (Roland et al., 1990). Furthermore, techniques that involve ionizing radiation exposure to subjects preclude the sort of repetitive studies that would provide greater sensitivity. Functional images are then often produced by pooling data collected on multiple subjects. Any gross variation in individual anatomy and mental imagery strategy would decrease the chance to see activation of a specific cortical region. Indeed, a survey of the PET/SPECT literature on mental imagery showed that twelve out of nineteen published studies report activation of V1 in mental imagery. With the recent advances in functional magnetic resonance imaging (fMRI), it has been made feasible to produce functional images at a temporal resolution of seconds and spatial resolution of millimeters. FMRI is a technique that images intrinsic blood signal changes accompanying variations of cerebral blood flow (CBF), cerebral blood volume (CBV), and oxygenation during mental activity. An important advantage that accounts for fMRI's increasing popularity for brain activation studies is its ability to acquire, within the same individual, repeated, multiple scans in a noninvasive manner. Although the basic design of most studies centers on comparison of baseline to an active (test) condition, as with positron emission tomography, fMRI allows an important departure from the single scan per condition study-design into more flexible paradigms of multiple scans over varying time intervals and multiple conditions. This completely noninvasive procedure provides a powerful means to reinvestigate the question of the role of primary visual cortex in the generation of mental imagery. Using fMRI we showed clear evidence that the primary visual cortex in the calcarine fissure can be activated during both visual perception and visual recall (Le Bihan et al., 1993).

In this study brain activation maps calculated with actual photic stimulation were compared with those obtained when the subject was later asked to recall the same visual stimulus. Seven normal subjects (five males, two females), ranging in age from twenty-six to forty-six years, underwent dynamic MRI. Studies were performed on a clinical 1.5T whole-body MRI scanner. Images were obtained in coronal orientation, approximately perpendicular to the calcarine fissures. In two of the responding subjects, another sequence was used, which allowed an in-plane resolution of 1.5 mm × 0.8 mm^2 and acquisition of images in an axial-oblique orientation, following the calcarine fissures and giving a better identification of striate cortex. The visual stimulation was provided by a light-proof binocular, fitted with red light–emitting diodes geometrically arranged as two square patterns flashing at 16 Hz. With these goggles, the stimulus was diffuse and excited both visual fields within a large angle. The task sequence consisted of a single prestimulation of the visual cortex for thirty seconds, during which time the subjects were asked to memorize the stimulus. The stimulus was then switched alternately on and off twice for periods of twenty-four seconds. Between these two actual photic stimulation episodes, the subjects were asked instead to recall the previously seen stimulus for twenty-four seconds, controlled by vocal command. The subjects were in complete darkness during the experiment and were asked to keep their eyes open for the duration of data acquisition. Regions of interest (pixel-by-pixel irregular regions) were placed on the areas of maximum response during actual stimulation on the medial surface of the occipital lobe in the bank of the calcarine fissure. The exact position and shape of each region of interest was defined for each individual from the activation map calculated during actual stimulation. Typical size for regions of interest was 10–20 mm^2. The same regions of interest were used to determine the amplitude of the response during the recalled stimulus as well.

In the functional activation images, regions in the primary visual cortex showed highly localized changes of intensity during actual stimulation, in agreement with previous studies (Belliveau et al., 1991; Frahm et al., 1992; Kwong, Belliveau, and Chesler, 1992; Ogawa et al., 1992; Bandettini et al. 1992). The recalled stimulus activation maps clearly showed that primary visual cortex was also activated,

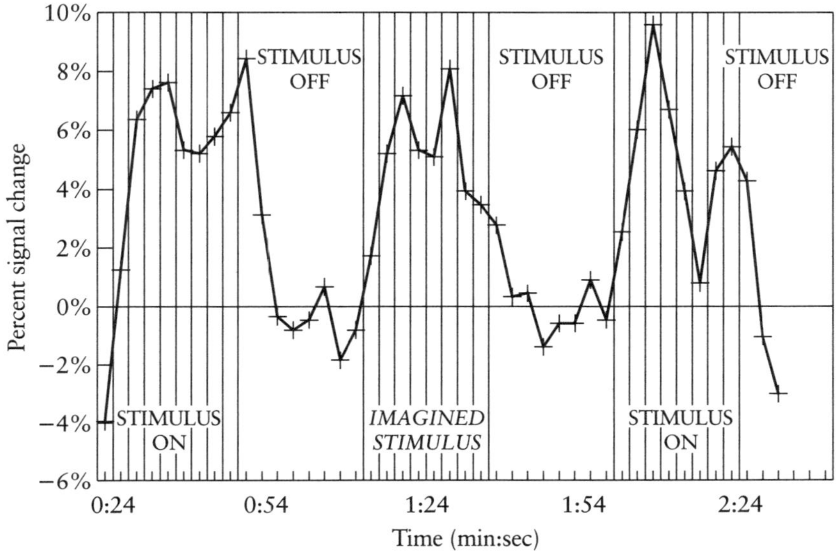

Figure 14.1. Plot of the relative MRI signal time course for primary visual cortex during perception and imagination of a pattern of flashing red dots.

though with less intensity, when the subject was asked to recall the stimulus. Figure 14.1 displays the measured MRI signal changes in a region of interest in the striate cortex in one of our subjects during visual stimulation conditions and when asked to recall the stimulus between the two actual stimulation episodes. During actual photic stimulation, each of our seven subjects showed a significant increase in MRI signal, occurring bilaterally within the calcarine fissure (unpaired Mann-Whitney test, $p < .004$). More interestingly, significant signal increases were also observed in five of our seven subjects in the same regions when the subject was recalling the stimulus (unpaired Mann-Whitney test, $p < .01$). The amplitude of the response to the recalled stimulus, when present, was, however, not as large as the response to the actual stimulus. In two subjects, otherwise unremarkable, no significant signal increase from baseline could be demonstrated during the recall condition, although a brief signal increase could be seen. However, the subject attention and the quality of the visual recall performance could not be screened. Measurements within the visual cortex, but beyond V1 and probably V2, showed no significant response.

Although there was little spatial variability among subjects in the response to stimulation, important differences in the magnitude of the response were observed. However, repeated measurements indicated that intra-individual variations were also important for both the perceptual and the recall conditions. Such variations may reflect slightly different locations of the image slice and partial volume effects in different parts of the visual cortex. It is also worth noting that in some of our subjects the end of the measured response sometimes occurred too early or too late with respect to the expected end of the recall interval, as if the subject had difficulty in maintaining or terminating the recall task. The subject's attention may be an important factor to consider in the quality of the mental imagery.

Using a very similar flashing-light paradigm and another task where subjects were asked to image objects that they could see when walking in their hometowns, the fMRI group of the University of Minnesota has confirmed activation of V1 (Chen et al., 1996) as well as bilateral activation of the lateral geniculate nuclei. In total, seven out of eight fMRI studies have reported activation of V1 in mental imagery. The results, combined with those of Kosslyn et al. using PET (Kosslyn et al., 1995; Kosslyn, Thompson, and Alpert, 1998), seem to resolve a debate in the literature about whether imagery activates early visual cortex: visual perception and visual imagery share common pathways down to the earliest visual areas.

Unfortunately the debate may be not over: an early fMRI study has not been able to detect activation in V1 during visual imagery (D'Esposito et al., 1997). In these conditions, studies of the factors contributing to the activation in V1 are of the highest importance, since we have to accept the fact that perhaps not all kinds of mental images activate V1. Indeed, several types of mental images can be produced. Some are more related to spatial properties (such as orientation and navigation) and do not seem to activate V1. Other mental images refer more to the properties of the object (such as complexity and details). According to Kosslyn, "lower" visual areas may be more specifically activated during mental imagery involving "depictive" representation where "high resolution" is present (Kosslyn et al., 1995; Kosslyn, Thompson, and Alpert, 1998).

Another study conducted by our group may support the idea that V1 activation could be linked to visual complexity (Mellet et al., 1998). Japanese readers offer a unique opportunity to address this question, since the written Japanese language is distinct from most of the Western world languages in the duality of its writing system, composed of Kanjis and Kanas. The Kanji characters, of which 45,000 are known, correspond to the morphemes of the Japanese language. These morphograms (which originated from Chinese characters during the sixth century) are complex drawings (made of one to twenty-three strokes) which, separately or combined, are associated with one object or one idea. Kanjis have both phonetic and semantic values. The second system, called Kana, consists in two sets of forty-six signs (Hiragana and Katakana) which are syllabograms (or phonograms), allowing the construction of syllables in Japanese words. The Kanas are oversimplified cursive forms of Kanjis and have only one pronunciation without any particular meaning. All Japanese words can be written with Kanas, but Kanjis are more conventionally used for nouns, adjectives, or verb stems, everything else being written with Kanas. In practice Kanas often supplement Kanjis, even for nouns, as there are about 45,000 known Kanjis and only 1,945 must be learned by the end of high school. Young children first use Kanas exclusively, and it is not uncommon to see Kanas printed atop of Kanji words to indicate pronunciation for unusual Kanjis. Hence a Japanese sentence is most often made of a combination of both Kanjis and Kanas.

Nine neurologically normal native Japanese right-handed females were studied. The mean age was thirty-one years (range of age 26–43). Experiments were performed on a 3T whole-body system. After localization on sagittal scout images, twelve axial contiguous slices of 6 mm thickness and 20 cm field of view were selected. This set of twelve slices was then scanned every six seconds during the task. The task paradigms used in our studies were composed of five epochs of sixty seconds each. The "active tasks" occurred during the second and the fourth epochs; the other epochs were in a resting (control) condition. At the beginning of each of the two "active" epochs, one Japanese sound cue *(mora)* was given and subjects were asked to covertly generate words beginning with that Japanese sound (for sixty seconds) and to mentally visualize them using either Kanas (paradigm 1) or Kanjis (paradigm 2). Hence the word generation part of the task was common to both Kana and Kanji paradigms, while the main difference between paradigms lay in the mental imagery of the words using either writing system. The order of the task (that is, Kana and Kanji paradigms) was counterbalanced across subjects. Sound cues were randomly drawn from a pool of *mora* most commonly found at the beginning of Japanese words, and were never used twice with the same subject, in order to avoid any bias in word selection. Of course, *mora*s were balanced between Kanas and Kanjis over our subjects. The subject's eyes were closed for the duration of the paradigm and subjects were debriefed afterward to ensure that they had followed instructions. Because we wanted to investigate the processes involved in the mental manipulation of the two symbol systems, no visual presentation was used, so as to avoid interference with actual perceptual processing. All subjects were new to the task, but, to ensure adequate performance, subjects practiced with a word generation and mental reading test before undergoing the experiment in the magnet. Subjects were also evaluated after completion of the experiment.

To increase statistical power, regions found activated over the twelve slices of our nine participants were then pooled for analysis. In this study, because of intersubject variability in the magnitude of the response, the average number of activated pixels in each region (activated surface) was used as a measure of the level of activation for any pair comparison, that is, Kana versus Kanji or left versus right hemisphere activation. Statistical significance was tested using a paired Student's t-test.

A preliminary analysis shows that more than half of the activated regions are found in the frontal lobe (inferior frontal gyrus, supplementary motor area, dorsolateral prefrontal cortex, premotor and motor complex), predominantly in the left hemisphere, in agreement with previous PET and fMRI word generation studies performed in English (McCarthy, Blamire, and Rothman, 1993; Rueckert et al., 1994; Cuenod et al., 1995). Left hemispheric dominance is also clearly visible ($p < .05$), both for Kanjis and for Kanas, in most of the parietal, temporal, and occipital areas. However, comparing Kanjis and Kanas, it appears that, although the regions activated with the

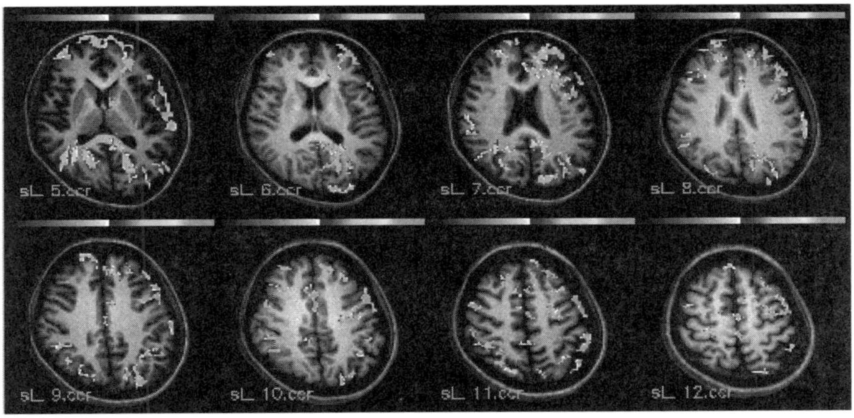

Figure 14.2. Set of fMRI slices obtained in a Japanese participant performing a covert word generation task while mentally visualizing words written using the Kanji Japanese writing system. Activation of visual cortex near the calcarine fissure can be seen.

Kana and the Kanji paradigms overlap most of the time, the areas activated with Kanjis are often significantly more numerous and wider than those activated with Kanas, in both left and right hemispheres.

Activated regions encompass those areas traditionally considered to be critical for word generation studies. Bilateral activation of visual regions, which have not been pointed out in previous simple word generation tasks performed in English, is found with Kanas and Kanjis. Both the associative cortex and V1 are found activated, but activation was larger in the associative cortex (Figure 14.2). The finding of the visual regions' activation may not be surprising considering that, in our paradigm, subjects had to mentally read words in addition to producing them. Furthermore, the size of the activated foci was about two times larger with Kanjis than with Kanas, but no significant hemispheric dominance could be seen. Participation of topographically oriented visual areas may be especially necessary for mental imagery with detailed spatial features (Kosslyn et al., 1995), as may be necessary for complex drawings such as Kanjis.

Discrepancies between studies may also result from a difference in the activation paradigm and from the difficulty of evaluating the performance of the mental imagery task. In the work of D'Esposito et al. (1997) using fMRI, subjects were alternatively presented concrete and abstract words and instructed to produce mental images of these words. Words were presented at a rate of one word per second. Contrast in the resulting functional images related to a difference in the activation produced by the concrete and the abstract words. Results showed activation of the left infero-temporal region and the associative cortex, but not in V1. There are three potential pitfalls with this paradigm, which may explain why the authors failed to see V1 activated. First, only differences in activation patterns could be detected with the described paradigm, as there was no "control" state. If V1 was equally activated with concrete and abstract words, activation could not be detected. Second, words were presented at a rather high rate. It might be that activation of V1 during mental imagery requires time. A similar study (based on concrete and abstract words) using PET, but where subjects were given more time to generate mental images, did not show activation in V1 (Mellet et al., 1998). Finally, the authors could not control the mental imagery performance of their subjects. This is, of course, a general problem with mental imagery. The way subjects are instructed to perform mental images, as well as the kind of mental images they have to produce is of the highest importance in the design of such experiments.

To better understand conditions leading to V1 activation, we recently implemented a slightly different fMRI experiment, aiming at differential V1 activation by concrete and abstract words (Klein et al. 2000). Our study design was based on the detection of individual trials using Event-Related (ER) fMRI (Buckner 1996). This approach allows one to mix stimuli of different types and to record images and response times for each stimulus individually. Images may be grouped by stimulus type after the acquisition to maintain an adequate signal:noise ratio. In our experiment, animal names were presented orally. Subjects were instructed to mentally image these animals for several seconds. Then a question was given involving either concrete (for example, pointed ears) or abstract (for example, affectionate) features of the animal, implying a true/false response. Again subjects were instructed to use a mental image to covertly answer the question and to press a button (left or right, according to the response). The response time was recorded. Beside this control of the performance, there were two major differences with the paradigm of D'Esposito et

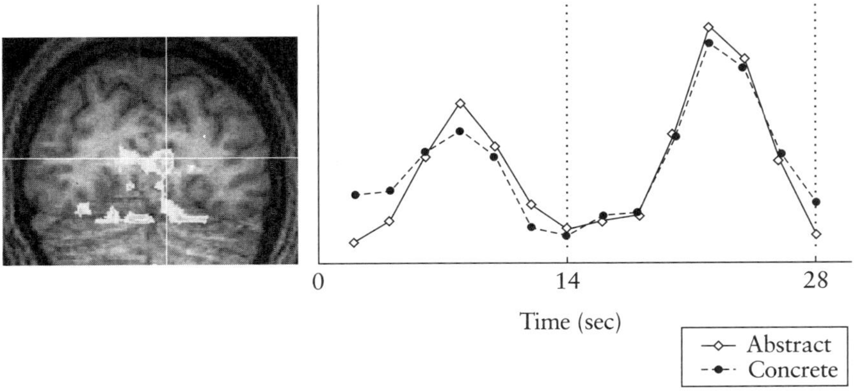

Figure 14.3. Concrete/abstract animal feature ER-fMRI experiment. (A) Activation map (coronal slice) of one participant showing the location of strongest activated voxels in striate cortex (centered on white cursor) during mental imagery. (B) Average response in these voxels during sixty trials of "Concrete" and "Abstract" imagery. The response in relation to the two events (formation/evaluation of the mental image) is represented during one 28-second imagery trial. The similarity of responses between "Concrete" and "Abstract" conditions is striking. In addition, the mental image "evaluation" event triggers a larger response than the mental image "formation" event.

al. First, the subjects were given a large time interval in which to form their mental images. Second, subjects were primed by the nature of the question (details or abstract feature) that would follow each animal name when they formed the first mental image. Eight healthy volunteers (aged twenty to twenty-five) were imaged on a 3 Tesla MRI. ER-fMRI images were obtained while subjects were to perform, given auditory instructions, the following two back-to-back events of fourteen seconds: (1) generating the visual image of an animal; (2) deciding whether or not the animal has a particular feature, either "concrete" or "abstract." The fMRI time series were analyzed using SPM96. All eight subjects showed significant activation in V1 during all mental imagery conditions ($p < 10^{-3}$). Not only could neural activity be measured for each averaged trial type, but also a single BOLD (blood oxygen level dependent) contrast response was detected in this region during individual imagery events. Surprisingly, similar amounts of activation in V1 were observed in the "concrete" and "abstract" trials (Figure 14.3). Furthermore, activation was larger in the "deciding" task than in the simple "generating" task. It took about two seconds after subjects began to form the image or use it before a response in V1 was detectable.

To our knowledge, this study is the first to report transient signal changes along the calcarine sulcus when participants, with eyes closed and in complete darkness, form images and evaluate imaged objects. ER-fMRI thus appears to be significantly more sensitive than fMRI based on block designs. Not only could neural activity be measured for each averaged trial type, but also a single response could be monitored in this region during single visual imagery events, indicating that in the absence of retinal input the formation of a single visual mental image can induce a response in the earliest stages of the visual system. These ER-fMRI data also highlight the importance of individual variability, even within a single imagery session; such variability may have influenced previous results, particularly when data were averaged across long imagery periods (such as with block paradigm fMRI or PET studies).

Although our data strongly suggest that methodological issues may be responsible for the previous "negative" results of V1 activation, our results indicate that selective neural mechanisms may modulate the activity of primary visual cortex during visual imagery. Indeed, in seven out of eight participants the amount of activation in calcarine cortex was robustly larger (in terms of size of activation and in terms of magnitude of response) when participants evaluated either a concrete or an abstract characteristic than when they simply formed an image. These mechanisms presumably are related to those used in attention; in fact, researchers have found that attention can modulate activation in V1 during visual perception (Martinez et al., 1999; Somers et al., 1999).

Although understanding the precise nature of neural mechanisms that causally link activity in V1 to visual imagery requires further investigation, these findings of transient and enhanced neural activity in calcarine cortex provide strong evidence that visual mental imagery recruits the earliest stages of the visual system.

Conclusion

These studies demonstrate that activation of brain regions by mental imagery may be mapped completely noninvasively with unmatched combined spatial and temporal resolution using MRI. Such high resolution allows us to demonstrate that some of the same "low level" cortical areas that are active during visual perception are also activated during internal imagery, at least in some conditions. The existence of such early common pathways suggests that strong interactions between perception and imagery may occur in particular conditions and give us an internal representation of the world which is not unbiased, but may be influenced by our present mental condition, our history, and our learning experience. The spatial resolution of fMRI, however, does not allow us to eliminate the possibility that different subsets of neurons in this region may be activated. The exact mechanism underlying activation of the V1 region is still not understood, as apparently all kinds of mental imagery do not activate V1. Large subject differences also exist, probably reflecting varying strategies in the production of mental images. Finally, one has to remember that visual imagery is part of a more general mental "imagery" process that involves many other regions besides V1. Whether these regions are specific to imagery remains to be shown. The ease and noninvasiveness of this technique, which can be repeated at will on the same subject, should significantly improve our understanding of the mechanisms and the conditions involved in visual imagery.

References

Bandettini, P. A., Wong, E. C., Hinks, R. S., et al. 1992. *Magn. Reson. Med., 25,* 390–397.

Belliveau, J. W., Kennedy, D. N., McKinstry, R. C., et al. 1991. *Science, 254,* 716–719.

Buckner, R. L., Bandettini, P. A., O'Craven, K. M., Savoy, R. L., Petersen, S. E., Raichle, M. E., Rosen, B. R. 1996. *Proc. Natl. Acad. Sci. (USA), 93,* 14878–14883.

Charlot, V., Tzourio, N., Zilbovitius, M., et al. 1992. *Neuropsychologia, 30,* 565–580.

Chen, W., Kato, T., Zhu, X'H., et al. 1996. *International Society of Magnetic Resonance in Medicine (abs.), 3,* 1858.

Cuenod, C. A., Bookheimer, S. Y., Hertz-Pannier, L., Zeffiro, T. A., Theodore, W. H., and Le Bihan, D. 1995. *Neurology, 45,* 1821–1827.

D'Esposito, M., Farah, M. J., et al. 1997. A functional MRI study of mental image generation. *Neuropsychologia, 35* (5), 725–730.

Farah, M. J. 1984a. *Cognition, 18,* 245–272.

——— 1984b. *J. Exp. Psychol. Gen., 114,* 91–103.

——— 1988. *J. Exp. Psychol. Gen., 117,* 248–257.

Frahm, J., Bruhn, H., Merboldt, K. D., et al. 1992. *JMRI, 5,* 501–506.

Goldenberg, G., Podreka, I., Steiner, M., et al. 1989. *Neuropsychologia, 27,* 641–664.

Hebb, D. O. 1968. *Psychol. Rev., 75,* 466–477.

Kaufman, L., Schwartz, B., Salustri, C., et al. 1992. *J. Cogn. Neuroscience, 2,* 124–132.

Klein, I., Paradis, A. L., Poline, J. B, Kosslyn, S. M., Le Bihan, D. J. 2000. *J. Cognitive Neurosci., 12,* 15–23.

Kosslyn, S. M., and Pomerantz, J. R. 1977. *Cognitive Psychology, 9,* 52–76.

Kosslyn, S. M., Thompson, W. L., and Alpert, N. M. 1998. *Neuroimage, 6,* 320–334.

Kosslyn, S. M., Thompson, W. L., and Kim, I. J., et al. 1995. *Nature, 378,* 496–498.

Kwong, K. K., Belliveau, J. W., and Chesler, D. A. 1992. *Proc. Natl. Acad. Sci. (USA), 89, 5675–5679.*

Le Bihan, D., Turner, R., Zeffiro, T. A., et al. 1993. *Proc. Natl. Acad. Sci. (USA), 90,* 11802–11805.

Martinez, A., Anllo-Vento, L., Sereno, M. I., Frank, R., Buxton, R. B., Dubowitz, D. J., Wong, E. C., Hinrichs, H., Heinze, H. J., and Hillyard, S. A. 1999. *Nature Neuroscience, 2,* 364–369.

McCarthy, G., Blamire, A., and Rothman, D. L. 1993. *Proc. Natl. Acad. Sci. (USA), 90,* 4952–4956.

Mellet, E., Tzourio, N., Denis, M., and Mazoyer, B. 1998. Cortical anatomy of mental imagery of concrete nouns based on their dictionary definition. *NeuroReport, 9,* 803–808.

Ogawa, S., Tank, D. W., Menon, R. S., et al. 1992. *Proc. Natl. Acad. Sci. (USA), 89, 5951–5955.*

Roland, P. E., Eriksson, L., Stone-Elander, S., et al. 1987. *J. Neurosci., 7,* 2373–2389.

Roland, P. E., Gulyas, B., Seitz, R. J., et al. 1990. *NeuroReport, 1,* 53–56.

Rueckert, L., Appollonio, I., Grafman, J., Jezzard, P., Johnson, R., and Le Bihan, D. 1994. *Neuroimaging, 4,* 67–70.

Somers, D. C., Dale, A. M., Seiffert, A. E., and Tootel, R. B. H. 1999. *Proc. Natl. Acad. Scie. (USA), 96,* 1663–1668.

Developing Knowledge of Space: Core Systems and New Combinations

15

Elizabeth S. Spelke

Three Intuitions about Human Intelligence

People who reflect on their own cognitive capacities often share three intuitions. First, human thinking appears to be qualitatively different from the thinking of other animals. Second, human thinking appears to change qualitatively over development. Third, human thinking appears to depend in some way on language: our unique system for expressing thoughts somehow seems to make those thoughts possible.

In contemporary cognitive science, these intuitions have fallen on hard times. Behavioral biologists, comparative psychologists, and neuroscientists have found homologies between the representational systems of humans and other animals in numerous domains, including vision, object recognition, attention and working memory, and action planning. These homologies challenge those who believe any gulf divides human from nonhuman cognition. Studies of children have revealed striking continuities over human development: constant, core capacities to represent space and number, reason about objects and people, and engage in coordinated, goal-directed acts. These findings suggest that developmental changes in children's thinking stem more from the elaboration of core knowledge systems than from the emergence of new systems. Finally, studies of people with language impairments reveal rich and elaborate representations of the environment, indicating that the capacity to think does not depend on the capacity to express one's thoughts with words.

Conceptual challenges also face those who embrace the three intuitions, raising doubts about the possibility that human cognition could differ fundamentally from nonhuman cognition, change qualitatively over development, or depend on language. The evolution of humans was a recent event, and evolutionary change works by modifying existing structures, not by creating new ones from whole cloth. How, then, could humans have evolved wholly new ways of thinking? Learning plays a large role in the development of human knowledge, and it is constrained by the learner's preexisting representational capacities. How, then, could children's conceptions undergo radical change? One can only come to understand the words and expressions of a specific language if one can relate each word or expression to preexisting conceptual representations. How, then, could language learning result in an increase in the learner's conceptual resources?

Despite the evidence and arguments to the contrary, I suggest that there is something right about all three of the initial intuitions: human cognition does have unique properties, those properties emerge over the course of human development, and they relate to the acquisition of language. In this chapter, I defend these intuitions by presenting a case study in comparative, developmental cognitive science. The case lies in the domain of spatial memory and concerns the process by which one reorients oneself after losing one's sense of position and heading. We will see that human reorientation depends in part on processes that are homologous to those in other animals, constant over much of human development, and independent of language—just as those skeptical of the three intuitions would expect. Nevertheless, human navigation also depends on spatial representations that are unique to humans, emergent over development, and related to the acquisition of a specific natural language. The case study provides a perspective on the development of thought and language that may meet the conceptual challenges facing the three intuitions. In closing, I suggest other aspects of human cognition that might usefully be approached from the same perspective.

Comparative Studies of Reorientation

Mobile animals who return to fixed places within the environment have mechanisms for representing their changing position in relation to those places. One set of mechanisms, found in animals from ants to humans, accomplishes this task through a process of "dead reckoning" or "path integration": a moving animal continuously updates a representation of its position relative to its starting point by combining information about its position at the start of the updating step and its velocity over that step. Dead reckoning is subject to cumulative errors, however, and animals from ants to humans have mechanisms for correcting them. When an animal finds itself in a familiar environment, it draws on its memory for the positions and directions of features of that environment to correct errors in its current reckoned position and heading. My case study focuses on this process of error correction, or reorientation.

Because reorientation requires some form of spatial memory, comparative cognitive scientists can investigate the nature of the information that enters this representation and the processes that operate upon it. Cheng and Gallistel (Cheng, 1986; Margules and Gallistel, 1988) studied reorientation in rats in a rectangular chamber with a rich array of visual and olfactory landmarks. Hungry rats were shown the location of partially buried food, they were taken from the environment and disoriented, and then they were returned to the environment and allowed to search for the food. To the investigators' surprise, rats searched the two geometrically appropriate locations within the room with equal frequency, despite the fact that the locations bore different relations to the nongeometric features of the environment (Figure 15.1). This search pattern was obtained only when rats were disoriented; rats readily used nongeometric landmarks in other spatial memory tasks.

Cheng and Gallistel concluded that rats reorient by comparing the shape of their current surroundings to a geocentric representation of the shape of the environment they had previously encountered when oriented. Because this comparison is task-specific (it is invoked only for purposes of reorientation) and informationally encapsulated (it operates only on information about the shape of the environment), Cheng and Gallistel concluded that reorientation in rats is accomplished by a "geometric module." Although their claim for modularity is controversial, research from other laboratories has confirmed Cheng and Gallistel's central findings of a task-specific reliance on geometric information (Biegler and Morris, 1993; Dudchenko et al., 1997).

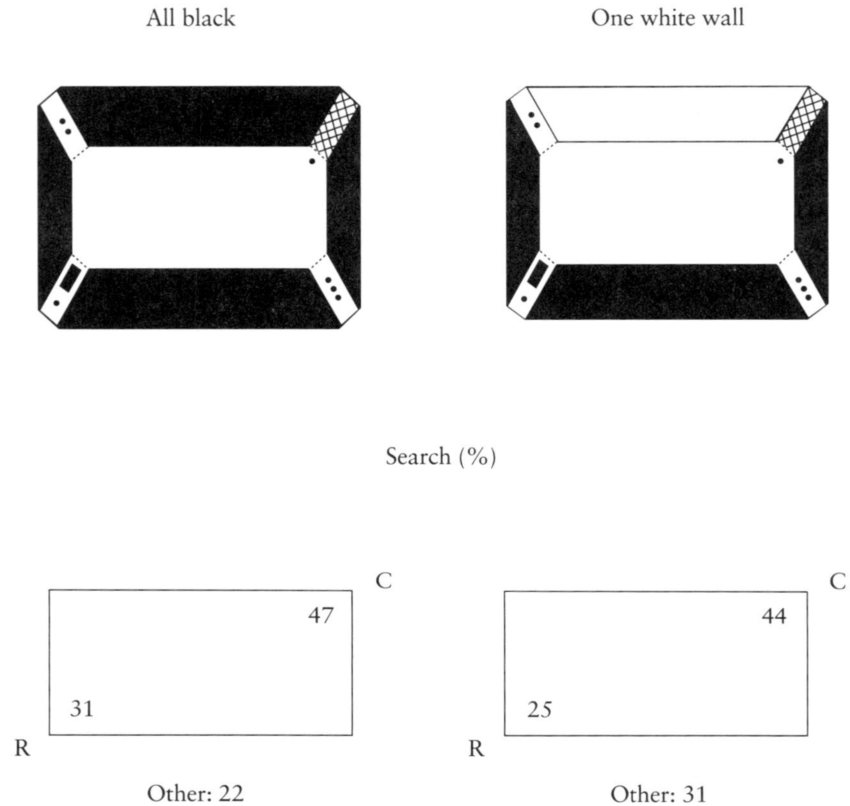

Figure 15.1. Testing environments and search patterns in two studies of reorientation and spatial memory in rats (Cheng, 1986). Rats searched at high levels at both geometrically appropriate corners of each chamber. Although they appeared to search the corner with appropriate nongeometric properties more than the opposite corner, this tendency was not significant (Cheng, 1986) and may be an artifact of incomplete disorientation (Margules and Gallistel, 1988).

The "Geometric Module" in Humans

Do humans have a homologous reorientation mechanism? Linda Hermer-Vazquez, Ranxiao Frances Wang, and I attempted to answer this question by adapting Cheng and Gallistel's experiments for young children (Hermer and Spelke, 1994, 1996; Wang, Hermer-Vazquez and Spelke, 1999). In our studies, 1.5- to 2-year-old children were brought individually into an experimental chamber by a parent, who hid a toy in one of the chamber's corners. Then the children were lifted and turned slowly with their eyes covered to induce a state of

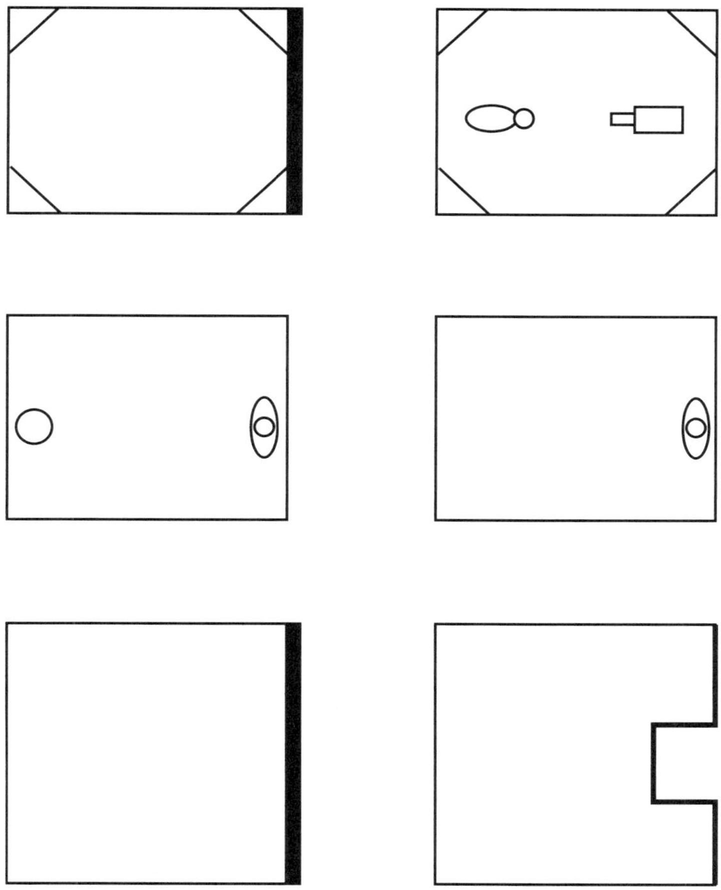

Figure 15.2. Testing environments used in studies of reorientation and spatial memory in young children (Hermer and Spelke, 1994, 1996; Wang, Hermer-Vazquez, and Spelke, 1999). Children searched with high and equal frequency at the two geometrically appropriate corners of the rectangular chamber, the four corners of the square chamber, and the single correct corner of the square chamber with the protuberance. The children's search did not accord with the colors of walls, or the presence or identities of movable objects.

disorientation (but not dizziness). Finally, they were released in a standing position facing one of the walls of the chamber, their eyes were uncovered, and they were encouraged to find the toy. In different experiments and conditions, we varied the properties of the chamber so as to determine the information children used to guide their search for the object (Figure 15.2).

In one condition, children were tested in a rectangular room with entirely white walls and no distinctive landmarks. These children searched the two geometrically appropriate corners equally, indicating that they were truly disoriented and that no inadvertent cues in the environment served to guide them to the object. Moreover, the children searched those two corners markedly more than the other two, geometrically inappropriate corners, indicating that they were sensitive to the geometric information used by rats. In a second condition, children were tested in the same room with a single, distinctively colored wall. Like rats, children continued to search the two geometrically appropriate corners with high and equal frequency, indicating that they failed to use the colored wall to relocate the object. In further experiments, we presented distinctive toys as symmetry-breaking landmarks, drew children's attention to the landmarks in various ways, allowed children to play in the chamber for several hours so that nongeometric landmarks became highly familiar, and reduced the informativeness of room geometry by testing children in a square or circular environment (Wang, Hermer-Vazquez, and Spelke, 1999; Gouteux and Spelke, 2001; see also Stedron, Munakata, and O'Reilly, 2000). None of these manipulations affected the findings: like rats, children searched for the hidden toy in correct relation to the shape of the room and without regard for the room's nongeometric landmarks.[1]

Was the children's search guided by a task-specific mechanism for reorientation? To investigate whether children truly reoriented by the shape of the room, Hermer-Vazquez (Hermer, 1997) investigated disoriented children's search for multiple landmarks (two hidden toys and the concealed chamber door) in a rectangular room with a single blue wall. When asked to point to each hidden object and to the door, children pointed with high and equal frequency to the correct location and to the geometrically equivalent, opposite location: once again, their search was guided by the shape of the room and not by the nongeometric landmark. Most important, however, children who pointed at the correct location for one of the objects pointed correctly for all of them, whereas children who pointed to the opposite location for one object showed the same reversal for the others. These findings provide evidence that children did not use local properties of the shape of the room to specify directly the individual locations of the objects. Instead, children evidently used the shape of the room to reorient themselves and, once oriented, searched for the objects in their remembered locations. Like rats, disoriented children locate objects in a familiar environment through a two-step process, in which they first reestablish their own geocentric orientation and then move to the remembered, geocentric positions of the objects.

Further experiments investigated whether children's reliance on room geometry stems from the "informational encapsulation" of the reorientation mechanism or from a more general, task-independent property of children's spatial memory. In a series of studies (Hermer and Spelke, 1996; see also Wang, Hermer-Vazquez, and Spelke, 1999), we compared children's search for a toy hidden in a corner of a rectangular environment under two sorts of conditions: in one condition, the toy remained in an apparently stable position and children were disoriented. In the other condition, the child remained oriented, with eyes closed, while the hiding places in the room were moved. Even when children viewed exactly the same environment in these two conditions, their search patterns were different: oriented children's search was guided by the nongeometric properties of the hidden object's container, but disoriented children's search was guided by the shape of the room (Figure 15.3). Search guided by geometry therefore appears to be specific to the task of reorientation. Like rats, children have a task-specific, encapsulated system for reorientation.

All these findings provide evidence for a close homology between the spatial representations and navigation processes of humans and rats: contrary to the first intuition with which I began, human navigation so far does not appear to depend on cognitive processes unique to humans. The plot thickens, however, when we turn from young children to older children and adults.

Developmental Changes in Spatial Representations

Adults were given the same reorientation task as young children in some of the same environments (Hermer and Spelke, 1994). When they were tested in a rectangular room with no distinctive landmarks, adults performed like young children and rats, searching the two geometrically correct locations with high and equal frequency. This find-

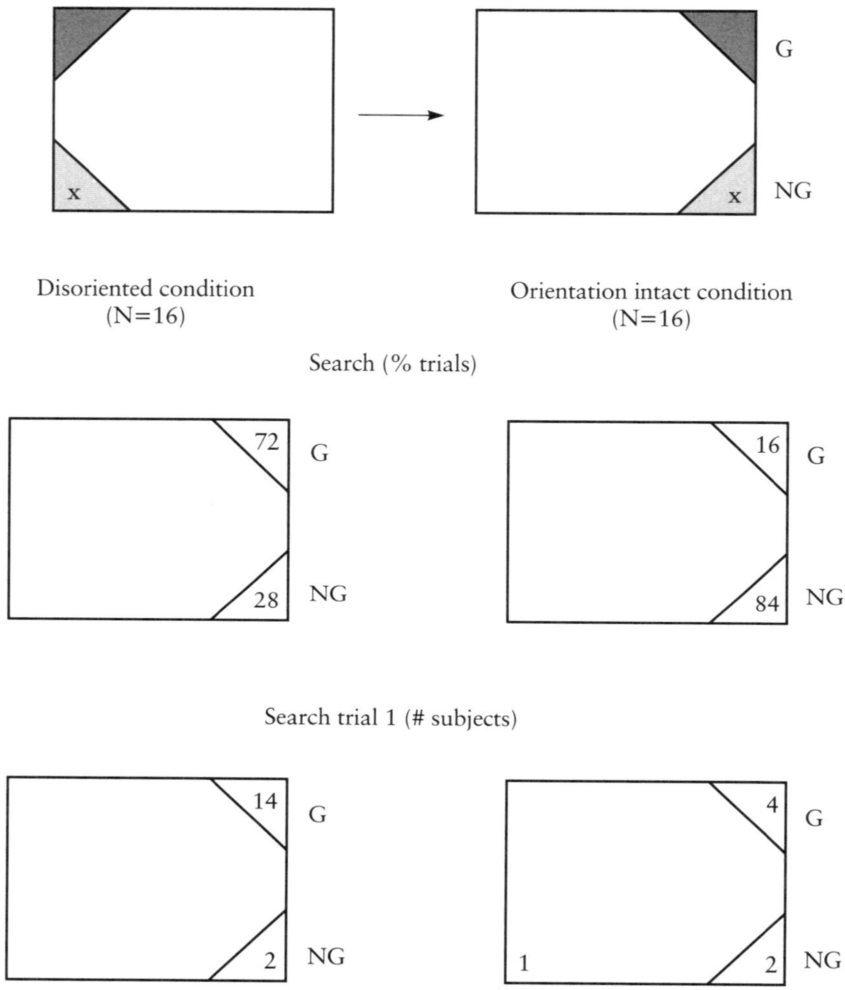

Figure 15.3. Testing environment and search patterns in a study of reorientation and object search by young children (Hermer and Spelke, 1996). For all children, an object was hidden in one of two distinctly colored and patterned boxes in adjacent corners, children's eyes were covered, and the boxes were moved to new locations that dissociated their geometric and nongeometric properties. Children who remained oriented during the boxes' displacement searched the box with the appropriate color and patterning, whereas those who were disoriented did not. Different search patterns were observed even on the first trial, before the children could know whether their task would be to locate a displaced object or to reorient themselves. Children evidently perceived and remembered both geometric and nongeometric properties of the hiding locations and used different properties selectively in different tasks.

ing suggests that the geometric reorientation system found in rats and children is present and functional in adults, a suggestion supported by new research using functional brain imaging (Epstein and Kanwisher, 1998). When a nongeometric landmark (a blue wall) was present in the rectangular environment, in contrast, adults outperformed young children and rats and confined their search to the single, correct corner of the environment. Sometime between two and twenty years of age, humans evidently come to locate objects under circumstances that defeat adult rats.

Further studies by Hermer-Vazquez, Moffet, and Munkholm (2001) investigated the development of this ability by testing children of various ages in the same environment. Children began to perform like adults, confining their search to the single correct location, at about six years of age. Those who succeeded at the task, moreover, often used spatial language to comment on their success.

To focus more directly on the transition from reorientation by pure geometry to the use of nongeometric landmarks, Hermer-Vazquez, Moffet, and Munkholm (2001) conducted a further study of six-year-old children, asking what other cognitive changes accompany the transition. In one session, children were given the reorientation task. In that session and a second session, a different investigator gave the children a battery of tests of spatial and verbal working memory, IQ, vocabulary size, comprehension of spatial expressions using the terms "above," "below," "front," "back," "left," and "right," and production of spatial expressions using the same terms. About half the children were found to reorient as adults do, using a colored wall to break the room's symmetry and specify the object's location. Stepwise regressions, with chronological age, sex, and performance on each of the other tests as predictor variables, revealed that the only factor associated with success on the reorientation task was performance on the language production task with expressions involving "left" and "right." Successful use of the nongeometric landmark was associated with successful production of spatial language.

These studies suggest that humans form spatial representations not found in other animals, and that these representations emerge over the course of human development. Do the representations depend on language? For familiar reasons, correlational research cannot answer this causal question, and so our last studies have taken a different approach. If uniquely human patterns of navigation depend on human language, then those patterns should disappear in any situation that prevents the normal exercise of the language faculty. We have tested this prediction in studies with normal human adults, using a dual-task method (Hermer-Vazquez, Spelke, and Katsnelson, 1999).

Turning Humans into Rats: Dual-task Studies

In these studies, disoriented adults again searched for an object hidden in a square or rectangular environment with a single distinctively colored wall. In one condition, subjects searched with no interference, as in our previous studies. In a second condition, subjects engaged in a simultaneous task of verbal shadowing: throughout the reorientation test, they listened to and repeated a continuous prose passage. This demanding task was designed to occupy the language faculty throughout the study and to prevent adults from using language to encode properties of the environment. Unfortunately, verbal shadowing is also quite demanding of attention and working memory, and so a further condition was included in the experiments. In that condition, subjects engaged in a nonverbal, rhythm-shadowing task: throughout the reorientation test, they listened to a changing succession of rhythmic drumbeats and continuously reproduced the rhythms by clapping. In a separate experiment, the verbal and rhythm-shadowing tasks each were performed with the same output system, concurrently with an attention-demanding visual search task. As judged from performance on the visual search task, the rhythm-shadowing task was at least as demanding of attention and effort as verbal shadowing. Unlike verbal shadowing, however, rhythm shadowing placed no demands on the language faculty.

The findings of our experiments are simply summarized: adults who engaged in rhythmic shadowing performed like adults in our original studies and searched in the correct relation to the nongeometric landmark. In contrast, adults who engaged in verbal shadowing performed like young children and rats and searched equally in the two geometrically appropriate locations (Figure 15.4). Geometrically appropriate search was as high as it is for children and rats in both shadowing

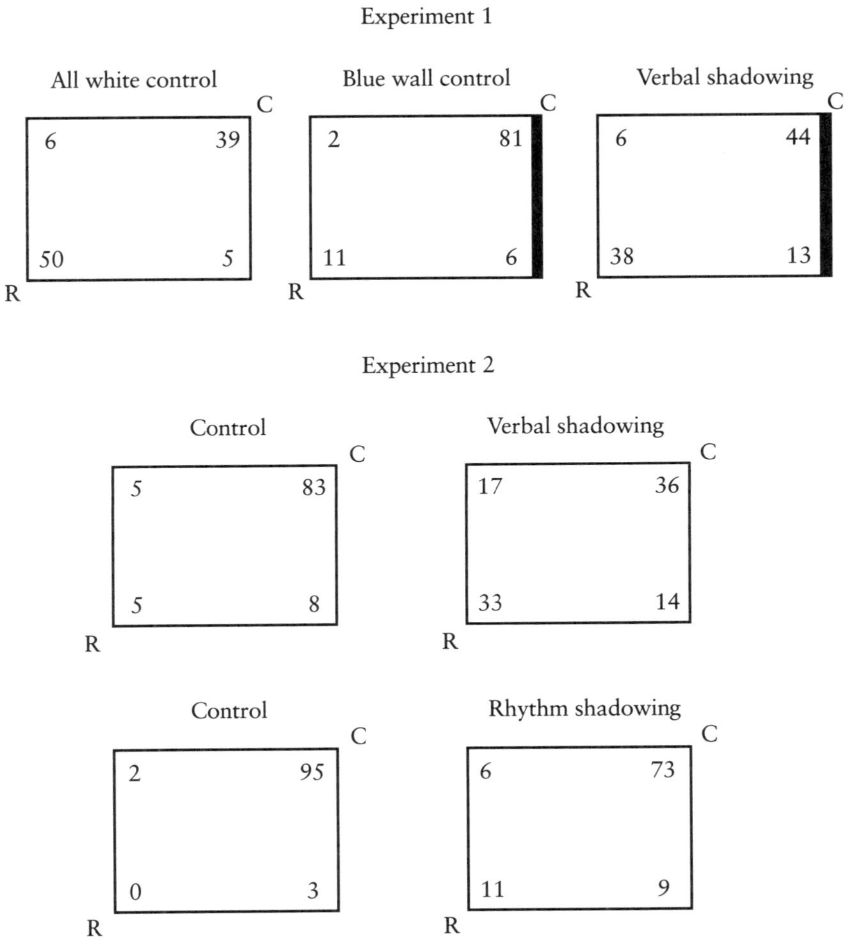

Figure 15.4. Testing environment and search patterns in a study of reorientation and spatial memory in adults (Hermer-Vazquez, Spelke, and Katsnelson, 1999). Adults searched in accord with both geometric and nongeometric information when they searched without distraction or performed a nonverbal distractor task. When engaged in a verbal distractor task, in contrast, adults searched in accord with geometric information alone.

conditions, suggesting that verbal shadowing did not interfere with memory for the object's location or with the geometric reorientation process. This finding provides evidence that Cheng's "geometric module" is alive and functioning in human adults. In contrast, adults' ability to search in the correct relation to the nongeometric landmark evidently depended on the use of language, for it was abolished by verbal shadowing.

Core Systems and New Combinations

This case study provides evidence both for and against the three intuitions with which we began. Contrary to claims that human thinking is unique, emergent over development, and dependent on language, we have found evidence for a system of representation—Cheng's "geometric module"—that is shared by humans and rats, constant over development, and impervious to verbal interference. This system allows both children and adults to reorient themselves and locate hidden objects. In accord with the initial intuitions, however, we have found evidence for a further system of representation that has not been observed in rats or other animals, that emerges over human development, whose emergence coincides in time with the acquisition of spatial language, and whose functioning is suppressed by verbal interference. What is the nature of the latter system, and in what ways might it depend on language?

To approach these questions, consider first what the language-dependent system does *not* do. Humans do not need language in order to notice, remember, or act on nongeometric information, because both infants and rats have all these abilities. Humans also do not need language in order to notice, remember, or act on the sense relationships encoded in language by the terms "left" and "right." Both Cheng's rats and Hermer-Vazquez's toddlers showed high sensitivity to sense relationships, for only those relationships distinguished the geometrically appropriate corners of the rectangular room (for example, the corners with a long wall on the *left*) from the inappropriate corners (those with a long wall on the *right*). Colors, patterns, lengths, and sense relations are all detectable and memorable independently of language, and all serve to guide the actions of nonverbal animals and preverbal children.

What rats and young children appear not to do is to combine these sources of information flexibly. Although rats and children represent the sense relations among walls of different *lengths,* they do not appear to represent the sense relations among walls of different *colors. Left, blue,* and *wall* are concepts available to the rat and the young child, but *left of the blue wall* is not.

This small example raises a larger possibility. Humans and other animals may share a common collection of innate, domain-specific cognitive systems, each of which gives rise to a set of core concepts. Distinctively human, developmentally emergent cognitive achievements may stem in part from our unique ability to form new combinations of these concepts, and that ability in turn may depend on the acquisition of a natural language.

How can a natural language be learned in the first place, if the concepts it expresses are not yet available to the child? Children may learn the words and expressions of a natural language by drawing on the concepts that their core, language-independent systems of representation make available. For example, the term "left" could be learned by relating the language-independent spatial representations used for navigation or object localization to expressions such as "turn left" or "look on the left." Terms for nongeometric landmarks and their properties could be learned by relating language-independent representations of objects or scenes to expressions such as "the blue box" or "the blue sky."

Once these terms are learned, natural languages may make new representations available, because of two of their most remarkable properties. First, a natural language is a combinatorial system: once terms have been learned in the context of one set of expressions, they can be used and understood in other sets of expressions with no further learning. Second, a natural language is a domain-general system of representation: its combinatorial rules concatenate entities only in accord with the syntactic properties of those entities and irrespective of their domain-specific content. Although nonverbal animals and preverbal children also have combinatorial representational systems, those systems operate in restricted domains. The present case study, for example, concerns a language-independent system that combines sense and distance relations (allowing rats and preverbal children to represent corners with a *short* wall on the *left*) but not sense and color relations. A speaker of English, in contrast, can combine sense relations not only with geometric properties but with nongeometric properties such as color ("the corner with the blue wall on the left"), number ("left of the first seven houses"), arbitrary associations ("left of the tunnel where Diana died"), or any other properties we have words to express.

The explosive, domain-independent combinatorial power of natural language may give human thinking its unique flexibility, and the acquisition of a natural language may underlie the emergence of new concepts and conceptual resources in children. Nevertheless, language is too powerful a combinatorial system, for it allows speakers to form bizarre and senseless combinations as well as useful and meaningful ones. Because nothing in the language faculty serves to distinguish potentially significant combinations from senseless ones, other selective processes are needed to guide children and adults toward useful combinations. Instruction, observation, and trial-and-error learning all may play this role (see Chapter 23).

Surveying the Landscape

These sweeping claims are a heavy burden for a small case study to bear; might they apply in other domains? Research on children's developing concepts of objects, of persons and their actions, and of number suggests other cases where uniquely human thinking may emerge through the acquisition of language. I sketch each case briefly.

Objects

Human infants and other primates have elaborate, and similar, abilities to perceive and represent objects. Young children nevertheless take a major step beyond the smartest nonhuman primates when they begin to learn about artifacts. On a single exposure, toddlers who view an adult using a tool develop new and enduring knowledge about the functional properties of that object. Human knowledge about objects comes to include a complex mix of information about an object's composition, parts, affordances, history, and culturally sanctioned functions. The ability to combine diverse sources of information into unitary object representations may be one source of the distinctively human propensity to surround ourselves with things of our own making.

What accounts for this ability? Human infants and nonhuman primates may be sensitive to many of the kinds of information that enter into mature representations of artifacts. Only verbal children and adults may combine these representations, however, so as to form concepts of objects with both physical properties and conventional functions, and natural language may provide the medium in which this combination of information is represented. The first steps of this process may occur when children learn their first words for kinds of objects (see Xu and Carey, 1996, for evidence and discussion).

Human Action

A wealth of research over the last two decades has investigated the emergence, in ontogeny and phylogeny, of a "theory of mind": a distinctive way of viewing, predicting, and explaining the actions of people and other animals as guided by their intentions, tempered by their emotions, and planned in accord with their perceptions and representations of their surroundings. Although early observations suggested that this intentional view might be common to humans and other primates (Premack and Woodruff, 1978; Whiten and Byrne, 1988), subsequent studies have provided very limited evidence for theory of mind reasoning in any nonhuman primate (Premack, 1988; Cheney and Seyfarth, 1990; Povinelli and Eddy, 1996; compare Hare et al., 2000). Similar research with children provides evidence for marked developmental changes in reasoning about human action. Very young children appear to represent human actions as directed to goals (Gergely et al., 1995; Woodward, 1998), as responsive to events perceived at a distance (Spelke, Phillips, and Woodward, 1995; Hood, Willen, and Driver, 1998), and as guided by desires (Wellman, 1990). In contrast, two-year-old children fail to reason about actions as guided by states of knowledge, and three-year-old children consistently fail to predict a person's actions from knowledge of her beliefs when the beliefs are false (for example, Perner, 1991). These findings suggest that an understanding of actions as guided by mental states develops slowly over the preschool years.

If "theory of mind" reasoning is distinctively human and emergent over development, what are its origins? The research described above suggests that young children understand desires and thoughts as directed to simple objects and actions. For example, young children can represent a given individual as *wanting an apple, wanting to jump,* or *thinking about Fred.* These language-independent representations may allow children to learn the meanings of verbs such as "want" and "think" when they appear in corresponding expressions. Studies of young children's spontaneous use of the verbs "want" and "think" are consistent with this possibility (Bartsch and Wellman, 1997). Further language-independent representations of states of affairs (for example, *Fred is late* or *John cut the apple*) would allow children to learn simple expressions describing those states of affairs. Once children have learned these expressions, the syntactic rules of their language allow for the construction of more complex expressions with embedded complements: for example, "I want John to cut the apple," "I think Fred is late." The syntax of embedding may provide the combinatorial machinery needed to represent propositional attitudes, which in turn may allow for the development of a theory of mind.

Recent research by de Villiers and de Villiers (1999) is consistent with this hypothesis. Their studies of normal and language-delayed children provide evidence that the emergence of the ability to express and understand sentences with embedded complements—sentences such as "John said that it's raining" or "Mary thinks we're crazy"—precedes and predicts success on false belief tasks. The acquisition of a natural language therefore might play a role in the development of an understanding of false beliefs and other propositional attitudes.

Number

Although many have proposed that knowledge of number is dependent on language, this claim remains problematic (see Chomsky, 1986; Bloom, 1994; Gallistel and Gelman, 1992; Dehaene, 1997). How could language be the source of our "number sense"? If it were, then how could knowledge of counting and arithmetic ever develop in children? Could abstract properties of the language faculty (recursion, discrete infinity) be harnessed for other domains?

A view of human cognition as founded on core systems, linked by language to form new combinations, suggests an approach to these questions (Spelke and Tsivkin, 2001). A language-independent number sense may arise from core systems for representing discrete, small numbers of objects and for representing approximate quantities: systems found in human infants and other animals (Dehaene, 1997; Scholl and Leslie, 1999). Children may learn the meanings of the first words in the counting sequence by mapping the words both to object representations (for example, "two apples" refers to *an apple and another apple*) and to magnitude representations (for example, "two apples" refers to *a very small quantity of apples* or *the next-to-smallest quantity of apples*). Because all the counting words follow a single sequence, children who have learned the meanings of "one," "two," and "three" may come to realize that each word in the sequence denotes both a distinct, discrete set of entities and a distinct magnitude (Wynn, 1992). Number words, on this view, serve as links for combining representations that exist independently of language but that have no privileged relation to one another.

This view predicts that mature representations of large, exact numerical magnitudes will show language dependence, whereas mature representations of small sets and of approximate numerical magnitudes will not. Studies of bilingual arithmetic and of numerical processing in language-impaired neurological patients provide some support for these predictions (Dehaene, 1997; O'Kane and Spelke, 2001; Spelke and Tsivkin, 2001).

Languages of the Brain

My case study in comparative, developmental cognitive science suggests a set of tasks for cognitive neuroscientists. We need, first, to chart the homologies between human and nonhuman cognition: to find and decipher the languages of the brain that are common to humans and other primates, and even to more distant animals. There are likely to be many such languages, in my view, embodied in distinct brain systems. If that hunch is correct, then cognitive neuroscientists can use the increasing array of tools at our disposal to study these systems at multiple levels and in multiple species.

The task of cognitive neuroscience will not end, however, with the charting of these homologous systems, for we need also to explore the distinctive ways in which humans combine their systems to form new concepts and new solutions to problems. I am speculating that each monolingual person may have just one language of the brain for combining expressions for his or her diverse mental languages. When humans solve problems that only we can solve, or think thoughts that only we can entertain, the multiple languages of the brain may communicate with one another by means of a single language that we also use to communicate our thoughts to one another. Discovering how this internal communication takes place in the fluent adult, and how it emerges in the developing child, could challenge cognitive neuroscientists for some time.

Note

I thank Linda Hermer-Vazquez and Raoxiao Frances Wang for their collaboration and the participants of the Harvard/IPSEN conference for bracing discussion. Supported by a grant from NIH (HD23103).

1. Young children do reorient by a nongeometric landmark, such as a wall of a distinctive color, when they are tested in a much larger environment such that the landmark appears at a considerable distance (Learmonth, Newcombe, and Huttenlocher, in press). Room size appears to be the critical variable, for such children fail to reorient by the same nongeometric landmark when tested in an otherwise identical environment of the size of the room used by Hermer and Spelke (Learmonth and Nadel, personal communication, 2000). In a large room, it is possible that a distant, asymmetrically placed surface that contrasts with its surroundings in brightness will serve as a compass signal for humans and for other animals (Mittelstedt, personal communication, 1996; Wang and Spelke, 2000).

References

Bartsch, K., and Wellman, H. M. 1997. *Children talk about the mind.* New York: Oxford University Press.

Biegler, R., and Morris, R. G. M. 1993. Landmark stability is a prerequisite for spatial but not discrimination learning. *Nature* 361, 631–633.

Bloom, P. 1994. Generativity within language and other cognitive domains. *Cognition, 51,* 177–189.

Cheney, D. L., and Seyfarth, R. M. 1990. *How Monkeys See the World.* Chicago: University of Chicago Press.

Cheng, K. 1986. A purely geometric module in the rat's spatial representation. *Cognition, 23,* 149–178.

Chomsky, N. 1986. *Knowledge of language: Its nature, origin, and use.* New York: Praeger.

Dehaene, S. 1997. *The number sense.* New York: Oxford.

de Villiers, J. G., and de Villiers, P. A. 1999. Linguistic determinism and false belief. In *Children's Reasoning and the Mind,* ed. P. Mitchell and K. Riggs. Hove, UK: Psychology Press.

Dudchenko, P. A., Goodridge, J. P., Seiterle, D. A., and Taube, J. S. 1997. Effects of repeated disorientation on the acquisition of spatial tasks in rats: Dissociation between the appetitive radial arm maze and aversive water maze. *Journal of Experimental Psychology: Animal Behavior Processes, 23,* 194–210.

Epstein, R., and Kanwisher, N. 1998. A cortical representation of the local visual environment. *Nature, 392,* 598–601.

Gallistel, C. R., and Gelman, R. 1992. Preverbal and verbal counting and computation. *Cognition, 44,* 43–74.

Gergely, G., Nadasdy, Z., Csibra, G., and Biro, S. 1995. Taking the intentional stance at 12 months of age. *Cognition, 56,* 165–193.

Gouteux, S., and Spelke, E. S. 2001. Children's use of geometry and landmarks to reorient in an open space. *Cognition, 81,* 119–148.

Hare, B., Call, J., Agnetta, B., and Tomasello, M. 2000. Chimpanzees know what conspecifics do and do not see. *Animal Behavior, 59,* 771–785.

Hermer, L. 1997. Internally coherent spatial memories in a mammal. *NeuroReport, 8,* 1743–1747.

Hermer, L., and Spelke, E. S. 1994. A geometric process for spatial reorientation in young children. *Nature, 370,* 57–59.

——— 1996. Modularity and development: The case of spatial reorientation. *Cognition, 61,* 195–232.

Hermer-Vazquez, L., Moffet, A., and Munkholm, P. 2001. Language, space, and the development of cognitive flexibility in humans: The case of two spatial memory tasks. *Cognition, 79,* 263–299.

Hermer-Vazquez, L., Spelke, E. S., and Katsnelson, A. 1999. Sources of flexibility in human cognition: Dual-task studies of space and language. *Cognitive Psychology, 39,* 3–36.

Hood, B. M., Willen, J. D., and Driver, J. 1998. Adults' eyes trigger shifts of visual attention in human infants. *Psychological Science, 9,* 53–56.

Learmonth, A. E., Newcombe, N. S., and Huttenlocher, J. In press. Toddlers' use of metric information and landmarks to reorient. *Journal of Experimental Child Psychology.*

Margules, J., and Gallistel, C. R. 1988. Heading in the rat: Determination by environmental shape. *Animal Learning, 16,* 404–410.

O'Kane, G. C., and Spelke, E. S. 2001. Language dependence in representations of number, space, and time. Poster presented at the meeting of the Psychonomic Society, Orlando, Fla. November.

Perner, H. 1991. *Understanding the representational mind.* Cambridge: MIT Press.

Povinelli, D. J., and Eddy, T. J. 1996. What young chimpanzees know about seeing. *Monographs of the Society for Research in Child Development, 61,* serial no. 247.

Premack, D. 1988. "Does the chimpanzee have a theory of mind" revisited. In *Machiavellian intelligence,* ed. R. Byrne and A. Whiten. New York: Oxford University Press.

Premack, D., and Woodruff, G. 1978. Does the chimpanzee have a theory of mind? *Behavioral and Brain Sciences, 1,* 515–526.

Scholl, B. J., and Leslie, A. M. 1999. Explaining the infant's object concept: Beyond the perception/cognition dichotomy. In *What Is Cognitive Science?* ed. E. Lepore and Z. Pylyshyn. Oxford: Blackwell.

Spelke, E. S., Phillips, A., and Woodward, A. L. 1995. Infants' knowledge of object motion and human action. In *Causal cognition: A multidisciplinary debate,* ed. D. Sperber, D. Premack, and A. J. Premack. New York: Oxford University Press.

Spelke, E. S., and Tsivkin, S. 2001. Language and number: A bilingual training study. *Cognition, 78,* 45–88.

Stedron, J. M., Munakata, Y., and O'Reilly, R. C. 2000. Spatial reorientation in young children: A case of modularity? Poster presented at the 2000 meeting of the International Conference on Infant Studies, Brighton, U.K., July.

Wang, R. F., Hermer-Vazquez, L., and Spelke, E. S. 1999. Mechanisms of reorientation and object localization by children: A comparison with rats. *Behavioral Neuroscience, 113,* 475–485.

Wang, R. F., and Spelke, E. S. 2000. Updating egocentric representations in human navigation. *Cognition, 77,* 215–250.

Wellman, H. 1990. *The child's theory of mind.* Cambridge: MIT Press.

Whiten, A., and Byrne, R. W. 1988. Tactical deception in primates. *Behavioral and Brain Sciences, 11,* 233–244.

Woodward, A. L. 1998. Infants selectively encode the goal object of an actor's reach. *Cognition, 69,* 1–34.

Wynn, K. 1992. Addition and subtraction in infants. *Nature, 358,* 749–750.

Xu, F., and Carey, S. 1996. Infants' metaphysics: The case of numerical identity. *Cognitive Psychology, 30,* 111–153.

Discussion: Section 4

DAVID CAPLAN: This is for Bernard Mazoyer. Can I ask about your interpretation of the visual effects? It seems to me that in both experiments in which there is emphasis on exploration of space you're activating a high parietal/frontal system that's very similar to the dorsal visual system. And in the object imagery or concrete noun definition task, where you're presumably activating object features, you're activating an inferior temporal system that's similar to the ventral visual system. I didn't think you put that kind of interpretation on your results. And I am wondering whether I misunderstood or whether you had considered it?

BERNARD MAZOYER: No, I think you're right. I didn't put that as a major result because I think the fact that mental imagery relies on the two visual routes has been so strongly established that it isn't news. If you're doing spatial mental imagery you activate the dorsal route, and if you're doing object mental imagery you activate the ventral route. I wanted to emphasize our finding that when you do mental imagery, there is a strong component of working memory, with the spatial working memory for visual spatial tasks—which activates the parietal/frontal network—and the object working memory for shape-based imagery tasks—which is more ventral. But you're right. We have the two routes involved also in mental imagery.

ALBERT GALABURDA: Bernard, how is it possible to know that the subject is not imaging something even though the content of the word is not imageable, like "justice" or "truth?" For instance, if I can't image the object, I image the written word itself, or a symbol for the word, such as the blindfolded lady holding the scales in the case of "justice."

MAZOYER: Well, there is no on-line control for what they're doing. But we asked them what they were doing, and you ask the words they've been hearing, and you actively control the number of words they can recall. But I will agree, that there is no direct on-line control of what the people are doing.

JEAN-PIERRE CHANGEUX: Just as a naive listener: When we are discussing, such as has just been occurring as you were speaking to us, is mental imagery being stimulated or not?

MAZOYER: I think, most likely yes. People often generate mental images when hearing a discussion.

CHANGEUX: Is there is some kind of objective test for this, or must we just rely on introspection?

MAZOYER: That's one difficulty in all these tasks. If we have a very formal and abstract debate, like we had when we discussed the papers on language, it is very hard to form mental images for some of the things that are said. But for researchers who use neuroimaging, for example, I think mental imagery is very common when one reads the data.

STEPHEN KOSSLYN: There is good behavioral technology for documenting that people use imagery in a particular task. Probably the most straightforward relies on selective interference between imagery and perception in the same modality. Seeing selectively disrupts visual mental imagery more than auditory imagery (such as of a phone ringing), but vice versa for hearing. In fact, researchers, such as Lee Brooks and people like Bob Logie who study working memory, have documented dissociations between spatial (location-based) interference and visual (shape-based) interference for different kinds of imagery tasks—which fits nicely with what Bernard was saying, that there are at least two different types of imagery.

MICHEL DENIS: There is no doubt that imagery may be involved when you are listening to the speech of another person or reading written material. But in conversation, in dialogue, my answer would be that first it depends on the content, obviously. Some contents are more amenable to visualizations than others. But it also depends on another factor, which is sometimes underestimated, namely: do people involved in the dialogue in the conversation, do they need to build a common representation of the object they are speaking about? Frequently people have partial representations that do not exactly overlap and it's part of their first objective to build common representation before conversing about it. We are conducting some studies on how people provide route directions in familiar environments. And part of this research involves several people working together to produce such route directions. It's very impressive that the first step is for them to build a common representation, frequently by drawing the route before conversing about it. So the notion of joint or common representation seems to be important in this respect.

BARBARA GROSZ: Is the image simply the result of the conversation?

DENIS: It is difficult for me to say that language contributes to imagery or imagery to language. They both jointly contribute to the building of representations. They contribute to understanding the environment, or the intentions, or the descriptions from other people. So I would favor the notion of a joint operation, or joint mechanisms designed to create a higher order of representations.

DENIS LE BIHAN: I agree, but think the situation is even more complex. Let me give you an example. I don't know if you've seen the movie, a French movie, *All the Morning of the World,* which is about this musician from the sixteenth century, Marien Marie, who has lost his wife and is an exceptional musician. And by playing music, which is a kind of language—right?—he is able to reproduce his wife, living, in front of his eyes. The message is that there are different kinds of languages that we use in order to produce internal images, which can make us happy or lead us to think about something in particular. So we need language, but different kinds of languages in order to help us to build the representations we need at the given time.

ELIZABETH SPELKE: Here's a naive one for Denis Le Bihan. It seems to me that, on the one hand, your results accord well with the intuition that when we're imagining something there is something qualitatively like what's going on when we're perceiving. On the other hand, we don't mistake our images for perceptions most of the time. Imagining something doesn't feel like perceiving something in a dark room or with difficulty and so forth. Why not?

LE BIHAN: That's a good question. Although there are some people who confuse reality and their mental images, perception and imagery probably differ in the sheer amount of stimulation.

SPELKE: If fMRI, and other techniques, are getting better temporal resolution, it might be nice to explore the time course in which different regions are activated, and see where the representations are coming from.

LE BIHAN: That's a very good idea.

KOSSLYN: I'm wondering whether your assumption is correct, Liz. There's a literature that goes under the name of Reality Monitoring, a term coined, I believe, by Marcia Johnson. These findings show that in fact people commonly confuse having visualized something for seeing it; we do in fact mistake our images for perceptions. Moreover, there is a growing literature showing that visualizing something interferes with seeing it, particularly if the image overlaps with what one is looking at. However, I think Denis is right: there are cues that allow us usually to distinguish between imagery and perception. Think of how inconvenient life would be if this were a major chore!

ALFONSO CARAMAZZA: I'd like to introduce a variant of the question Liz asked. Why does it take time, so much time, to generate an image, when in visual perception we don't have that feeling of effort and perceiving?

LE BIHAN: In my experience, we don't really need a long time to produce mental images. Nevertheless, if you want the activation to go all the way down to V1, if it comes from a region like the temporal lobe, it has to go through the temporal pathway up to V1. This may require time.

CARAMAZZA: I guess that's what I find bizarre, in the sense that in vision, in language, and whatever, that time is minuscule by comparison to the time we're talking about here.

LE BIHAN: It might be that first you are dealing with some properties and say, well, that's not enough, so now you have to go on to another step. And here you need to repeat the entire process, to add the necessary information.

KOSSLYN: It might be useful to pause for a moment to consider the neuroanatomy of the visual system. It turns out that virtually every area that is connected to another one with an afferent (downstream) connection also receives an efferent (backward) connection. But crucially, the backward connections are not as precise as the forward; they're quite diffuse. So it is not so simple to form a pattern in early visual cortex by using the backward connections. One does not simply "paint" an image on early cortex, such as V1. Rather, it is very much a constructive process in a way that bottom-up processing isn't, which may be why it takes so much time to form many types of mental images.

PIERRE JACOB: I have a question for Liz Spelke, and for people who study aphasic patients. Is it conceivable to find adults with Broca's aphasia who have trouble naming spatial relations or using such relations either in comprehension or in production? If so, your theory would predict that they should have more trouble reorienting themselves than normal adults, right?

SPELKE: Right. There's also a normal population that will be interesting to look at, and that's people who speak languages that don't have terms for left and right in them. Now I wouldn't expect to see noticeable disabilities in navigation in these people—in the same way that we don't see disabilities in animals, which can be very good at navigating around the environment. And I would expect these people will too. The key prediction is that there will be disabilities if we set up these special tasks where you can't use your natural navigation systems, where you have to bring together information in new ways. The prediction is yes, if there were an aphasia that radical, we'd expect not to see the normal adult pattern in these cases.

CARAMAZZA: Is language needed for representing the information or for remembering the information? Your experiments required that you disorient the child, the rat, and so on, but when they're not disoriented they can use the information. So presumably they must be able to encode it as an object and as a relation, perhaps. But perhaps language is not needed then for encoding information but only for remembering it. Is that a possibility?

SPELKE: Yes, except for the following. We can show in the studies of animals and also in the studies of young children that their inability to bring together information about sense relations with these arbitrary other things, like wall coloring, is not due to a memory limit. If you take the subjects outside the task of navigation and ask them in another way, was there a blue wall there, what was the blue wall, they can tell you. So the limit that we see in the language-independent systems is not a memory limit. On the other hand, what you're really asking is, is the ability to conjoin, to bring together information into new combinations, without language, versus being able to make these combinations, but they are just so fleeting that it's there one second and gone the next. I'm inclined to think that it's not simply a memory problem. Because if it were simply a memory problem, then you have to ask, how do these arbitrary sets of information get combined together?

STANISLAS DEHAENE: I have both a comment and a question. The comment is that there are patients with left parietal lesions who cannot speak about left and right very well, and so you could readily test this idea on those patients, I think. The question is, do you really need language to make this convergence? Or is it more like a global work space, which is available in humans, and that actually makes it possible to acquire language—but it's not really language by itself that's doing the convergence?

SPELKE: I think your second question is the key question. I hope I can hold it in working memory while I answer the first. The problem with the parietal lesions is that they may knock out the core language, in these people who can't distinguish left from right. What we need is people who still can distinguish left from right within the core language–independence system, who would succeed, for example, in the Cheng and Gallistel task as well as rats do, distinguishing the corner with a long wall on the left from the one with the long wall on the right—but who simply can't conjoin it together. So depending on what those patients are like, that might or might not be a critical case here. About the second question, I would like to push the idea that natural language and the language faculty is the system of representation that allows us to combine things together. And that the other systems that we clearly use as adults, that artists use, the system that your subjects use with Arabic numerals, and so forth, develop out of the initial combinations made possible by the language faculty. But at this point, that's a religious belief on my part. I have no data that bear on it.

MARC JEANNEROD: Consider the distinction between the huge number of words that we have to describe the intrinsic attributes of objects, such as color and shape and so on, versus the very few words that we have to describe spatial relationships, no more than ten or twelve. So, is there a dissociation in terms of learning those words and manipulating those concepts, respectively, intrinsic and extrinsic attributes?

SPELKE: Yes. I think that one of the central questions for this whole meeting, and for people studying language and language acquisition, is how do children choose which of the many conceptual distinctions they can make in the world to be mapped onto language. And what are the properties of the language-independent systems of representation that make some properties, some entities in those representations, not available at all? For example, take retinal size, we don't really have words for that. Other entities are available but only with difficulty. Left versus right is an example of that. Although it looks like the underlying sense relationship is easily available to a rat or a young child, in the language system it's very slow to be acquired. And then other terms come in very, very rapidly. I have one suggestion about this. I don't know if it will work. But the idea is that in some cases terms transparently map onto entities in particular privileged domains. I think this is true for names for kinds of objects, for example. In other cases, the relationship is more indirect and a single term may map to entities in several representations. I think this may account for children's problems in learning the number words and the count sequence—if they don't have a unitary representation of number but rather two distinct representations and they have to map these terms to both of them. But whether that will account for all of the phenomena of why some things are hard in language learning and others things are easy, why the adult language seems to be rich in some conceptual domains and much poorer in others, probably not.

KOSSLYN: It is known that there are a large number, thirty-two at last count, of visual areas in the monkey cortex. Many of these areas appear to have distinct types of visual representations. Do you think language is needed to coordinate all of these representations?

SPELKE: I think there is good reason to believe that there are multiple kinds of visual representations and that some of them have privileged connections to one another which are quite independent of language. You see them in young children, you see them in other animals. Not all "binding" of representations requires language. But in other cases, the connections among distinct representations may in fact not be privileged in the architecture of the visual system. In particular, the coming together of those things that may be critical for developing representations underlying tool use and things like that, may be at least facilitated by language and possibly made possible by it.

ANNE CHRISTOPHE: What you could have is several specialized modules like the geometric modules, object representation, and so forth, and the combinatorial ability in the language faculty. But that one doesn't work from the start, it needs some language input to start working. So there is some parameterization of the syntax. And then once you start acquiring the vocabulary for the specific domains, you can use the combinatorial ability to these domains.

SPELKE: Thank you. You said that so much better than I did. That's exactly what I think. Not that the combinatorial ability somehow falls out of the sky, but that it inheres in the language faculty. And becomes available to combine information across other domains once terms and expressions of the language are learned. And the language faculty itself undergoes whatever development it does.

CHRISTOPHE: Another question on this. I wondered whether you had any idea about how left and right were represented in sign languages? And whether maybe it might be easier to learn because it would be closer to the original domain?

SPELKE: I've been told something about that. I don't know if this is right. That in sign languages there is more tendency to represent spatial relationships geocentrically. And there are some spoken languages that do that as well. There are languages that don't have terms for left and right. And would describe this, for example, as my northern arm, if that happened to be north. Interesting that speakers of left/right–type languages tend not to know whether that happens to be north or not. These ideas lead to predictions about differences that you'll get between speakers of those languages and speakers of left/right–type languages. And if it's right that sign language tends to preserve geocentric relations, then there are predictions there as well. As yet, those predictions haven't been tested. By the way, these predictions don't take the form of assuming inferiority or superiority of conceptions in one language community over another. But rather qualitative differences under just the conditions under which things will be combined and the ways in which they'll be combined.

EDGAR ZURIF: I have some information on this. If you have a right-sided lesion and you're deaf, you lose the ability to refer to things in space, left versus right, and so on. But you can still use the language to do that. And vice versa if you have a left-sided lesion. That is, your ability to deal with arguments goes even though you can refer to those same things in space in the nonlanguage mode. Clearly, different systems of representation are at work, even in the deaf.

Section 5
Visual and Motor Representations

This section follows naturally from Section 4. Images are not just visual; as Denis Le Bihan and his colleagues pointed out, they occur in multiple modalities. Not only can we visualize, but we can imagine hearing something, as occurs, for example, if we're asked whether the first three notes of "Three Blind Mice" go up or down. Try to do this. Notice that in addition to having an auditory image, you may also have a motoric image: your throat may seem to mimic the movements made when singing the song. This is a good example of the sort of working memory representation that Baddeley included in his "articulatory loop." Each sensory modality probably has its own short-term memory system. But short-term memory is more than transient perceptual representations: the motor system is intimately involved in such perceptual systems.

For reasons that are not clear, the motor system is often neglected in cognitive psychology (and cognitive science) texts, but it is clear that the motor system is intimately involved in mental representation. The motor system is interesting from the present perspective for at least two general reasons. First, the representations used in guiding movements are part of the "toolbox" of the mind, and can be used more generally. For example, motor processes are sometimes involved when we manipulate objects in visual mental images. One can imagine an object rotating, for example, by imagining what one would see if one twisted it in a certain way—and the ease of performing the transformation depends on the actual ease with which one could perform that movement. In addition, motor representations play crucial roles in our representations of where we are presently located and where other objects are located. Second, the motor system intimately interacts with the perceptual systems. For example, one typically is moving around in the world, encoding different things; depending on how one is oriented, one encodes different stimuli. Moreover, one is not simply passively registering what one perceives. Rather, as one moves, one continually generates expectations about what one will next encounter, and such top-down priming clearly influences that which one does in fact register.

In this section we begin by considering the idea that imagery depends on the confluence of different forms of mental representations. Stephen Kosslyn argues not only that these mental representations are used together in various ways, but also that in some sense they are constructed as needed (rather than simply drawn from a preexisting collection). Following this, Alain Berthoz and his colleagues focus on the role of motor processes in setting up representations of space. Berthoz argues that "topokinetic" representations exist in memory, and that movement and action are always involved in mental events; indeed, Berthoz goes so far as to argue that the organization of action is the fundamental language of the brain. Next, Marc Jeannerod emphasizes the role of processes that predict subsequent actions and their consequences. Jeannerod garners insights in part by observing the types of errors made by schizophrenics, who often have delusions that involve being influenced by other people. Finally, Nalini Ambady and Mark Hallahan consider how information about actions is encoded and recognized. They note that we have representations of very specific aspects of human behavior. In particular, Ambady and Hallahan examine how well people can detect telltale cues from very small "slices" of behavior. In this case, they investigate the ability to detect sexual orientation when one views very short videoclips, and reveal the key role of motion in conveying such information.

Einstein's Mental Images: The Role of Visual, Spatial, and Motoric Representations

16

Stephen M. Kosslyn

> The psychical entities which seem to serve as elements in thought are certain signs and more or less clear images which can be "voluntarily" reproduced and combined . . . This combinatory play seems to be the essential feature in productive thought—before there is any connection with logical construction in words or other kinds of signs which can be communicated to others. The above-mentioned elements are, in my case, of visual and some muscular type. Conventional words or other signs have to be sought for laboriously only in a secondary stage, when the mentioned associative play is sufficiently established and can be reproduced at will.
>
> —*Albert Einstein, 1945*

Although there is no guarantee that Albert Einstein would have made as good a psychologist as he made a physicist, let's assume that he was correct in his introspection that imagery comes before language-based thoughts. After all, if thoughts were based on language, why would we ever have trouble putting our thoughts into words? In this chapter I want to focus on the ways images can vary; not just visual images, but motoric as well.

The brain evolved in the service of basic needs of survival: the organism needed to be able to eat and survive long enough to find a mate and reproduce. Perceptual and motor systems play major roles in these most basic games of life. Indeed, systems that subserve perception and motor abilities are present even in the most primitive single-cell organisms. I argue that once the mechanisms were in place to register the environment and to program appropriate responses, these mechanisms could be used for other things—in particular, imagery. This is an example of what Gould and Lewontin (1979) called an "exaptation." By analogy, our noses evolved to warm air, direct scents, and so on. But once you've got a nose, you can use it to hold up glasses. Similarly, once you've got perceptual and motor systems, you can use them in thinking.

An understanding of imagery, then, would lend insight into the nature of our fundamental mental processes. We will look first, therefore, at a theory of imagery processing that is consistent with much data (see Kosslyn, 1994). Next we consider some of the distinct ways in which this system can operate, and finally we explore a few of the implications of these modes of operation.

A Modular View

Perhaps the most striking advance of contemporary cognitive science and cognitive neuroscience is the differentiation of mental faculties. Virtually all faculties that we name with a single word, such as memory, language, perception, and imagery, have turned out not to be a single "thing" but, rather, to have a complex underlying structure. The theory of imagery I summarize here is built on a theory of visual object identification and motor control. The theory posits a set of subsystems, each of which performs one part of the complete information-processing task. The subsystems are outlined in Figure 16.1, and briefly summarized below.

Visual Buffer

One of the most striking things about imagery is the sense that objects are extended in space. Part of the reason for this, I claim, is that images occur in a structure I call the visual buffer. The visual buffer corresponds to a set of retinotopically mapped areas in the occipital lobe (for example, see Van Essen, 1985; Felleman and Van Essen, 1991). The earliest (that is, the first to receive input from the eyes) cortical structure is area 17, followed by area 18. These structures represent spatial variations with high resolution; other areas, which extend up into the occipital-temporal junction, represent shapes with lower resolution (for example, Van Essen, 1985). According to the theory, a visual mental image is a pattern of activation in the visual buffer that is imposed from stored information, not on-line perception.

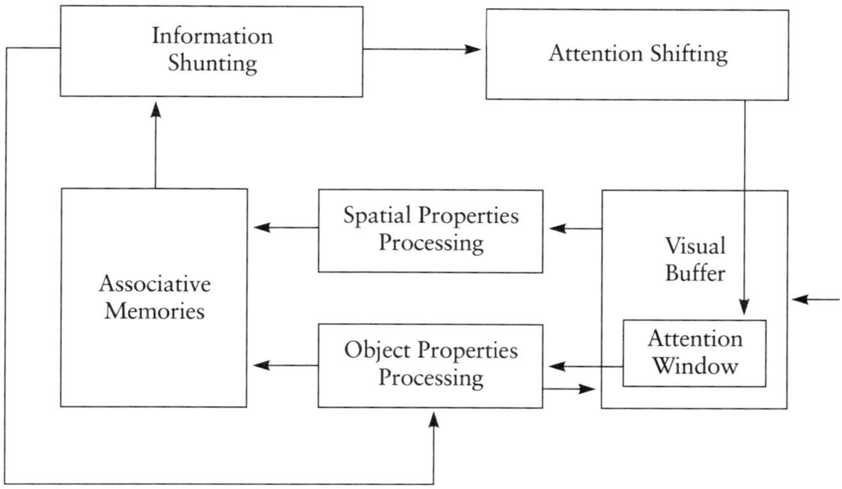

Figure 16.1. Functions used in late visual perception and visual imagery.

Attention Window

There is much more information in the visual buffer than can be processed in detail. Attention is the selective aspect of information processing, and one of its mechanisms is an "attention window." This mechanism selects a region of the visual buffer for further processing (Treisman and Gelade, 1980; Cave and Kosslyn, 1989; Posner and Petersen, 1990). One can scan over images, or focus on parts, during both imagery and perception in part by adjusting the attention window.

Object-Properties Processing

Two major neural pathways lead from the occipital regions that implement the visual buffer. One runs down to the lower portions of the temporal lobe, and is involved in visual recognition. These areas store visual memories and play crucial roles in both visual recognition and visual imagery (for example, Ungerleider and Mishkin, 1982; Mishkin, Ungerleider, and Macko, 1983; for review, see Kosslyn, 1994). During the process of visual recognition, input is compared with stored visual memories, and if a match is found the stimulus is recognized (Haxby et al., 1991; Sergent, Ohta, and MacDonald, 1992; Kosslyn, 1994). In imagery, stored visual representations are activated, forming the basis for constructing a visual image in the visual buffer (see Kosslyn, Thompson and Alpert, 1997). Critically, pathways run backward from the temporal lobe areas involved in visual memory to the occipital areas that make up the visual buffer (for example, Van Essen, 1985; Douglas and Rockland, 1992). These connections allow stored information to be used to reconstruct a shape.

Spatial-Properties Processing

The other major pathway leading from the occipital lobe runs up to the rear portions of the parietal lobes (Ungerleider and Mishkin, 1982). These areas are involved in registering spatial properties of stimuli during perception, such as the location and size of an object (for example, Andersen, 1987). Moreover, these mechanisms play a special role in guiding movements (Goodale and Milner, 1992) and also represent a "map" of the locations of objects in space (Mesulam, 1990). Processing in these regions plays three roles in imagery: first, such processing can register previously unnoticed aspects of imaged objects (for example, as will probably occur if you try to decide in which hand the Statue of Liberty holds the torch). Second, spatial information can be used to amalgamate two or more parts or objects into a single image (of a complex object or scene). And third, one can form "spatial images" by setting up locations and spatial properties of named objects, without needing to represent shape in the image. For example, if you look at a tiled floor, you can probably "see" shapes (such as letters of the alphabet) even though all you are doing is picking out which tiles to pay attention to at the same time. This task requires spatial organization and relies in part on parietal mechanisms.

Associative Memory

The *recognition* of shape is sometimes not enough to *identify* an object; recognition takes place when visual input matches a stored visual representation in the object-properties-processing subsystem, but all you get out of this is a feeling of familiarity. Identification occurs when you know the name of the object, categories to which it belongs, common contexts in which it occurs, and the rest of the wealth of information associated with it. The feeling of "knowing that face" but having no idea who it is occurs when one recognizes but doesn't identify. Identification takes place when the appropriate representation is activated in associative memory, which cross-indexes various sorts of information. As is evident in Figure 16.1, the output from both the object-properties-processing and the spatial-properties-processing subsystems converge on associative memory. Sometimes a black cat is only a black cat and sometimes it is a black panther; a major difference is that panthers tend to be larger (a spatial property) than black cats. The information in associative memory is used during perception to guide the visual search for additional information about a stimulus and is used in imagery to construct images of objects from parts. I assume that associative memory stores descriptions of how parts are arranged to form an object, or where high-resolution details belong on objects; this information is used to guide the construction of images, as noted below.

My colleagues and I have reported evidence that long-term associative memory is implemented in the angular gyrus area 19 (for example, see Kosslyn, Thompson, and Alpert, 1995). In addition, the dorsolateral prefrontal cortex appears to store a short-term associative memory structure, where shape and object properties are "held on-line" in perception, so that one can make decisions about the input (see Goldman-Rakic, 1987; Rao, Rainer, and Miller, 1997; Smith and Jonides, 1999). This buffer also plays a role in the process of setting up an image from parts, if the parts need to be arranged in a novel way.

Information Shunting

In perception, the information-shunting subsystem registers the most highly activated representation in associative memory. If an object cannot be immediately identified, the most highly activated representation in associative memory is used to guide one to examine potentially important aspects of the stimulus. In this case, the corresponding object is treated as a hypothesis about what the stimulus may be. The information-shunting subsystem uses this information in two ways: first, it sends information about location to the mechanisms that shift attention, leading them to focus on the location where a salient part or characteristic should be present; and second, the specification of the identity of the part or characteristic is used to "prime" the corresponding visual representation in the object-properties-processing subsystem. I call this sort of priming *anticipatory priming* because one is anticipating seeing a particular shape or characteristic. For example, if you see an apple and think it might be a Delicious apple, you might look up the fact (in associative memory) that Delicious apples have little bumps on the bottom. This information in turn would lead you to look at that location, while at the same time priming you to see the bumps.

In perception, anticipatory priming makes it easier for one to encode an expected part or characteristic. In imagery, anticipatory priming is carried to an extreme, forcing a pattern of activation in the visual buffer, which is the representation of the image itself. That is, one anticipates seeing something so strongly that one actually does see it (compare Neisser, 1976). The information-shunting subsystem is implemented in dorsolateral prefrontal cortex (DLPFC) (for example, Damasio, 1985; Luria, 1980; see also Kosslyn, Thompson, and Alpert, 1995).

Attention Shifting

Finally, another subsystem actually causes attention to shift to a new location. In both perception and imagery, these mechanisms allow one to focus on a specific part or characteristic. This subsystem is remarkably complex, and relies on a host of areas, including those that implement voluntary control of attention shifting (for example, the frontal eye fields), disengaging attention from its current location (superior parietal lobes), actually shifting the eyes, head, and body (as well as the attention window) to a new location (superior colliculus), and engaging attention at a new location (which relies on the thalamus; for example, see Posner and Petersen, 1990).

In perception, once one has shifted attention a new part or characteristic is encoded, which may be recognized and identified. Encoding the new part or characteristic may be enough to identify the object as a whole. In imagery, the same mechanisms are used to scan over imaged objects and add details. In this case, when one has focused on a particular location, a new part or characteristic is added (via the priming mechanism). For example, if asked to visualize a cat, one probably visualizes an overall shape, with relatively low resolution. If then asked whether the front claws are curved, one probably scans to that part and then "zooms in" (increases the visual angle of the part) and adds the claws to the image, and then categorizes their shape. The claws were not part of the image until one was asked about them (for evidence, see Kosslyn, 1980). Once the image is formed in the visual buffer, it can be "inspected" using the object-properties-processing and spatial-properties-processing mechanisms as they are used during perception, except that the image is very short lived.

Image Transformations

Not only do images of objects seem less vivid than percepts of objects (typically, but there are exceptions; for example, Perky, 1910), but they also can be modified at will. One can add or delete parts, as well as imagine the object expanded, shrunken, stretched, rotated, and so on (Shepard and Cooper, 1982). According to the theory I've developed (Kosslyn, 1994), objects in images can be transformed in two general ways. In one, the motor system plays a key role. Such image transformations occur when one *anticipates* what one will see if one manipulates an object in some way. This anticipation modulates the mapping function from the object-properties-processing subsystem to the visual buffer. In the other method, one anticipates what one would see if someone (or something) else manipulated an object. In this case, the motor system is not directly involved in modulating the mapping function, but rather one relies on memories of previous events to form the anticipation (see Kosslyn, 1994).

Modes of Operation

The flowchart of Figure 16.1 might seem to imply a rigid order of processing, akin to that in a computer. However, the system clearly operates differently in different circumstances. Figure 16.1 suggests ways to think about these differences.

Stored Information

First, if images are often built up a part at a time on the basis of information stored in associative memory (Kosslyn, 1980), one can ask what sort of information is stored to specify how the parts are to be arranged. Kosslyn et al. (1989) provided evidence that two kinds of spatial relations can be encoded. *Categorical* spatial relations (such as above/below, left/right, on/off) specify categories of relations, whereas *coordinate* spatial relations specify metric distance from an origin. This and other research (for example, Hellige and Michimata, 1989; Laeng, 1994; for review, see Chabris and Kosslyn, 1998) has shown that the left cerebral hemisphere encodes categorical spatial relations better than the right, whereas the right cerebral hemisphere encodes coordinate spatial relations better than the left.

Kosslyn et al. (1995a) reasoned that if the two kinds of representations could be encoded, then they should also be stored. If so, then when one later constructs mental images, it should be possible to arrange the parts in two ways: using either categorical or coordinate spatial relations. Kosslyn et al. (1995a) provided behavioral evidence for this, but we have provided much more compelling evidence in recent neuroimaging work. In this study, subjects memorized figures in one of two ways before the study proper. In one condition, they memorized a verbal description of how segments were arranged to form a novel shape. This method forced them to encode and store categorical spatial relations. In another condition, they saw segments one at a time within a frame, and were to "mentally glue" them together to form a single novel shape. This method forced them to encode and store coordinate spatial relations.

The subjects' brains were then scanned as they visualized each complete form as if it were within a set of four corner brackets (which defined a rectangular space), and decided whether an X mark would have fallen on or off the form. In this task, the left hemisphere was more strongly activated if the form had been learned via a description, whereas the right was more activated if it had been learned by memorizing the precise positions of segments. The same shapes were visualized equally often in the two ways, and thus the differences had nothing to do with the final images themselves. The conclusion I want to draw from this is straightforward: depending on the information stored in memory, the brain uses different techniques to form images.

Task Requirements

In Figure 16.1, the information-shunting subsystem looks up stored descriptions, which guide the system to begin forming an image and to flesh out details of the imaged object. But what determines how much detail is added? Consider a study in which the task required the subjects to visualize objects with high resolution. Kosslyn et al. (1995b) asked people to memorize line drawings of common objects. Later, they were to close their eyes and listen to stimuli such as "guitar . . . right higher." These stimuli cued them to visualize a particular drawing, and then to wait for a question; the question required them to classify the shape in some way (such as by deciding whether the right side was higher than the left). In this study, the subjects visualized the drawings at three different sizes (very small, medium, or large). In a control condition, the same auditory cues were presented, but the subject was not to visualize objects (this condition was presented first, before the subjects had seen the drawings or knew about the imagery task). The results showed that not only did area 17 become more activated during the imagery task than during the baseline task, but the precise location of the activation in area 17 depended on the size of the image: as occurs in vision, objects seen at smaller sizes activated more posterior portions of area 17.

These results are in striking contrast to those reported by Mellet et al. (1996), who asked subjects to listen to sets of directions. The directions indicated how cubes were to be arranged into shapes. Brain activation during this task was compared with activation in a control task in which subjects listened to abstract words (which sounded like the directions). No judgments were required, but the imagery task clearly did not require visualizing detailed shapes. In this task, there was activation not of area 17 but, rather, of higher-level areas in the inferior temporal lobe and areas in the parietal lobe (among other areas). The task required only imagery of sequences of locations, and hence did not recruit areas implementing the visual buffer. A later study, Mellet et al. (2000), required high-resolution mental images in order to make judgments about the relative heights of geometric forms arranged along a bar—but did not require visualizing detailed shapes. No area 17 activation was found here. In contrast, in another subsequent study, Klein et al. (2000), area 17 was activated whenever images of animals were visualized from long-term memory.

The contrast between these results was captured by meta-analyses we have conducted (Kosslyn and Thompson, 1999; Thompson and

Kosslyn, 2000), which showed that area 17 is activated in studies that required the subjects to visualize parts of objects with high resolution, but not in studies that did not require them to "see" parts with high resolution. In short, the task requirements appear to affect which brain areas are involved in imagery.

Strategy

According to the theory summarized in Figure 16.1, mental image transformations can be accomplished in two general ways: one either visualizes what one would see if one performed an action, or one visualizes what one would see if someone else performed the action. In the former case, motor processes should be involved. To examine this hypothesis, Kosslyn et al. (1998) asked people to participate in two types of mental rotation tasks. One was the classic Shepard and Metzler (1971) task, in which subjects see pairs of three-armed angular shapes, which are identical or mirror-images. In the test condition, the shapes are presented at different relative orientations, and the subjects are asked to decide whether the shapes are identical or mirror-images. We compared brain activation in this condition to that in a baseline condition, which was identical to the test condition except that the shapes in each pair were always presented at the same orientation. The second mental rotation task required the subjects to rotate images of drawings of pairs of hands. In these conditions, the task was to decide whether each pair had pictures of the same hand (both left, or both right), or whether a left and right hand were present. Again, in the test condition the stimuli were presented at different relative orientations, whereas in the baseline condition they were presented at the same orientation.

In our publication, we reported that motor processes were used for hands, but not for the Shepard and Metzler stimuli; this finding provided support for the idea that there are two distinct ways to imagine objects rotating. Further analyses and additional experimentation have revealed what I believe are more interesting results. Each person did both types of rotation, with half receiving the hands before the Shepard and Metzler task, and vice versa for the other half. When the Shepard and Metzler task came first, we found activation in inferior parietal and dorsolateral prefrontal cortex, as well as in the right angular gyrus. These results were in sharp contrast to those obtained when this same task followed the hands task: now we found activation in over ten areas, many of which are involved in motor control. Indeed, we found activation in area M1, primary motor cortex. These results for the Shepard and Metzler task were in many ways more similar to what we found in the hands rotation task than to what we found when the same task was presented at the outset. We later extended this study, and the results remained solid. Apparently, the subjects imagined moving their own hands in the hand rotation task (as has previously been found; for example, see Parsons et al., 1995), and continued to use a motor-based strategy for the Shepard and Metzler task (imagining what they would see if they physically twisted the objects) if it followed on the heels of the hands task. In short, we had evidence that very different strategies could be used for the same task.

In addition, in a more recent study (Kosslyn et al., 2001) we asked whether these two strategies are under voluntary control. In this study, before neuroimaging the participants watched Shepard-Metzler stimuli being rotated in one of two ways. In one condition, they viewed an electric motor rotating a wooden model of a Shepard-Metzler object; in the other condition, they grasped the model and physically rotated it. Following this, they participated in the standard mental rotation task, but were asked to visualize the figures rotating as they had just seen the model rotate. We found that motor cortex was activated when they imagined the rotations as if they were physically turning the objects, but not when they imagined an electric motor rotating the objects. Clearly, the two strategies could be adopted at will.

Emotion

It has long been fashionable to view emotion as distinct from cognition (for a review, see LeDoux, 1996). Kosslyn and Koenig (1995) develop a different view, in which emotion is seen as a mechanism that primes some specific goals and processes while at the same time inhibiting other goals and processes. For example, to "like" an object typically means that one wants to approach it, protect it, and so on; in contrast, to "dislike" an object means that such goals—and the processes that will help accomplish them—are inhibited, and other goals and processes are primed (such as those involved in avoiding it). Kosslyn et al. (1996) studied the effects of negative emotion on imagery. In one condition, subjects began by memorizing a set of aversive pictures, such as a picture of a baby with a large tumor growing out of one eye and a picture of a battered woman; these pictures were taken from Lang and Greenwald's (1988) set of stimuli, which had previously been validated as producing an emotional response. In another condition, subjects began by memorizing a set of neutral pictures, such as a truck and a lamp. In both conditions, the subjects' brains were scanned as they closed their eyes and heard the names of each picture in the set. After each name, they were to visualize the object and hold the image until the computer read a statement aloud, such as "The tumor is over the right eye." The subject had to decide whether the statement was true or false.

My colleagues and I found a number of areas to be activated when one visualized aversive stimuli, including a region in dorsolateral prefrontal cortex. However, this region was not the same as that found in the previous experiments. We also found more activation in areas 17 and 18 when one visualized aversive stimuli than when one visualized neutral stimuli. Moreover, we found that aversive emotion produced activation in additional regions, most particularly the anterior insula—which is known to be the major cortical site that receives input from the autonomic nervous system. The emotional content clearly recruited new areas, and seemed to modulate activity in previously observed areas.

Modules Reconsidered

The subsystems that produce and use images operate differently in at least four circumstances: if one has encoded different information, has different task requirements, adopts a particular strategy, or the material has emotional content. It turns out that Einstein probably would have made a decent psychologist after all; as he reported (in this chapter's epigraph and elsewhere), images can be visual (with high or low resolution), spatial, or motoric.

If you looked at the overlap in areas activated during our various imagery experiments, a large portion of the brain would turn out to be involved in imagery. These findings can be interpreted in two ways. First, it is possible that there are many highly specialized processors, and different ones are recruited in different circumstances. If so, then it should be possible to identify very specific coordinates in the brain with very specific processes. I myself doubt that this will come to pass, except in the earliest perceptual and motor areas. Second, a more intriguing possibility is that many of the modules are not predefined. Rather, depending on the information that was encoded, on the requirements of the task, and on the strategy that was adopted, different "modules" are created on the spot. On this view, *what the brain does depends on what the organism wants.* For present purposes, we can take the boxes in Figure 16.1 as functional descriptions of operations the brain performs during visual mental imagery and late visual perception, not as hard-wired functions that are determined by the genes. Indeed, in a recent review of the literature on brain development, Huttenlocher (2002) summarizes evidence that only a minority of brain circuits are defined by the genes; the rest are initially configured randomly, and only via experience are specific circuits formed. I am going one step further here, suggesting that in the adult brain at least some of these circuits are "general purpose" and that the pattern of activity within them defines different modules in different circumstances (functionally, not structurally—the connections themselves are not changed, only the patterning within them).

The notion that modules are created as needed would explain why the precise locations of activation in dorsolateral prefrontal cortex during imagery, for example, vary so much from experiment to experiment. Indeed, Bly and Kosslyn (1997) reviewed the neuroimaging literature on activation of inferotemporal cortex during object recognition, and found that activation had been observed in a very wide range of loci even in such basic tasks.

Why does it matter whether modules are predefined or created as needed? At least three general reasons come to mind. First, if modules are created as needed rather than predefined (like special registers in a computer), then we will never be able to catalog them all and should stop trying to do so. Second, if modules are created as needed, then we should focus on the principles that lead to their definition. Surely the wiring constrains the possibilities, but in what ways? Finally, the current enthusiasm for "evolutionary psychology" (for example, Pinker, 1997) relies on the idea that modules have been produced via natural selection. If many modules for higher-level cognitive functions are not predefined by the genes, then this story will require modification.

Conclusion

The brain appears to have evolved using a strategy of "divide and conquer." Different parts of the brain do different things, and different parts work together to accomplish tasks. Moreover, depending on which processes work together, different strategies emerge. Even in a process as seemingly well defined as mental imagery, there clearly is more than one type and more than one way to accomplish the same ends. However, not all of the distinct processes may be predefined. It is possible that at least some "modules" are functionally defined only at the time they are required.

References

This report was supported by a grant from the Fogarty programs of the NIH and by NIH grant ROI-MH60734-01.

Andersen, R. A. 1987. Inferior parietal lobule function in spatial perception and visuomotor integration. In *Handbook of physiology,* Section 1: *The nervous system,* ed. V. B. Mountcastle. Volume 5: *Higher functions of the brain,* ed. F. Plum, 483–518. Bethesda, Md.: American Physiological Society.

Bly, B. M., and Kosslyn, S. M. 1997. Functional anatomy of object recognition in humans: Evidence from PET and fMRI. *Current Opinion in Neurology, 10,* 5–9.

Cave, K. R., and Kosslyn, S. M. 1989. Varieties of size-specific visual selection. *Journal of Experimental Psychology: General, 118,* 148–164.

Chabris, C. F., and Kosslyn, S. M. 1998. How do the cerebral hemispheres contribute to encoding spatial relations? *Current Directions in Psychological Science, 7,* 8–14.

Damasio, A. R. 1985. The frontal lobes. In *Clinical neuropsychology,* K. M. Heilman and E. Valenstein, 339–402. New York: Oxford University Press.

Douglas, K. L., and Rockland, K. S. 1992. Extensive visual feedback connections from ventral inferotemporal cortex. *Society of Neuroscience Abstracts, 18,* 390.

Einstein, A. 1945. A testimonial from Professor Einstein (Appendix II). In *An essay on the psychology of invention in the mathematical field,* ed. J. Hadamard, 142–143. Princeton: Princeton University Press.

Felleman, D. J., and Van Essen, D. C. 1991. Distributed hierarchical processing in primate cerebral cortex. *Cerebral Cortex, 1,* 1–47.

Goldman-Rakic, P. S. 1987. Circuitry of primate prefrontal cortex and regulation of behavior by representational knowledge. In *Handbook of Physiology,* Section 1: *The nervous system,* ed. V. B. Mountcastle, Volume 5: *Higher functions of the brain,* ed. F. Plum. Bethesda, Md.: American Physiological Society.

Goodale, M. A., and Milner, A. D. 1992. Separate visual pathways for perception and action. *Trends in Neurosciences, 15* (1), 20–25.

Gould, S. J., and Lewontin, R. C. 1979. The spandrels of San Marco and the Panglossian paradigm: A critique of the adaptationist programme. *Proceedings of the Royal Society of London, Series B, 205,* 581–598.

Haxby, J. V., Grady, C. L., Horwitz, B., Ungerleider, L. G., Mishkin, M., Carson, R. E., Herscovitch, P., Schapiro, M. B., and Rapoport, S. I. 1991. Dissociation of object and spatial visual processing pathways in human extrastriate cortex. *Proceedings of the National Academy of Sciences of the United States of America, 88,* 1621–1625.

Hellige, J. B., and Michimata, C. 1989. Categorization versus distance: Hemispheric differences for processing spatial information. *Memory and Cognition, 17,* 770–776.

Huttenlocher, P. 2002. *Neural plasticity.* Cambridge: Harvard University Press.

Klein, I., Paradis, A.-L., Poline, J.-B., Kosslyn, S. M., and Le Bihan, D. 2000. Transient activity in human calcarine cortex during visual imagery. *Journal of Cognitive Neuroscience, 12,* 15S–23S.

Kosslyn, S. M. 1980. *Image and mind.* Cambridge: Harvard University Press.

——— 1994. *Image and brain: The resolution of the imagery debate.* Cambridge: MIT Press.

Kosslyn, S. M., DiGirolamo, G. J., Thompson, W. L., and Alpert, N. M. 1998. Mental rotation of objects versus hands: Neural mechanisms revealed by positron emission tomography. *Psychophysiology, 35,* 1–11.

Kosslyn, S. M., and Koenig, O. 1995. *Wet mind: The new cognitive neuroscience.* New York: Free Press.

Kosslyn, S. M., Koenig, O., Barrett, A., Cave, C. B., Tang, J., and Gabrieli, J. D. E. 1989. Evidence for two types of spatial representations: Hemispheric specialization for categorical and coordinate relations. *Journal of Experimental Psychology: Human Perception and Performance, 15,* 723–735.

Kosslyn, S. M., Maljkovic, V., Hamilton, S. E., Horwitz, G., and Thompson, W. L. 1995a. Two types of image generation: Evidence for left- and right-hemisphere processes. *Neuropsychologia, 33,* 1485–1510.

Kosslyn, S. M., Shin, L. M., Thompson, W. L., McNally, R. J., Rauch, S. L., Pitman, R. K., and Alpert, N. M. 1996. Neural effects of visualizing and perceiving aversive stimuli: A PET investigation. *NeuroReport, 7,* 1569–1576.

Kosslyn, S. M., and Thompson, W. L. 1999. Shared mechanisms in visual imagery and visual perception: Insights from cognitive neuroscience. In *Handbook of Cognitive Neuroscience,* 2d ed., ed. M. S. Gazzaniga. Cambridge: MIT Press.

Kosslyn, S. M., Thompson, W. L., and Alpert, N. M. 1995. Identifying objects at different levels of hierarchy: A positron emission tomography study. *Human Brain Mapping, 3,* 107–132.

——— 1997. Neural systems shared by visual imagery and visual perception: A positron emission tomography study. *NeuroImage, 6,* 320–334.

Kosslyn, S. M., Thompson, W. L., Kim, I. J., and Alpert, N. M. 1995b. Topographical representations of mental images in primary visual cortex. *Nature, 378,* 496–498.

Kosslyn, S. M., Thompson, W. L., Wraga, M. J., and Alpert, N. M. 2001. Imagining rotation by endogenous and exogenous forces: Distinct neural mechanisms for different strategies. *NeuroReport, 12,* 2519–2525.

Laeng, B. 1994. Lateralization of categorical and coordinate spatial functions: A study of unilateral stroke patients. *Journal of Cognitive Neuroscience, 6,* 189–203.

Lang, P. J., and Greenwald, M. K. 1988. The International Affective Picture System standardization procedure and initial group results for affective judgments. *Technical report 1A.* Gainesville, Fla.: Center for Research in Psychophysiology, University of Florida.

LeDoux, J. 1996. *The emotional brain.* New York: Simon and Schuster.

Luria, A. R. 1980. *Higher cortical functions in man.* New York: Basic Books.

Mellet, E., Tzourio, N., Crivello, F., Joliot, M., Denis, M., and Mazoyer, B. 1996. Functional anatomy of spatial mental imagery generated from verbal instructions. *Journal of Neuroscience, 16,* 6504–6512.

Mellet, E. M., Tzourio-Mazoyer, N., Bricogne, S., Mazoyer, B., Kosslyn, S. M., and Denis, M. 2000. Functional anatomy of high resolution visual mental imagery. *Journal of Cognitive Neuroscience, 12,* 98–109.

Mesulam, M.-M. 1990. Large-scale neurocognitive networks and distributed processing for attention, language, and memory. *Annals of Neurology, 28,* 597–613.

Mishkin, M., Ungerleider, L. G., and Macko, K. A. 1983. Object vision and spatial vision: Two cortical pathways. *Trends in Neurosciences,* 6(10), 414–417.

Neisser, U. 1976. *Cognition and reality.* San Francisco: W. H. Freeman.

Parsons, L. M., Fox, P. T., Downs, J. H., Glass, T., Hirsch, T. B., Martin, C. C., Jerabek, P. A., and Lancaster, J. L. 1995. Use of implicit motor imagery for visual shape discrimination as revealed by PET. *Nature, 375,* 54–58.

Perky, C. W. 1910. An experimental study of imagination. *American Journal of Psychology, 21,* 422–452.

Pinker, S. 1997. *How the mind works.* New York: W. W. Norton.

Posner, M. I., and Petersen, S. E. 1990. The attention system of the human brain. In *Annual Review of Neuroscience,* ed. W. M. Cowan, E. M. Shooter, C. F. Stevens, and R. F. Thompson, 25–42. Palo Alto, Calif.: Annual Reviews.

Rao, S. C., Rainer, G., and Miller, E. K. 1997. Integration of what and where in the primate prefrontal cortex. *Science, 276,* 821–824.

Sergent, J., Ohta, S., and MacDonald, B. 1992. Functional neuroanatomy of face and object processing: A positron emission tomography study. *Brain, 115,* 15–36.

Shepard, R. N., and Cooper, L. R. 1982. *Mental images and their transformations.* Cambridge: MIT Press.

Shepard, R. N., and Metzler, J. 1971. Mental rotation of three-dimensional objects. *Science, 171,* 701–703.

Smith, E. E., and Jonides, J. 1999. Storage and executive processes in the frontal lobes. *Science, 283,* 1657–1661.

Thompson, W. L., and Kosslyn, S. M. 2000. Neural systems activated during visual mental imagery: A review and meta-analyses. In *Brain mapping II: The systems,* ed. A. W. Toga and J. C. Mazziotta, 535–560. San Diego: Academic Press.

Treisman, A. M., and Gelade, G. 1980. A feature integration theory of attention. *Cognitive Psychology, 12,* 97–136.

Ungerleider, L. G., and Mishkin, M. 1982. Two cortical visual systems. In *Analysis of visual behavior,* ed. D. J. Ingle, M. A. Goodale, and R. J. W. Mansfield. Cambridge: MIT Press.

Van Essen, D. C. 1985. Functional organization of primate visual cortex. In *Cerebral cortex,* ed. A. Peters and E. G. Jones. New York: Plenum Press.

Spatial Memory during Navigation: What Is Being Stored, Maps or Movements?

17

Alain Berthoz, Isabelle Viaud-Delmon,
and Simon Lambrey

It has been known since the time of the pre-Socratic Greeks that the brain uses memory of environmental space, such as cities or palaces, to store words, events, or eventually objects. This memory of space includes a process of *mental navigation* through memorized cities, palaces, houses, and so on in order to retrieve these important elements of language or objects. To perform this interaction between memory and space, the brain can use several types of spatial knowledge.

For instance, we can remember the route we followed from the door of a hotel to a conference room or from our house to our office by two ways, as proposed by Tolman (1948). One, which we shall call a "route strategy," would be to remember the turns, the movements, and the associated landmarks that we make when we navigate along the route (Amorim et al. 1997). The other, which we shall call a "survey strategy," would consist in evoking a map of the environment (the hotel or the city) and looking down mentally "from above" on this map of the route (Mellet et al. 1995). According to a recent study (Mellet et al. 2000), the "route" and "survey" strategies would have some neural correlates in common, but would also imply specific neural structures.

A third hypothesis has been proposed which, by contrast with a "route strategy" or a "survey strategy," we could name an "architectural strategy," a concept supported by the observation that when we think about the building in which we are working, for instance, and try to imagine the office of a colleague, we have a kind of transparent inner perception of the building that, keeping only in mind only the structure, crosses walls as if we were in a glass building (Thorndyke and Hayes-Roth, 1982).

The survey strategy, which is to mentally view or make a propositional description of a map, is indeed used particularly when we want to think about long distances. It has been the subject of many imagery studies. The theory proposed by O'Keefe and Nadel (1978) suggests that the hippocampus is a crucial area of the brain involved in this kind of performance, because it is the location of a "cognitive map." This concept is challenged by other authors, however. Recent evidence (Hermer and Spelke, 1994; Epstein and Kanwisher, 1998) suggests indeed that there are geometrical modules in the brain, which may actually be located in the para-hippocampus, according to the latter study. A clear dissociation has been found between these different strategies ("route" versus "survey") in patients with brain lesions. Several studies have demonstrated the impairment in the topographic memory, and a dissociation has been claimed between the (a) the ability to recognize familiar landmarks (Whiteley and Warrington, 1978; Incisa della Rocchetta, Cipolotti, and Warrington, 1996), sometimes leaving the capacity to describe well-known routes relatively intact, and (b) the ability to describe routes with recognition of landmarks relatively unaffected (Pallis, 1955; Paterson, 1994). Sometimes patients can also describe routes and recognize landmarks but they still lose their way because landmarks no longer convey directional information (Hécaen, Tzortzis, and Rondot, 1980). The hippocampus is not necessarily the only area involved in these spatial memory deficits; Habib (1987) has shown that the lesions in their patients with topographic memory loss were restricted to the para-hippocampus and the subiculum but not extending to the hippocampus. By contrast patient R.B., who had a severe anterograde amnesia following selective damage to the hippocampus, did not report getting lost in his neighborhood (Zola-Morgan, Squire, and Amaral 1986).

The patient studied by Incisa della Rocchetta, Cipolotti, and Warrington (1996) had a severe deficit in describing familiar routes in her environment but no difficulty in identifying countries from outline maps and in naming a city within a country when it was identified by a dot. Both episodic and semantic memory was impaired in this patient. The suggestion is that this patient has a specific deficit for category-specific knowledge of inanimate objects (hills, buildings, and so on). There seems to be a specific coding of topographic objects distinct from other classes of object and a separation between the objects that require locomotion to reach them, and other objects.

One should therefore be careful before ascribing to any particular area or to the cortex a crucial role in spatial memory. It seems more likely that this function is distributed in several areas, implying that each makes a distinct contribution. For example, the frontal cortex seems to be involved in visual spatial memory (Courtney et al. 1996) and in mental recall of complex environments (Guariglia et al. 1993).

We will consider here mainly what we have called the "route" strategy. We believe that the mental simulation of one's movement in space during navigation is a fundamental component of the cognitive foundations of geometry. Henri Poincaré, the great mathematician, wrote that "to localize a point in space is simply to represent the movement which has to be made to reach it." He continues: "When I say that we represent the movement, I mean to represent the *muscular sensations* which are associated with this movement which have no geometrical character, and therefore do not suppose a preexisting representation of space" (1970, p. 67). Therefore, Poincaré proposed that the basic origin of geometry and of our representation of space is motor function and action. Einstein approved this view, which has been criticized by logicians like Hilbert and by the theories that have formalized logic and dominated mathematics in the last three or four decades. We need to rehabilitate the views of Poincaré and Einstein (Berthoz 1997, 1998). We have to reinsert the "body in action" in the theories concerning the representation of space and keep in mind that movement is a language of the brain even in the representation of space.

With Droulez (1990, 1991), we have proposed the idea that the brain actually does not represent space solely in so-called spatiotopic maps. In order to control goal-oriented movements, the brain may use a process of *dynamic remapping,* employing a "dynamic memory" mechanism, which actually consists in permanently updating the location of visually evoked activity on the map by "reentering" feedback or corollary signals from the motor output stages. According to this theory, the brain does not need to reconstruct a representation of space in spatial coordinates to control a saccade, a hand reaching, or a locomotor pointing task, because the movement feedback (eye velocity, for example) will reorganize the sensory maps and automatically bring the eye on target. We have tried to test this hypothesis of a dynamic memory mechanism by several psychophysical methods during navigation tasks designed to study *movement memory*.

Previous Results Suggesting Dynamic Memory of Movement during Navigation

Comparison of the Brain Areas Activated by Mental Route Strategy and Mental Map Exploration

Brain areas activated during a route memory task. The first experiment was designed to study the differences in the areas of the brain that are activated during route memory and map memory, respectively. The details of the experiments are given in Ghaem et al. (1997), and we shall therefore only summarize the main features of this task.

Subjects were driven to a totally unfamiliar urban environment and were asked to walk along a previously selected route about 800 meters long. The subjects walked the route three times and were asked to remember it and, in particular, seven prominent visual landmarks (tower, gas station, public telephone, and so on). The first two times they were guided by the experimenter and the third time they walked under supervision. The time of locomotion was recorded from landmark to landmark. The day after this learning session and four to six hours before the PET (positron emission tomography) session, the subjects executed two tasks, which were repeated in the PET:

- A mental simulation of routes task. The subject was instructed verbally to indicate the name of two landmarks, chosen by the experimenter, between which he was supposed to walk mentally while sitting in total darkness. The subject pressed a button upon mentally arriving at the second landmark, and the sequence was

repeated with another set of two landmarks. This allowed us to measure the mental locomotion time and compare it with the previously recorded actual time in the real environment.
- A visual imagery of landmarks task. The subject was instructed to mentally visualize a landmark and keep it in memory upon hearing its name through the earphones.

The results indicate, first, that there was a strong correlation between the real time of locomotion in the city and the time needed to walk mentally, in total darkness, between two segments during both the training session and the PET session. This correlation suggested that the subjects were indeed doing the required task. During the tasks performed in total darkness, the following main areas were activated, in comparison with the rest condition. During the mental simulation of routes task, there was bilateral activation of the dorsolateral cortex, posterior hippocampal areas, posterior cingulate gyrus, supplementary motor area; right middle hippocampal areas; left precuneus, middle occipital gyrus, fusiform gyrus, lateral premotor area. During the visual imagery of landmarks task, there was bilateral activation of the middle hippocampal regions; left inferior temporal gyrus, left posterior hippocampal regions, precentral gyrus; right posterior cingulate gyrus. When these two conditions were subtracted (mental simulation of routes minus visual imagery of landmarks) only activation of the left hippocampal regions, precuneus, and insula was significant.

The activation seen in the hippocampal areas is important, because it was not activated in previous studies addressing the question of spatial memory using a "delay-matched-to-sample" memory task concerning the location of objects (Aguirre et al., 1996; Maguire, Frackowiak, and Frith, 1996; Ghaem et al., 1996). The activation of the insula may also have been related to the fact that subjects had to remember the turns of their body during the memorized locomotor task. Activation of the insula has been found during tasks requiring mental repositioning of the body with respect to external objects (Bonda et al., 1995).

Brain areas activated during mental exploration of a map. The second set of experiments concerned the mental exploration of an environment learned from a map (Ghaem et al., 1998). The main task involved mental exploration of a map that had been learned twenty-four hours before and scanning for the shortest route between two landmarks specified on the map (similar to the visual landmarks in the route task experiment described above). Three other tasks were performed by the subjects: (a) a rest condition; (b) visual imagery of landmarks, in which the subject had to visualize a landmark upon hearing its name; and (c) gaze and attention displacement in which the subjects, when hearing a landmark name, had to move their gaze from the center of the map to the imagined location of the landmark.

Several brain areas were activated by these tasks, but the main result is that the hippocampus was not activated, in contrast to the previous memorized-route task. In addition, several areas that had not been activated in the route experiment were found to be active in the map memory task.

These studies confirm the idea that there is a class of spatial memory that could be called "topokinetic" memory (Berthoz 1997), which involves several brain structures (parietal and parieto-insular cortex, insula, cingulate cortex, hippocampal formation, dorsolateral frontal cortex, and so on) involved in the processing of self-generated navigation. By topokinetic memory we mean a memory of the movements made during the navigation associated with a set of events or visual landmarks. This motor memory is akin to an ongoing episodic memory but is not limited to an episode. The self-generated nature of this memory is probably essential, as it has been shown that place cells, for instance, are only well specified when rats actually move in space. The limit of brain imagery, however, is that it does not provide any information about the nature of the neural processes that underlie memory. These can be studied by a psychophysical approach, and our laboratory has designed several new methods for this purpose. We shall here give only one example relevant to the problem of topokinetic memory.

Reproduction of Passively Imposed Linear Motion on a Mobile Robot

Subjects were placed on a computer-controlled mobile robot to reproduce a passively imposed movement (Berthoz et al., 1995). This robot could be passively moved forward by the computer and therefore impose on the subjects a passive linear translation. But subjects could also take control and move the robot with the help of a joystick, which controlled robot velocity. Subjects were seated on the robot with their eyes closed and therefore were without any visual cues concerning their motion. The robot would first move forward by a few meters (0 to 10 meters). This was the "imposed distance." After a few seconds during which subjects had to remember their displacement (memory period) they were asked to "reproduce" the traveled *distance* by controlling the robot's velocity forward with a joystick. They had to use vestibular information about their movement stored in spatial memory and somehow retrieve this information from memory to perform a distance task. Precautions were taken, such as taking the same traveling time for different distances, to ensure that subjects could not use time as a measure of distance. The reproduction was quite accurate.

The brain can therefore derive, from linear acceleration information (which is what is being measured by the vestibular receptors responsible for the detection of linear acceleration: the otoliths), some measure that allows the reproduction of distance. The more trivial explanation of this process is that there are, in the brain, mechanisms performing this "integration," in the mathematical sense, between acceleration and displacement. A value representing displacement would then be stored as a distance, retrieved during the reproduction task and compared with another integrated measure of displacement detected by the otoliths.

The more interesting question, however, is whether the brain really stores distances on "look-up tables" of numbers or whether what is being stored is *movement*. In other words, as Poincaré proposed, what is being stored may be the movement one has to make to go from one point in space to another, and not a Cartesian distance number. Indeed if we vary the velocity profile of the imposed passive movement during robot motion (for example, by changing the duration of acceleration and deceleration phases), subjects tend to reproduce the velocity profile as if what they had memorized was the velocity profile of the linear motion and not a distance per se. If this is the case, the fact that they reproduce distance is a secondary effect of an accurate reproduction of the velocity profile. Movement memory may be a crucial memory for distance reproduction.

A New Paradigm: Reproduction of Memorized Trajectory Following Navigation in a Virtual Corridor

We tried to overcome some of the limits of the passive displacement on robots by designing a new paradigm in order to study the nature of stored information during navigation. In addition, we have been interested in the integration of space-related multisensory information in anxious patients. Indeed, it has been shown that subjects with symptoms of panic and agoraphobia were destabilized by conflictual sensorial conditions while maintaining an upright posture (Yardley et al., 1994, 1995; Jacob, Redfern, and Furman, 1995; Jacob et al., 1996). It has then been hypothesized that dizziness symptomatology could be linked to a strategy for maintaining balance or orientation relying on visual dependence. Even if this hypothesis is not confirmed by all the studies (Jacob et al., 1997), an altered visual-vestibular interaction has often been demonstrated in anxious patients, illustrating the possible role of multisensorial integration in space-related anxiety disorders. We have developed a new paradigm in order to study the adaptation to incoherent visual-vestibular stimulation, in which subjects had to control their whole-body rotations with a joystick (Ivanenko et al., 1998; Viaud-Delmon et al., 1998, 1999). In the present experiment, we wanted to observe the effect of sensory conflict both on sensorimotor control and on the stored representation of a path.

The basic purpose of the experiment was then threefold: first, to build a device that can allow us to manipulate independently visual and idiothetic (vestibular, proprioceptive, and efferent motor commands) cues. Second, to avoid a purely passive navigation and involve the subject in an active process during the acquisition period. Third, to obtain a condition of recall of the memorized path allowing the objective measurement of output in order to compare the experienced navigation with the remembered one.

Experimental Setup

Subjects ($N = 20$) were seated on a rotating chair (a simple nonmotorized chair that could be turned by the subject like any office chair). Visual images were presented in a head-mounted visual display that had a monocular field of view of 48° by 36°. The orientation of the sub-

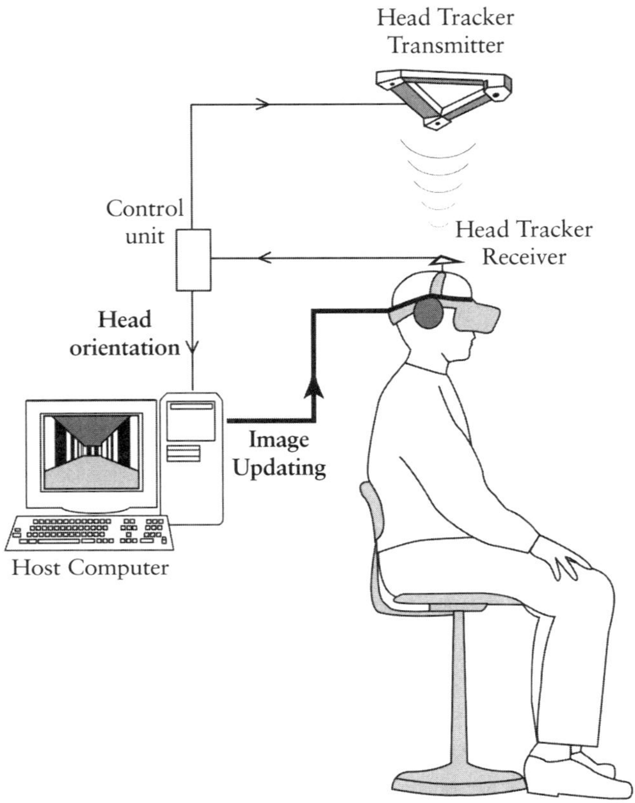

Figure 17.1. Experimental setup. The subject was seated on the chair, which he could rotate. He was immersed in a virtual environment by means of a head-mounted display. The subject's head direction was sensed by an ultrasound system. Custom-written software took the head angular position information from the tracker and output the corresponding visual image.

ject's head was sensed by an ultrasound tracker and computed by the software that output the corresponding image on the display. Visual images were thus coupled with the movements of the subject (Figure 17.1).

Subjects were first shown a virtual corridor and were passively advancing forward in this virtual world according to the linear velocity imposed by the computer. When the subject passively arrived at the end of a straight segment of virtual corridor, he had to negotiate a turn by rotating his head and body in the chair. The software did not allow subjects to cross the walls of the corridors, and therefore if a collision occurred, the trajectory slid along the walls.

The information concerning the horizontal angular displacements of the head during chair rotations was used to update the virtual images in the helmet through the computer graphics system, which generated the images. This was thus a "seated locomotion," in which the feet were still in charge of the rotations and the computer imposed the translations. This was the condition of "visual navigation."

Design of the Experiment

The subjects performed two tasks. In the "visual navigation" task the subjects could see the corridor and control their turns. They were instructed to control their direction, trying to go around corners as if they were in a real corridor, without coming too close to the walls and staying as close as possible to the middle of the corridor.

In a second task the subjects were asked to remember the previous "visual navigation" task and to reproduce the navigation in darkness without any visual cues, by imagining the trajectory. During the imagined linear segments they had to stay still in the chair, but when a turn was remembered they had to turn their body in the chair by the same amount as would have been necessary to update the computer in the previous case of visual navigation. This was the "memorized navigation" task.

The original quality of this paradigm is that it allows us to "see" what the subjects have stored in their brain by recording the movements on the chair. The angle of active rotation during mental turns gives an estimation of the accuracy with which rotations were measured, stored, and could be reproduced.

We have tried to break the coherence between the visual information, on the one hand, and on the other, the somatic, motor outflow and vestibular information by changing the ratio r of visual scene rotation V to body rotation B ($V = r \times B$). This ratio is normally 1. We have used two experimental conditions, during which the ratio was respectively 1.5 and 0.66. For a ratio of 1.5, a whole-body rotation of 90° would induce a rotation in the visual display of 135° ($V = 1.5 \times 90$). Thus when the angle of the corner in the corridor was 90°, the subjects would have to turn the chair by 60°. For a ratio of 0.66, if they rotated the chair by 90°, they would see in the corridor a rotation of 59.4°; they would then have to turn the chair by 136° to have a 90° rotation in the visual display.

This conflict condition allows us to use the "visual navigation" task to study the adaptation to a sensory conflict during a navigation task, a question that has not been addressed yet although numerous such investigations have been performed concerning the adaptive mechanisms of vestibular and visual reflexes (see Berthoz and Melvill Jones, 1985, for a review). The conflict condition also allows us to study, with a "memorized navigation" task, the transformation of sensory information (visual, vestibular, somato-sensory information, and motor outflow) into the stored representation of the path.

Four types of corridors (C1, C2, C3, and C4) were used to carry out the experiment. The first one was a training corridor made of eight segments of straight path and seven right angles (four to the right and three to the left). The three other corridors were made of four straight segments and three angles (45, 90, and 135 degrees) combined differently in each corridor. Additionally, subjects were asked to draw the last corridor on a sheet of paper at the end of the experiment.

Data Analysis

The computer recorded the virtual trajectory of the path followed by the subject in the corridor. A graphical plot of these trajectories was constructed by setting an initial direction, which corresponded to the initial angular position of the subject in the chair. Each point on the path was calculated by taking into account the instantaneous angular position of the subject. The amplitude and direction of each turn in the trajectory were computed. Trajectories could be displayed as shown in Figure 17.2A in the case of a "visual navigation task" and in Figure 17.2B for a "memorized navigation" task.

Results

Visual navigation task. In both the normal condition and the conflict condition most subjects could easily perform the "visual navigation task." Nevertheless, all of the subjects but one came into collision with a wall at least once during the experiment. The number of colli-

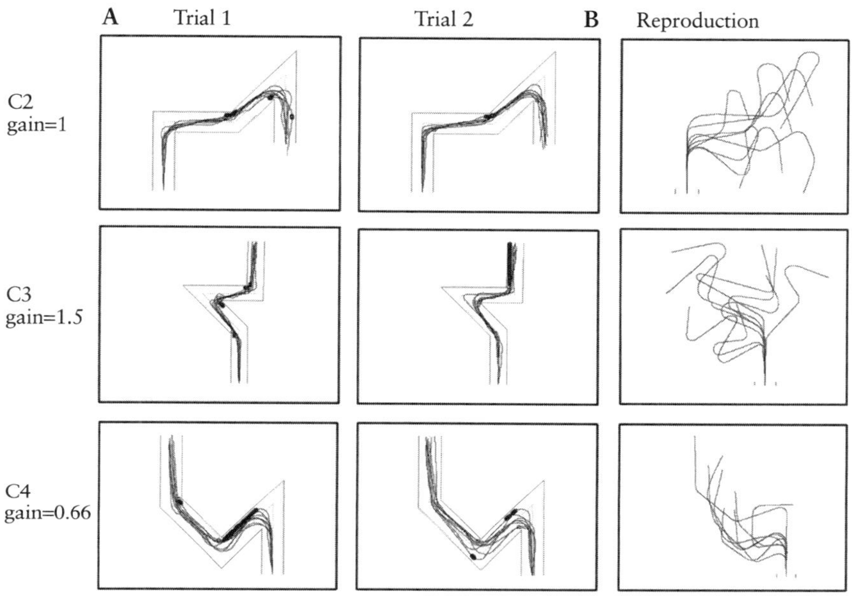

Figure 17.2. Example of trajectories of several subjects (N = 8) plotted together.

(A) Visual navigation task: two conditions were used, normal (corridor C2, ratio = 1) and conflicting (corridors C3 and C4, ratios = 1.5 and 0.66, respectively). Subjects had to navigate through the corridor twice (Trial 1 and Trial 2) before performing memorized navigation with eyes closed. In the conflict condition (corridors C3 and C4), the angles of the plotted trajectories were the real whole-body angles performed by the subject on his chair, multiplied by 1.5 and 0.66, respectively.

(B) Memorized navigation task: Trajectories reproduced with eyes closed, represented in the reference frame of the virtual world. Same conventions as in (A).

sions was always larger during the first trial than in the second. The imposed constant linear velocity made negotiation of turns more difficult than in a natural task, and could therefore induce hits, which always occurred when negotiating turns. In the conflict condition, subjects managed to navigate accurately in the corridors in spite of the difference between visual and nonvisual information. Standard deviations of the performed angles were nevertheless larger in the conflict condition when the ratio was set to 0.66 than when the ratio was set to 1.5.

A remarkable result of this experiment is that out of twenty subjects, only one was consciously aware of the conflict between vision and somato-sensory cues. It is indeed possible that the induced dis-

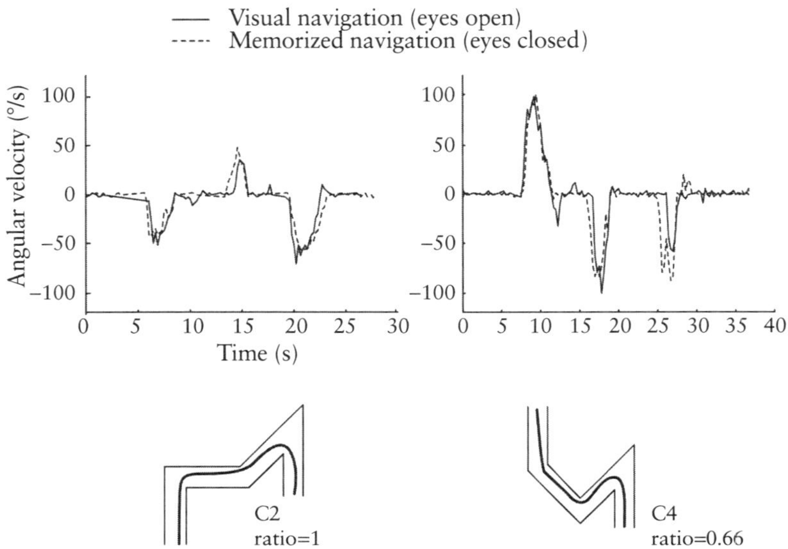

Figure 17.3. Example of angular velocity during visual (dashed line) and memorized navigation for two different subjects, in corridor C2 and C4, respectively. The map of the corridor corresponding to the trajectory is represented below each graph.

crepancy between sensory modalities did not exceed a physiological range requiring the intervention of an aware processing.

Memorized navigation task. When asked to reproduce from memory, subjects reproduced the approximate shape of the visual navigation task in all types of corridors. This shows that subjects could memorize the trajectory and reproduce its essential features, yet with some errors (Figure 17.2). It appears, however, that in these results the reproduction of the path in Cartesian coordinates, though similar to the original path, was not truly accurate.

The variations in the Cartesian map-like tracings of the path can come from several sources, both at the encoding of the path and at its reproduction. For example, active rotations have to be perceived, encoded, and retrieved. Our paradigm does not allow us to distinguish between these different components. Yet the fact that at least three sources of errors may have distorted the reproduction of the velocity profile renders the accuracy of this reproduction even more striking.

Interestingly, we noted that, for some subjects, the angular velocity profiles of the visual and memorized navigation tasks were remark-

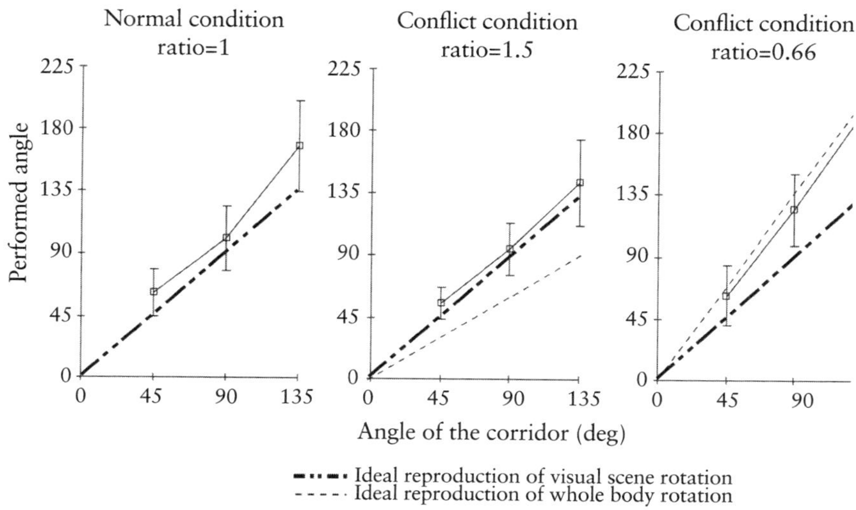

Figure 17.4. Real whole-body angles performed in the memorized navigation task and according to the conditions ($N = 20$). The darker dashed lines indicate the ideal reproduction of whole-body rotation in the conflict condition; the lighter dashed lines indicate the ideal reproduction of visual scene rotation.

ably similar (see Figure 17.3). Such an observation is in accordance with our hypothesis that what is being stored could be a velocity pattern of movement (Berthoz et al., 1995).

Results of the conflict condition did not exhibit a clear dichotic situation in which subjects would have reproduced either body rotations or visual rotations. Nevertheless, when the ratio was set to 0.66, in which body rotations had to be very large in order to correspond to the visual angle (corridor C4), subjects tended to reproduce whole-body motion rather than visual motion (see Figure 17.4). Subjects' drawings of the corresponding corridor were, however, very accurate when compared with the virtual trajectory, which suggests that the construction of a map might be dependent upon visual information (Figure 17.5). This suggests that the brain can store both movements and visual maps, and can even use them independently according to the envisaged action.

In conclusion we believe that this experiment is in accordance with our previous suggestion that the brain uses dynamic patterns of movement for the memory of routes, and not only static coordinates on cognitive maps. This suggestion is in accord with the proposal by

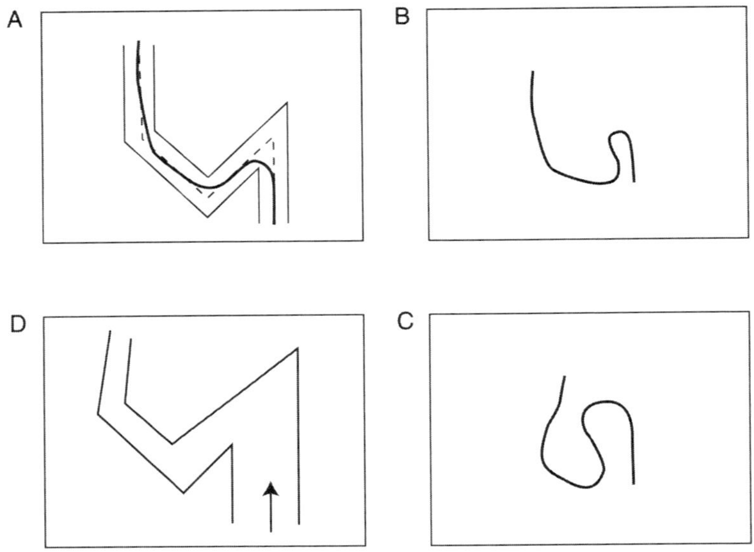

Figure 17.5. Example of performance obtained in corridor C4 (conflict condition, ratio = 0.66) for one subject. In this corridor, real body rotation had to be 1.5 times larger than rotation of the visual scene in order to navigate around the corners. This means that this subject performed 205 degrees in order to go through the first corner of 135 degrees, for example.

(A) Trajectory of the visual navigation task (second trial) in the reference frame of the virtual world, as in Figure 17.2.

(B) Same trajectory of the body in space coordinates. In this case, we plotted the real body rotation of the subject on the chair.

(C) Representation of the memorized trajectory in whole-body coordinates. The amplitude of the reproduced angles tends to correspond to the amplitude of whole-body rotations during the visual navigation task (panel B) rather than to the amplitude of visual scene rotation (panel A).

(D) Drawing of the corridor. The subject may have used the reference frame of the virtual world in order to draw the corridor. His drawing represents indeed quite accurately the angles he has seen.

Droulez and Berthoz (1990, 1991) that the brain uses dynamic remapping processes to perform spatial tasks that have been thought to be performed by coordinate transformations on Cartesian-like cognitive maps. We believe that the data presented here, as well as results obtained in the same experiment with standing subjects (Lambrey et al., in press), support the idea that the subjects will reproduce a trajectory corresponding to *either* visual *or* nonvisual information. In fact it may be that both types of cues are stored in parallel and can be chosen during retrieval depending on the task.

Conclusion

We can draw from these experiments and theories several conclusions. First, we need to study not only topographic memory but also "topokinetic memory." The organization of action is a fundamental language of the brain. The hippocampal formation is probably involved not only in static visual memory but also in the mental imagination of our own actions in space.

Second, although most models of multisensory interactions are based on the idea that the brain performs a weighting between these cues, our experiments suggest that one should also include the idea that separate parallel memories using either visual or nonvisual cues can be used and that the brain can switch between these models of movement memory.

These new paradigms may be useful in the future for studies of patients with functional deficits of dynamic spatial memory. As for question that we asked initially, "What is being stored, movement or maps?"—the answer is movement *and* maps, or rather movement *on* maps, or even maybe action *with* maps. Movement memory is a language of the brain.

References

Aguirre, G. K., Detre, J. A., Alsop, D. C., and D'Esposito, M. 1996. The parahippocampus subserves topographical learning in man. *Cerebr. Cortex,6*, 823–829.

Amorim, M. A., Glasauer, S., Corpinot, K., and Berthoz, A. 1997. Updating an object's orientation and location during nonvisual navigation: A comparison between two processing modes. *Percept. Psychophys., 59*, 404–418.

Berthoz, A. 1997. Parietal and hippocampal contribution to topokinetic and topographic memory. *Philos. Trans. Roy. Soc. Lond. [Biol.], 352*, 1437–1448.

——— 1998. Parietal and hippocampal contribution to topokinetic and topographic memory. In *The hippocampal and parietal foundations of spatial cognition*, ed. N. Burges et al. Oxford: Oxford University Press.

Berthoz, A., and Melvill Jones, G. 1985. *Adaptive mechanisms in gaze control: Facts and theories.* Amsterdam: Elsevier.

Berthoz, A., Israël, I., Georges-François, P., Grasso, R., and Tsuzuku, T. 1995. Spatial memory of body linear displacement: What is being stored? *Science, 269,* 95–98.

Bonda, E., Petrides, M., Frey, S., and Evans, A. 1995. Neural correlates of mental transformations of the body-in-space. *Proc. Natl. Acad. Sci. USA, 92,* 11180–11184.

Courtney, S. M., Ungerleider, L. G., Keil, K., and Haxby, J. V. 1996. Object and spatial visual working memory activate separate neural systems in the human cortex. *Cerebr. Cortex, 6,* 39–49.

Droulez, J., and Berthoz, A. 1990. The concept of dynamic memory in sensorimotor control. In *Motor control: Concepts and issues,* ed. D. R. Humphrey and J. R. Freund, 137–161. Chichester, U.K.: Wiley.

——— 1991. A neural network model of sensoritopic maps with predictive short term memory properties. *Proc. Natl. Acad. Sci. USA, 88,* 9653–9657.

Epstein, R., and Kanwisher, N. 1998. A cortical representation of the local visual environment. *Nature, 392,* 598–601.

Ghaem, O., Mellet, E., Crivello, F., Tzourio, N., Mazoyer, B., Berthoz, A., and Denis, M. 1996. Functional anatomy of mental stimulation of memorized routes. *NeuroImage, 3,* S249.

——— 1997. Mental navigation along memorized routes activates the hippocampus, preuneus, and insula. *NeuroReport, 8,* 739–744.

Ghaem, O., Mellet, E., Tzourio, N., Bricogne, S., Etard, O., Tirel, O., Beaudoin, V., Mazoyer, B., Berthoz, A., and Denis, M. 1998. Mental exploration of an environment learned from a map: A PET study. *NeuroImage, 7,* S115.

Guariglia, C., Padovani, A., Pantano, P., and Pizzamiglio, L. 1993. Unilateral neglect restricted to visual imagery. *Nature, 364,* 235–237.

Habib, M. 1987 Pure topographical disorientation: A definition and anatomical basis. *Cortex, 23,* 73–85.

Hécaen, H., Tzortzis, C., and Rondot, P. 1980. Loss of topographical memory with learning deficits. *Cortex, 16,* 525–542.

Hermer, L., and Spelke, E. S. 1994. A geometric process for spatial reorientation in young children. *Nature, 370,* 57–59.

Incisa della Rocchetta, A., Cipolotti, L., and Warrington, K. 1996. Topographical disorientation: Selective impairment of locomotor space? *Cortex, 32,* 727–735.

Israël, I., Grasso, R., Georges-François, P., Tsuzuku, T., and Berthoz, A. 1997. Spatial memory and path integration studied by self-driven passive linear displacement. 1. Basic properties. *J. Neurophysiol., 77,* 3180–3192.

Ivanenko, Y. P., Viaud-Delmon, I., Siegler, I., Israël, I., and Berthoz, A. 1998. The vestibulo-ocular reflex and angular displacement perception in darkness in humans: Adaptation to a virtual environment. *Neurosci. Lett., 241,* 167–170.

Jacob, R. G., Furman, J. M. R., Durrant, J. D., and Turner, S. M. 1996. Panic, agoraphobia, and vestibular dysfunction. *Am. J. Psychiatry, 153* (4), 503–512.

Jacob, R. G., Furman, J. M., Durrant, J. D., and Turner, S. M. 1997. Surface dependence: A balance control strategy in panic disorder with agoraphobia. *Psychosom. Med., 59,* 323–330.

Jacob, R. G., Redfern, M. S., Furman, J. M. R. 1995. Optic flow-induced sway in anxiety disorders associated with space and motion discomfort. *J. Anxiety Disorders, 5,* 411–425.

Lambrey, S., Viaud-Delmon, I., and Berthoz, A. In press. Influence of a sensory conflict upon the memorization of a path traveled in virtual reality. In "Multisensory Processing," special issue of *Cognitive Brain Research,* ed. C. Schroeder and J. Foxe.

Maguire, H., Frackowiak, R., and Frith, C. 1996. The activation of the hippocampal region during acquisition of topographical representations of a real-world environment. *NeuroImage, 3,* S589.

Mellet, E., Tzourio, N., Denis, M., and Mazoyer, B. 1995. A positron emision tomography study of visual and mental exploration. *J. Cogn. Neurosci., 7,* 433–445.

Mellet, E., Bricogne, S., Tzourio, N., Ghaem, O., Petit, L., Zago, L., Etard, O., Berthoz, A., Mazoyer, B., and Denis, M. 2000. Neural correlates of topographic mental exploration: The impact of route versus survey perspective learning. *NeuroImage, 12 (5),* 588–600.

O'Keefe, J., and Nadel, L. 1978. *The hippocampus as a cognitive map.* Oxford: Clarendon Press.

Pallis, C. A. 1955. Impaired identification of faces and places with agnosia for colors. *J. Neurol. Neurosurg. Psychiatr., 18,* 218–224.

Paterson, A. 1994. A case of topographical disorientation associated with a unilateral cerebral lesion. *Brain, 68,* 188–212.

Poincaré, H. 1970. *La valeur de la science.* Paris: Flammarion.

Thorndike, P. W., and Hayes-Roth, B. 1982. Differences in spatial knowledge acquired from maps and navigation. *Cognitive Psychology, 14,* 560–589.

Tolman, E. C. 1948. Cognitive maps in rats and men. *Psychological Review, 55,* 189–208.

Viaud-Delmon, I., Ivanenko, Y. P., Berthoz, A., and Jouvent, R. 1998. Sex, lies, and virtual reality. *Nature Neuroscience, 1,* 15–16.

Viaud-Delmon, I., Ivanenko, Y. P., Grasso, R., and Israël, I. 1999. Nonspecific directional adaptation to asymetrical visual-vestibular stimulation. *Cognitive Brain Research,* 7, 507–510.

Whiteley, A. M., and Warrington, E. K. 1978. Selective impairement of topographical memory: A single case study. *J. Neurol. Neurosurg. Psychiatr., 41,* 575–578.

Yardley, L., Britton, J., Lear, S., Bird, J., and Luxon, L. 1995. Relationship between balance system function and agoraphobic avoidance. *Behav. Res. Ther., 33,* 435–439.

Yardley, L., Luxon, L., Bird, J., Lear, S., and Britton, J. 1994. Vestibular and posturographic test results in people with symptoms of panic and agoraphobia. *J. Audiological Med., 3,* 48–65.

Zola-Morgan, S., Squire, L. R., and Amaral, D. G. 1986. Human amnesia and the medial temporal region: Enduring memory impairment following a bilateral lesion limited to field CA1 of the hippocampus. *J. Neurosci., 6,* 2950–2967.

Naturalization of Mental States and Personal Identity

18

Marc Jeannerod

Modern cognitive psychology tends to follow the idea that mental states have a causal role in behavior. Cognitive neuroscientists would add to this statement that the property of causing behavior is a consequence of its embodiment in brain states. This chapter will attempt to go one step further, by considering a specific dimension of human beings (as opposed to other information-processing devices, like computers): their inherently social nature. Attention will be focused on a category of mental states that pertain to the realm of communication between individuals and are crucial for understanding other people's minds. In the first sections, examples drawn from current research will be used to describe the mechanisms underlying the human ability to understand the behavior of other people and to infer their mental states from their behavior. It will be assumed that, during intersubjective communication, mental states are shared by several people, and that, because mental states are tightly related to brain states, the brain ultimately mediates social interactions. In the last section, the discussion will be focused on a major philosophical issue raised by these attempts at reducing mental states to brain states. Indeed, naturalization of mental states, especially in the context where these mental states are shared between several persons, questions the notion of individual identity. This will be an opportunity for discussing possible limitations to these attempts.

The Relationship of Mental States to Brain States in the Social Context

One of the possibilities for explaining how human beings can cope with their environment is that they are born with elementary rules for understanding external events. Such rules have been identified, among other domains, for language (how to parse speech sounds) and perception (how to organize a chaotic sensory world). These rules are started early by interaction with the external world, so that each individual can form representations about reality. In the domain of social communication, which is under discussion here, humans are known to be good at mind reading. They are born with mechanisms to attribute mental states to other individuals and with elementary skills for deciphering these states. This suggests that having mental states (intentions, and so on) is the precondition for reading and understanding the mental states of others. Going even further in this direction, one might postulate that the system we use for detecting intentions of other people is part of the system that generates our own intentions. The problems to be addressed, therefore, will be to understand how mental states are generated, how they can cause behavior, how they can be understood by others, and how the self can make a distinction between its own mental states and those of others.

Let us assume first that mental states are coextensive with brain states. In this section, some of the logical implications of this assumption, when applied to the context of communication between individuals, are examined. Social interaction during communication means that mental states can be shared by several individuals: the people who interact must have at least some intentions, beliefs, or desires in common, in order to understand each other. In line with the above propositions, it follows that the same intention, for example, may be simultaneously represented in several brains, with the intriguing possibility that the co-occurrence of a given brain state and a given mental state may not be unique to a particular individual. This possibility raises the obvious problem of how the intention can be attributed to its proper source, and suggests the existence of specific signals, the presence or the absence of which will determine attribution of the intention to the self or to another source, respectively. Producing a mental state and attributing this state to oneself are therefore two different processes that are not automatically linked. In other words, the brain has to inform itself about what it does, by using signals that are produced by its own activity: if this information is not present, not used, or not properly interpreted, the mental state can still be recognized but will be misattributed. Pathological examples will illustrate the fact that subjects can decipher thoughts they have produced and, at the same time, misattribute them to another person.

An essential aspect of social communication is to understand the meaning of overt behavior, which is the first step to accessing underlying mental states. For this reason, a large amount of our daily life is spent watching and interpreting the actions of others. Recognition of actions of conspecifics is a genuine ability, which seems to be highly developed in humans and nonhuman primates (Premack and Woodruff, 1978). Humans can easily distinguish biological motion from impulsions produced by mechanical devices, even when only a limited number of cues are available (Johansson, 1977; Dasser et al., 1989). Each individual builds up from this observation his or her own theory of the mind of others (for example, Leslie, 1987). In addition, observation of action is the first step of imitation, a powerful means of establishing contact with other individuals and acquiring new skills from them, which starts at birth and continues throughout life (Meltzoff, 1995).

These considerations raise key questions about the type of representation that is built while observing an action. It has been postulated that an observed action can be understood and imitated whenever it becomes the source of a representation of the same action by the observer: in other words, the observed action would have to be transformed into a potential action in order to be understood. This idea seems to be supported by recent experiments in the monkey, showing the existence of neuronal populations in several brain areas, which selectively encode postures and movements performed by conspecifics (Perrett et al., 1989; Carey et al., 1997). In the region of the premotor cortex a group of neurons are selective both for the monkey's active performance of a particular type of movement (for example, a hand movement) and for the monkey's observation of the same hand movement made by an experimenter or by another animal (mirror neurons, Rizzolatti et al., 1996).

A series of positron emission tomography (PET) experiments were recently performed in humans in order to explore brain activity during observation of actions performed by others. In these experiments, subjects are typically instructed to remain immobile and carefully observe simple actions displayed in front of them while their brain metabolism is monitored. Areas mostly located in the parietal and the frontal lobes, and clearly related to motor functions, were found to be activated (Grafton et al., 1996). Subjects' cognitive strategy during observation was also shown to influence the repartition of cerebral activation (Decety et al., 1997). When the subjects had received the instruction to memorize the actions with the purpose of later imitation, structures involved in motor functions (the supplementary motor area, the dorsolateral prefrontal cortex on both sides, premotor cortex) were activated. By contrast, when the instruction was to observe the actions with the purpose of simply recognizing them afterward, only the parahippocampal gyrus in the temporal lobe was activated. The pattern of activation also differed according to whether the observed actions were meaningful (that is, they referred to a recognizable goal) or meaningless sequences of movements. Observing a meaningful action activated areas that were mainly confined to the left hemisphere. The main structures involved were the inferior frontal (area 45), middle temporal (area 21), and parahippocampal regions. Activation of area 45 is of particular interest: according to Grafton et al. (1996), it could be functionally similar to the monkey ventral area 6, where mirror neurons are recorded. Indeed, the same region has been found to be activated during mental simulation of hand actions (Decety et al., 1994; Grafton et al., 1996) and during the recognition of man-made tools (Perani et al., 1995). Finally, by contrast with observation of meaningful actions, observation of meaningless sequences of movements primarily engaged the right hemisphere. Areas in the occipito-parietal region and the inferior temporal gyrus (areas 19–37) were activated.

These results reveal that, in many situations involving observation of an action (for example, observing meaningful movements to learn and replicate them), cortical areas that would be involved if one intended to perform that same action become active. It is tempting to generalize this finding to other situations where observation of conspecifics is a source of interindividual communication. The fact that several individuals can share the same representations (in neural terms) might provide a rationale for phenomena such as empathy, contagion of emotions, and so on.

Shared Representations and the Agency Problem: About Distinguishing One's Own Intentions from Those of Other People

The notion of shared representations in turn raises two related problems: First, how can one distinguish one's actions from those of other people? Second, how does one become aware of one's own actions? If one assumes that understanding actions implies representations that are common to several persons, then the possibility of attributing these actions to their real agent (the agency problem) should require the presence of specific signals at the level of these representations.

Barresi and Moore (1996) have attempted to specify the difference between conditions where an action appears. When the action is observed, the information available to the subject would carry a "third-person" knowledge, based on visual analysis of the movements of the agent toward objects, his gaze orientation, his facial expression, and so on. When an action is self-generated, by contrast, the available information would be of the "first-person" type, that is, based mainly on self-produced signals, such as proprioceptive signals. It is the presence or absence of the latter signals that would allow making a distinction between self-caused and world-caused effects on external objects, respectively. In addition, Barresi and Moore suggest, the fact that an action is taking place activates an "intentional schema," a structure internal to each agent with the capacity of coordinating first- and third-person information. According to the input signals available to the intentional schema, the action will be attributed to the self or to the other person. The theory has the advantage of explaining that, because the schema pertains to the subject, the action (self-generated or not) that is currently monitored can be readily understood by the subject. This mechanism may become critical in situations where the two types of information about the action are available at the same time, that is, when two agents are involved in situations such as joint attention, matched actions, or mutual imitation.

One way to deal with the problem of agency is to explore the degree of accuracy of subjects when they have to consciously determine the origin of an action. There are very few studies dealing with the subjective experience related to the execution of voluntary movements. In one of these investigations (Nielsen, 1963), subjects were presented with movements of an uncertain origin: they were shown the image of an alien hand visually superimposed to (and indistinguishable from) their own hand. Movements performed by the alien hand could be either in concordance or in discordance with the subjects' own movements. Even in the latter case, subjects experienced the alien hand as theirs, without regard for obvious discrepancies between the self-generated and the seen movements: they simply reported feelings of strangeness or, on some occasions, the impression of having their hand pushed by some external force, or having lost control of their movements. Normal subjects are thus poorly aware of their own movements. When placed in an ambiguous situation, they tend to experience movements of an alien hand as theirs. In addition, when required to make an agency judgment, they tend to privilege movement-related visual information over kinesthetic information.

This problem was systematically reexamined in a new experiment (Daprati et al., 1997). With the use of a closed TV circuit, the subject's hand and the experimenter's hand could be briefly displayed on the video screen seen by the subject. The two hands, covered with similar gloves, looked alike. In each trial, both the experimenter and the subject had to perform a given hand movement on command (for example, stretch thumb, stretch fingers 1 and 2): on some trials, however, the experimenter's movement departed from the instruction. As a result of this experimental arrangement, the subject was randomly shown either his own hand, or the experimenter's hand performing the same movement as he, or a different movement. At the end of each trial, a verbal agency judgment was recorded: the subject had to say whether the hand he had seen was his hand or another's hand. In the two "easy" conditions, normal subjects were able to unambiguously determine whether the moving hand seen on the screen was theirs or not: first, when they saw their own hand, they correctly attributed the movement to themselves; second, when they saw the experimenter's hand performing a movement that departed from the instruction they had received, they correctly denied seeing their own hand. By contrast, their performance degraded in the "difficult" trials, where they saw the experimenter's hand performing the same movement as required by the instruction: in this condition, they misjudged the alien hand as theirs in about 30 percent of cases.

The specific increase in the error rate observed in the difficult trials can be explained within the framework of the classical "comparator" model postulated by physiologists to account for how the central nervous system can distinguish between internally and externally generated changes of the external world. According to this popular theory (the corollary discharge model, Sperry, 1950; the efference copy model, von Holst, 1950), the comparator is a specialized structure which receives action-related signals from internal and external (sensory) sources. During a self-generated action, internal signals, which copy the commands sent to the effectors (and which therefore reflect the desired action), are sent to the comparator. These internal signals create therein an anticipation for the consequences of the action. When the action is effectively executed, sensory signals related to changes in the external world also reach the comparator. If these sensory signals match the anticipation of the comparator, the desired action is registered by the system; if they do not, a mismatch is registered between the desired action and the action that has been produced; finally, if sensory signals arrive in the absence of internal signals, a change in the external world independent from the agent is registered.

The pattern of responses that Daprati et al. (1997) recorded in their difficult condition can be better understood if one assumes that agency judgments made by the subjects are based on the state of the comparator. In the difficult condition, no obvious mismatch was likely to occur between the anticipated and the perceived final hand postures, because the subject's (invisible) hand and the experimenter's (visible) hand both executed very similar movements. Only slight differences in timing and kinematic pattern between the internal signals and the sensory signals arising from the visual and kinesthetic receptors were available to the comparator to give the correct agency response. This explanation also fits into the framework of Barresi and Moore. Indeed, in the ambiguous condition, the intentional schema was fed simultaneously with third-person signals (those from the seen experimenter's hand) and first-person signals (from the subject's unseen hand), and these signals, particularly those of visual origin, were partly confounded.

This result emphasizes the weakness of signals arising from the execution of one's own movements, with its obvious consequence on the perceived agency. Although the above mechanism may be sufficient for correct attribution of actions in everyday life, it may be insufficient in ambiguous situations. In addition, pathological conditions may produce specific alterations at one or the other level of the mechanism: the nervous system may fail to generate the proper signals, or they may be produced but remain unperceived, and so on. Using the same paradigm as in normal controls, Daprati et al. (1997) examined agency responses in schizophrenic patients. Although their responses were close to normal in the easy conditions of the task, they failed to give correct responses in the difficult condition, where they misattributed the experimenter's hand to themselves in more than 80% of trials (note that the fact they gave correct responses in all other conditions rules out a response bias in favor of a systematic self-attribution of all the hands they saw). This striking behavior is likely to reflect a dysfunction of the representations generated while observing actions. It is consistent with clinical reports showing that most hallucinating schizophrenic patients show a tendency to incorporate external events in their own experience, or to interpret environmental cues as specifically directed to themselves (see Georgieff and Jeannerod, 1998).

Personal Identity: A Limit to Mind Reading?

In positing that mental states can be the cause of behavior because they are brain states, it was assumed that the mechanism for transferring an intention into a behavior is inherent to the physical nature of the mental state. In addition, this property was considered a prerequisite for understanding the mental states of others, due to the construction of shared representations. These assumptions raise a critical point: how far can this attempt at naturalizing the mental content go? Trying to answer this question might reveal limitations in the amount of mental content that can effectively be shared between individuals. Consider, for example, the mental state of "intending." Assuming that this state corresponds to the activation of a given set of brain areas (as illustrated in the previous section), to what extent can this pattern of activation reveal what the "intention" is about? This distinction between a "vehicle" (the brain mechanism for intending) and its content (the semantic of the intention) has been elaborated in various contexts, the most typical example being the distinction, in language studies, between the syntax and the semantic content of a sentence. Another example borrowed from Dredske (see Dredske, 1988; see also Jacob, 1997) can be used for the sake of clarity: imagine a soprano singing an opera with an extremely high pitch so as to break the glass of a window. It is assumed that this effect is the result of the air vibration produced by the song at a high pitch. The semantic content of the song, however, could likely be altered without changing the effect: hence the idea that the causal effect of the vehicle (the air vibration) is unrelated to the semantic content of the opera.

This content/vehicle distinction, however, presents a number of difficulties. Because, as we suggest, an intention cannot have a causal effect on behavior without being implemented by brain mechanisms, both the vehicle for intending and the content of the intention should be neurally represented. This implies that for that intention to affect a specific part of the motor system, the content must at some point interact with the vehicle. If this is indeed the case, the consequence is that there should be no difference in nature between the vehicle and the content, because both would have to be implemented neurally. Imagine a situation where the same action can be caused by the same mental state of intending, but where this action has different purposes. For example, I can raise my arm at a meeting with the purpose of asking a question of the speaker or with the purpose of waving at someone who is leaving the room. Will the pattern of neural activity in my brain differ in the two situations? If yes, the difference in activity will reflect the covert, or private, aspect of my intention, that which cannot be accessed from outside. In this example, the speaker, who has access only to its overt aspect, may misinterpret the significance of the action. Note that the semantic content of an intention may also remain outside the subjective awareness of its own author.

This example, however, does not entirely rule out the possibility that the vehicle could exist independently from a content. Situations can be created by brain stimulation or by pathology, both of which illustrate this point. Brain stimulation of premotor cortex, for example, triggers a strong experience of "intending" or "wanting to move." Subjects feel the urge to raise their arm, for example, without being able to give any justification for this movement (see Jeannerod, 1997). In a similar vein, a single case was recently reported where a stimulation of the anterior cingular gyrus produced a pleasant experience with laughing, yet the subject felt unable to explain the reason for this feeling and could only find ad hoc justifications (Fried et al., 1998). In pathological conditions, epileptic fits with sensations of déjà vu also resemble an empty vehicle. It remains to be determined whether this dissociation could also appear in normal conditions.

Another way of discussing the content/vehicle distinction is to consider a difference of degree, not of nature, between the two. Accordingly, the vehicle would carry the public side of the mental state, the side that can be accessed and understood by other selves, because it is part of experience common to all individuals (for example, to experience pleasure or sorrow). By contrast, the content would represent the private side, that which cannot be accessed by other selves, because it relates to the history of a particular self. To illustrate, let us take an example drawn from everyday experience of communicating with others. I can share the sorrow of someone who lost a beloved person, because I know what sorrow is, that it creates sadness, that it is often manifested by crying, and so on. But the limit to my ability to share the sorrow of that person is that I cannot build exactly the same representation, because I have never experienced the same relationship with the person who died. It cannot be the case that sorrow is the same for all individuals who have lost a beloved person, and that there is an invariant pattern of sorrow for losing a mother, a wife, or a son.

The reason why full empathy and sympathy are impossible is that identical neural representations cannot be built by several persons, because of the fact that the private part of the mental states of a person cannot be accessed by others. The question arises whether this would become possible if all this private information became available. Imagine a situation where two persons had exactly the same brains and who experienced exactly the same events in their personal history (an extreme variety of monozygotic twins): will the content of their mental states be exactly the same? If the answer to this question were positive, then the public and the private sides of the mental state would be confounded, and the (private) contents of each mental state should be fully accessible to each of the two persons. A neurobiologist's critique to this example is that it is not possible that two brains will ever be the same, because of ontogenetic constraints (for example, Edelman, 1978). Similarly, it should not be possible that two individuals will ever share the same experience, because they will necessarily have different standpoints when facing the same external events. If the neurobiologist's critiques are correct, then mental states experienced by different persons about the same event will necessarily carry different contents. This would imply a negative answer to the above question and, as a consequence, content that is inaccessible to an observer who monitors the mental states of another person. Note that the answer would be negative, not because of some principle of incommensurability between content and vehicle, but because of the biological and physical constraints pertaining to individual development and interactions with the external world.

The facts that mental states have to be brain states, and that part of them remain uncommunicable, generate a false impression of dualism between what can be shared and what cannot. Ipseity, the property of having one's own identity and history, would therefore reside in that part of the mental/neural content for which representations cannot be built from observation. The paradox is that ipseity, although it is clearly in the realm of physics and biology, pertains to a category of facts that escape description and, because of that, may remain outside the aim of scientific inquiry.

References

Barresi, J., and Moore, C. 1996. Intentional relations and social understanding. *Behavioral and Brain Sciences, 19,* 107–154.

Carey, D. P., Perrett, D. I., and Oram, M. W. 1997. Recognizing, understanding, and reproducing action. In *Handbook of neuropsychology,* ed. F. Boller and J. Grafman, Vol. 11: *Action and cognition,* ed. M. Jeannerod, 111–129. Amsterdam: Elsevier.

Daprati, E., Franck, N., Georgieff, N., Proust, J. Pacherie, E., Dalery, J., and Jeannerod, M. 1997. Looking for the agent: An investigation into consciousness of action and self-consciousness in schizophrenic patients. *Cognition, 65,* 71–86.

Dasser, V., Ulbaek, I., and Premack, D. 1989. The perception of intention. *Science, 243,* 365–367.

Decety, J., Grezes, J., Costes, N., Perani, D., Jeannerod, M., Procyk, E., Grassi, F., and Fazio, F. 1997. Brain activity during observation of action: Influence of action content and subject's strategy. *Brain, 120,* 1763–1777.

Decety, J., Perani, D., Jeannerod, M., Bettinardi, V., Tadary, B., Woods, R., Mazziotta, J. C., and Fazio, F. 1994. Mapping motor representations with PET. *Nature, 371,* 600–602.

Dredske, F. 1988. *Explaining behavior.* Cambridge: MIT Press.

Edelman, G. M. 1978. Group selection and phasic reentrant signalling: A theory of higher brain function. In *The mindful brain: Cortical organization and the group-selective theory of higher brain function,* by G. M. Edelman and V. B. Mountcastle, 51–100. Cambridge: MIT Press.

Fried, I., Wilson, C. L., MacDonald, K. A., and Behnke, E. J. 1998. Electric current stimulates laughter. *Nature, 391,* 650.

Georgieff, N., and Jeannerod, M. 1998. Beyond consciousness of external reality: A "who?" system for consciousness of action and self-consciousness. *Consciousness and Cognition, 7,* 465–477.

Grafton, S. T., Arbib, M. A., Fadiga, L., and Rizzolatti, G. 1996. Localization of grasp representations in humans by positron emission tomography. 2. Observation compared with imagination. *Experimental Brain Research, 112,* 103–111.

Holst, E. von. 1954. Relations between the central nervous system and the peripheral organs. *British Journal of Animal Behavior, 2,* 89–94.

Jacob, P. 1997. *What minds can do.* Cambridge: Cambridge University Press.

Jeannerod, M. 1997. *The cognitive neuroscience of action.* Oxford: Blackwell.

Johansson, G. 1977. Studies on visual perception of locomotion. *Perception, 6,* 365–376.

Leslie, A. M. 1987. Pretense and representation: The origins of "theory of mind." *Psychological Review, 94,* 412–426.

Meltzoff, A. N. 1995. Understanding the intentions of others: Re-enactment of intended acts by 18-month-old children. *Developmental Psychology, 31,* 838–850.

Nielsen, T. I. 1963. Volition: A new experimental approach. *Scandinavian Journal of Psychology, 4,* 225–230.

Perani, D., Cappa, S. F., Bettinardi, V., Bressi, S., Gorno-Tempini, M., Matarrese, M., and Fazio, F. 1995. Different neural systems for the recognition of animals and man-made tools. *NeuroReport, 6,* 1637–1641.

Perrett, D. I., Harris, M. H., Bevan, R., Thomas, S., Benson, P. J., Mistlin, A. J., Citty, A. J., Hietanen , J. K., and Ortega, J. E. 1989. Framework of analysis for the neural representation of animate objects and actions. *Journal of Experimental Biology, 146,* 87–113.

Premack, D., and Woodruff, G. 1978. Does the chimpanzee have a theory of mind? *Behavioral and Brain Sciences, 4,* 515–526.

Rizzolatti, G., Fadiga, L., Gallese, V., and Fogassi, L. 1996. Premotor cortex and the recognition of motor actions. *Cognitive Brain Research, 3,* 131–141.

Sperry, R. W. 1950. Neural basis of the spontaneous optokinetic response produced by visual inversion. *Journal of Comparative and Physiological Psychology, 43,* 482–489.

Using Nonverbal Representations of Behavior: Perceiving Sexual Orientation

19

Nalini Ambady and Mark Hallahan

Ecological theories of perception (Gibson, 1977, 1979; McArthur and Baron, 1983; Zebrowitz and Collins, 1997) maintain that it is beneficial for people to be able to perceive quickly and accurately aspects of their environment that are relevant to their taking adaptive action. Consistent with this perspective, a growing body of evidence suggests that diverse aspects of the social environment can be perceived accurately from extremely minimal information. For instance, human observers are particularly sensitive to biological motion and can perceive the moving human form extremely rapidly on the basis of minimal information (Johansson, 1976). In addition, biological variables such as age and gender can be perceived accurately from sparse behavioral observations (Cutting and Proffitt, 1981; Johansson, 1975, 1976; Mather and West, 1993; Shiffrar, Lichtey, and Chaterjee, 1997). Thus moving point-light displays (small patches of lights attached to the joints) of only 200 msec provide sufficient information for naïve viewers to identify the locomotion of animals, types of human actions (such as pushups or jumping jacks), and the gender of walkers (Cutting and Kozlowski, 1977; Kozlowski and Cutting, 1977; Cutting, 1978; Runeson and Frykholm, 1983). Given the adaptive nature of this skill, it is not surprising that the perception of biological motion is believed to represent an intrinsic capacity of the visual system, one that is evident in infants three to six months in age (for example, Fox and McDaniel, 1982; Bertenthal, Proffitt, and

Cutting, 1984) and which appears to be subserved by a specific neural network (Bonda et al., 1996; Grezes et al., 2000).

Certain nonbiological variables can also be accurately judged from minimal information. But those variables most accurately judged from minimal information appear to be biologically relevant to the social perceiver. For instance, the ability to make rapid and appropriate interpretations of a target's affective state confers some survival value, so it is not surprising that the recognition of facial expressions from minimal information takes place spontaneously (Dimberg, Thunberg, and Elmehed, 2000) and without conscious intention (Whalen et al., 1998). Even personality traits such as extroversion can be judged accurately on the basis of extremely brief interactions with complete strangers (compare Albright, Kenny, and Malloy, 1988; Ambady, Hallahan, and Rosenthal, 1995; Funder, 1995). In this chapter we discuss accuracy in judging the important—and to some extent concealable—dispositional[1] (some might argue biological; compare Hamer, 1993; LeVay, 1993; Pattatucci and Hammer, 1995) variable of sexual orientation on the basis of brief observations of nonverbal behavior. Having conducted a series of studies investigating this issue, we will first summarize here our findings regarding the accuracy and efficiency of the use of nonverbal representations of behavior as well as preliminary investigations into the specific cues that mediate judgments of sexual orientation. Then we will discuss the extent to which the display of these cues can be consciously controlled.

Accuracy in Judging Sexual Orientation

A few previous studies investigating accuracy in judging sexual orientation have yielded somewhat inconsistent results. One study concluded that sexual orientation could not be judged accurately from 2–3 min videoclips (Berger et al., 1987; see Ambady, Hallahan, and Conner, 1999, for a discussion of the interpretation of Berger et al., 1987). Other studies have found that there seem to be identifiable cues that may convey information about sexual orientation. Thus men's sexual orientation was found to be judged accurately on the basis of 1.5 min audio clips (Linville, 1998). Further, lesbians were perceived to have more masculine speech than heterosexual women and gay men were perceived to have more feminine speech than heterosexual men (Travis, 1981).

Ambady, Hallahan, and Conner (1999) conducted a series of studies to examine the accuracy of judgments of sexual orientation from brief dynamic (10 sec and 1 sec silent video clips) as well as static cues (a series of still photos). Heterosexual and gay/lesbian targets (people whose sexual orientation was being judged) were recruited from various Harvard University graduate student organizations, including gay, lesbian, and bisexual student organizations. The final sample consisted of ten women (five lesbian, and five heterosexual) and fifteen men (eight homosexual and seven heterosexual) targets. To disguise the purpose of the research, information about targets' sexual orientation was obtained with a single question that was embedded in a longer questionnaire with a number of filler questions (such as questions about anxiety, alcohol consumption, and religiosity).

Targets later returned to the laboratory for what they were told was research investigating how students handle the competing demands of academic and extracurricular activities. They were videotaped for one minute as they discussed this issue. After being videotaped, targets were informed of the nature of the study and were asked to consent to have their videotape shown to people who would make judgments about their sexual orientation. At that point they were given the option of withdrawing and having the tape erased. Thus we ensured that the targets behaved as naturally as possible and were making no explicit attempt either to hide or to express their sexual orientation.

A silent 10 sec clip was created for each of the twenty-five participating targets by extracting the 25th through the 35th second of their videotape. Silent 1 sec clips were extracted from the middle of the 10 sec clip. Eight still photos were selected by freezing frames every 700 msec from the middle 5 sec of the 10 sec clip.

Ninety-six judges (people who made judgments of the targets' sexual orientation) were recruited from undergraduate residence halls as well as from various undergraduate organizations, including gay and lesbian organizations. Forty-eight of the judges were women (twenty-four homosexual and twenty-four heterosexual) and forty-eight were men (twenty-four homosexual and twenty-four heterosexual). All judges rated each of the three conditions (10 sec silent video, 1 sec silent video, 8 still pictures). Judges rated on a seven-point scale the extent to which they thought each target person was homosexual and, in a separate question, heterosexual. These two questions, which were strongly inversely related, were combined to obtain an overall measure of the judges' perception of the targets' sexual orientation.

Accuracy was significantly greater than chance for all three conditions, but was greatest for judgments based on 10 sec silent clips. In this condition, all (32/32) of the judges had greater-than-chance accuracy (that is, greater than 50 percent correct), and the typical judge correctly classified about 70 percent of targets (average = 69.97%, median = 72.00%). For the 1 sec silent clips, 97 percent (31/32) of the judges had greater-than-chance accuracy, and the typical judge correctly classified about 60 percent of targets (average = 61.13%, median = 60.00%). In the still-photo condition, 84 percent (27/32) of the judges had greater-than-chance accuracy, and the typical judge correctly classified about 55 percent of targets (average = 54.25%, median = 56.00%).

We computed a planned contrast to assess the extent to which accuracy was significantly greater in the two conditions with dynamic cues (10 sec and 1 sec) than in the static still-photo condition, $t\ (93) = 6.58$, $p < .05$. This trend supports previous work indicating that dynamic cues generally yield more accurate perceptual judgments than static cues (Barclay, Cutting, and Kozlowski, 1978; Valenti and Costall, 1997).

Clearly, targets' nonverbal behavior, particularly their dynamic behavior, conveys information that individuals use in making accurate judgments. Of course, although judgments of sexual orientation were more accurate than random guesses, this does not imply that any individual judgment of sexual orientation will be accurate in every case. The most accurate judges in this study judged sexual orientation accurately 80 percent of the time.

Individual Differences in Judgment Accuracy

In general, people are able to judge sexual orientation more accurately than chance. But are there individual differences in this ability? It is a common popular perception that some people are particularly good at perceiving sexual orientation. This perception is particularly strong among gay men. For example, in a study drawing on survey data, 71 percent of gay men versus 44 percent of lesbians reported that they could accurately judge sexual orientation (Sahgir and Robins, 1973). The ability to recognize sexual orientation without any discernible overt cues is sometimes called "gaydar" in popular culture. For example, DiLallo and Krumholtz (1994) in their self-proclaimed "Unofficial Gay Manual," define gaydar as "the instinctual ability to ascertain that another guy is gay, even in the absence of telltale signs" (p. 218). Gaydar is considered linked not to any cues involving dress or jewelry but, rather, to subtle nonverbal cues, and is often thought to be an ability unique to gay men.

We sought to test the extent to which popular beliefs about judging sexual orientation were supported under more controlled conditions by comparing the accuracy of gay/lesbian and heterosexual judges. Gay/lesbian and heterosexual judges were not significantly different in their accuracy in judging 10 sec clips, $F_{(1,28)} = 0.25$, $p = .62$. Gay and lesbian judges, however, were significantly more accurate than heterosexual judges in the 1 sec clip condition, $F_{(1,28)} = 5.90$, $p = .02$, though this difference was attributable more to the superior performance of lesbians than to that of gay men. Gay men and lesbians also judged sexual orientation on the basis of still photos more accurately than heterosexuals, $F(_{1,28}) = 4.14$, $p = .05$. This finding suggests that gay men and lesbians have an advantage in judging sexual orientation and that they seem to have the greatest advantage when the available information is relatively sparse.

Figural Outline Displays

The difference in accuracy based on dynamic information (10 sec and 1 sec silent videotapes) and static information (still photo) suggests that nonverbal communication channels, such as gestures, convey information about sexual orientation beyond what is available in more static aspects of appearance, such as hairstyle, clothing, or jewelry. To further examine the role of dynamic nonverbal behavior in conveying information about sexual orientation, we conducted an experiment investigating the judgment of sexual orientation from dynamic outlines of the targets. These figural outlines retained information about the targets' gestures and other nonverbal behavior, but obscured other more static aspects of their appearance.

Using a special-effects generator, nineteen of the original twenty-five 10 sec silent videoclips were altered to display the target persons as white silhouettes against a black background.[2] Additionally, the target persons' faces were obscured. The resulting images showed the targets' gestures and movement but did not show their facial expression or more static aspects of their appearances like their clothing, jewelry, or hairstyle. Sixteen judges rated targets' sexual orientation based on observations of these 10 sec figural outline displays. Overall, 94 percent (15/16) of the judges had greater-than-chance accuracy (that is, greater than 50 percent correct), and the typical judge correctly classified approximately 60 percent of targets (average = 59.76%), which was significantly above what would be expected by chance.

Cues Related to Sexual Orientation

In addition, we have been investigating accuracy in judging the gender of homosexual and heterosexual participants from point-light or biological motion displays (Ambady, Hallahan, and Dudkin, 2000). We hypothesized that gay men and lesbians would more often be misclassified in terms of their gender than would their heterosexual counterparts. Thirty-two participants (eight heterosexual females, eight heterosexual males, eight lesbians, and eight gay men) were videotaped walking, running, jumping, and pretending to pick up a heavy box. All participants were videotaped in a dark room wearing dark clothing. To obtain a saggital point-light display, we attached biker's personal safety lights to the shoulders, elbows, wrists, hips, knees, and lower ankles of the walkers. One light was attached to the hat each walker wore. Clips for each participant were approximately 50 seconds long.

Undergraduate judges were asked to rate the gender of each walker. Results indicated that lesbians were significantly more likely to be judged to be more male than heterosexual females, $t_{(15)} = 2.47$, $p < .01$. No significant differences were found, however, between heterosexual male and gay male walkers. This result suggests that, for women, subtle behavioral differences associated with sexual orientation are observable in point-light displays of dynamic movement. There was no clear evidence of a similar difference between gay and heterosexual men, though the sample for this preliminary investigation may not have been large enough to detect an existing effect. Thus the biological motion evidence indicates that lesbians are more likely to be misclassified as male from their gait than are heterosexual women.

Cues Related to Accurate Detection

Are there certain behaviors that provide clues to sexual orientation? To examine this issue, we had two coders rate a number of behaviors thought to be related to judgments of masculinity and femininity for each of the 10 sec clips of each of the twenty-five targets in the Ambady, Hallahan, and Conner (1999) study. The following behaviors were rated on a five-point scale: characteristics of gestures (fastness, smoothness, broadness, using the body to gesture); body position (elbows and hands away from body, arms symmetrical or crossed, limp wrist, fidgeting, leaning forward, shoulders kept erect, legs positioned apart, legs symmetrical or crossed, head tilt); overall style (smooth versus jerky, expressive, masculine, feminine); facial expression (gazing down, frowning, laughing, smiling, open smile, animated expression); and physical appearance (nontraditional dress, neatness of grooming, black clothing). Frequency counts per 10 sec were obtained for the following behaviors: number of gestures, head nods, head shakes, and touching clothing or hair. The mean reliability between the coders was $r = .64$.

For males ($n = 15$), there were a number of behaviors that were strongly related to sexual orientation. Gay men were judged to be more neatly groomed than heterosexual men ($r = .75$, $p = .001$). Heterosexual men were more likely to nod ($r = -.54$, $p = .04$) and to lean forward ($r = -.51$, $p = .05$) than gay men. A number of other correlations approached conventional significance levels: gay men were more likely to smile ($r = .48$, $p = .07$), to sit with shoulders erect ($r = .47$, $p = .07$), to have a smooth style ($r = .45$, $p = .09$), and to be perceived as expressive ($r = .45$, $p = .10$).

Among women ($n = 10$), heterosexuals were more likely to be perceived as having a smoother style than lesbians ($r = -.73$, $p = .02$). Lesbians were more likely to sit with their feet firmly on the ground ($r = .68$, $p = .03$) and were more likely to be perceived as being masculine ($r = .63$, $p = .05$) than heterosexual women. Additionally, heterosexual women were perceived to be more feminine ($r = -.61$, $p = .06$) than lesbian women.

Given the relatively small number of targets (ten women and fifteen men), these preliminary results must be interpreted with great caution. Although, at a general level, they suggest that some behavioral cues do convey information about sexual orientation, these sample correlations are not likely to provide especially precise estimates of the true size of the relationship between sexual orientation and specific nonverbal cues. More extensive data collection is needed to discern what specific cues tend to be associated with sexual orientation and precisely how strongly they are related to accurate judgments of sexual orientation.

Can Cues Associated with Sexual Orientation Be Consciously Controlled?

So far, this chapter has discussed research on the accuracy of judging sexual orientation that is based on observations of people who are neither explicitly attempting to conceal nor explicitly attempting to express their sexual orientation. However, we do not know the extent to which the cues that mediate accurate perception of sexual orientation can be consciously controlled. We are currently investigating whether sexual orientation can be judged accurately from dynamic nonverbal behavior when gay and lesbian participants explicitly attempt to conceal their sexual orientation (Ambady, Hallahan, and Dudkin, 2000). We present preliminary findings below.

Ten gay men and ten lesbians were recruited from the general community to serve as targets. Each target was videotaped in three different conditions: (a) behaving naturally, (b) trying to pass as heterosexual, and (c) exaggerating his or her sexual orientation (all targets did the behaving naturally condition first, and the order of the "exaggerate" and "pass" conditions was counterbalanced across targets). Twenty-two heterosexuals (eleven men, eleven women) were recruited to serve as targets and were videotaped behaving naturally. Brief videoclips (1 sec and 2 sec) were extracted for each target in each condition. For both the 1 sec and 2 sec clips, three different versions of a master videotape were created. Each version contained the twenty-two heterosexual targets behaving naturally and one of the three conditions for each of the twenty-two gay and lesbian targets. The master tapes were counterbalanced so that each gay and lesbian target appeared once in each of the three conditions across the three tapes.

Fifty-four people (fourteen gay men, one bisexual man, fourteen heterosexual men, ten lesbians, five bisexual women, and ten heterosexual women) were recruited to judge the sexual orientation of the targets from the 1 sec videoclips, and forty-nine people (twelve gay men, one bisexual man, eleven heterosexual men, eight lesbians, one bisexual woman, and sixteen heterosexual women) were recruited to judge the sexual orientation of the targets from the 2 sec videoclips. Each judge watched one version of the master videotape and rated the targets' sexual orientation.

Interestingly, accuracy in judgments of male targets did decrease when targets were trying to conceal their sexual orientation. On the basis of 1 sec clips, judges correctly discerned the sexual orientation of 48 percent of targets in the "pass" condition and 62 percent of targets in both the "normal" and the "exaggerate" conditions. Similar results were found in the 2 sec condition; judges correctly judged 38 percent of targets in the "pass" condition and 52 percent of targets in the normal and exaggerate conditions. Judges were similarly accurate at judging the sexual orientation of women targets regardless of whether they were trying to conceal their sexual orientation. On the basis of 1 sec clips, judges correctly judged the sexual orientation of 65 percent, 83 percent, and 78 percent of the women in the "pass," "normal," and "exaggerate" conditions, respectively. Similarly, on the basis of 2 sec clips, judges correctly judged the sexual orientation of 87 percent, 78 percent, and 83 percent of the women in the "pass," "normal," and "exaggerate" conditions respectively.

These results suggest that, to some extent, people are able to control the display of the cues that provide information about sexual orientation. However, our preliminary investigation suggests that men seem to be better able to control the display of cues than women.

Conclusion

Thus judgments regarding sexual orientation can be made accurately from a mere slice of behavior. Static information, however, yields considerably less accurate judgments than does dynamic information. Judgments of sexual orientation remain fairly accurate (more so for women than for men), even when participants explicitly attempt to conceal their orientation. These results suggest that sexual orientation is not an invisible, completely concealable category: information regarding sexual orientation is transmitted through subtle behavioral cues that can be detected accurately.

Previous research on motion perception has shown that the visual system is remarkably adept at identifying moving objects on the basis of very minimal information (Cutting and Proffitt, 1981; Johannson, 1975, 1976; Mather and West, 1993; Shiffrar, Lichtey, and Chaterjee, 1997). For example, information in a few successive frames of behavior are enough for the categorization and organization of information (Johannson, 1976). This study shows that even with an exposure of only 1 sec, naive judges can judge the very subtle category of sexual orientation at above-chance levels. Further, sexual orientation can be detected even from substantially degraded information such as figural outlines. The present results suggest that human beings can detect dispositional information from motion. This work highlights the effectiveness and efficiency of using representations of nonverbal behavior to make ecologically valid judgments.

Notes

Preparation of this article was supported by a PECASE award (Grant no. BCS-9733706).

1. By using the term "dispositional" we are not making any assertions about the etiology of sexual orientation. Rather, we use the term to indicate a behavioral pattern of arousal by members of the same, opposite, or both

sexes, in the same way that we might use the term "extroversion" to indicate a behavioral pattern of being outgoing.

2. Figural outline displays were not be generated for six of the original targets because they did not make any gestures or movements during their 10 sec clips.

References

Albright, L., Kenny, D. A., and Malloy, T. E. 1988. Consensus in personality judgments at zero acquaintance. *J. Pers. and Social Psychol., 55,* 387–395.

Ambady, N., Hallahan, M., and Conner, B. 1999. Accuracy of judgments of sexual orientation from thin slices of behavior. *J. Pers. and Social Psychol., 77* (3), 538–547.

Ambady, N., Hallahan, M., and Dudkin, D. 2000. On passing and the judgment of sexual orientation. Manuscript in preparation.

Ambady, N., Hallahan, M., and Rosenthal, R. 1995. On judging and being judged accurately in zero acquaintance situations. *J. Pers. and Social Psychol., 69,* 518–529.

Barclay, C. D., Cutting, J. E., and Kozlowski, L. T. 1978. Temporal and spatial factors in gait perception that influence gender recognition. *Percep. and Psychophys., 23,* 145–152.

Berger, G., Hank, L., Rauzi, T., and Simkins, L. 1987. Detection of sexual orientation by heterosexuals and homosexuals. *J. of Homosexuality, 13,* 83–100.

Bertenthal, B. L., Proffitt, D. R., and Cutting, J. E. 1984. Infant sensitivity to figural coherence in biomechanical motions. *J. Exp. Child Psychol., 37,* 213–230.

Bonda, E., Petrides, M., Ostry, D., and Evans, A. 1996. Specific involvement of human parietal systems and the amygdala in the perception of biological motion. *J. of Neurosci., 16* (11), 3737–3744.

Cutting, J. E. 1978. Generation of synthetic male and female walkers through manipulation of a biochemical invariant. *Perception, 7,* 393–405.

Cutting, J. E., and Kozlowski, L. T. 1977. Recognizing friends by their walk: Gait perception without familiarity cues. *Bulletin of the Psychonomics Soc., 9,* 353–356.

Cutting, J. E., and Proffitt, D. R. 1981. Gait perception as an example of how we may perceive events. In *Intersensory perception and sensory integration,* ed. R. D. Walk and H. L. Pick. New York: Plenum Press.

DiLallo, K., and Krumholtz, J. 1994. *The unofficial gay manual: Living the lifestyle (or at least appearing to).* New York: Doubleday.

Dimberg, U., Thunberg, M., and Elmehed, K. 2000. Unconscious facial reactions to emotional facial expressions. *Psychol. Sci., 11* (1), 86–89.

Fox, R., and McDaniel, C. 1982. The perception of biological motion by human infants. *Science, 218,* 486–487.

Funder, D. C. 1995. On the accuracy of personality judgment: A realistic approach. *Psychol. Rev., 102,* 652–670.

Gibson, J. J. 1977. The theory of affordances. In *Perceiving, acting and knowing: Toward an ecological psychology,* ed. R. E. Shaw and J. Bransford. Hillsdale, N.J.: Erlbaum.

——— 1979. *The ecological approach to visual perception.* Boston: Houghton Mifflin.

Grezes, J., Fonlupt, P., Bertenthal, B., Delon-Martin, C., Segebarth, C., and Decety, J. 2000. Does perception of biological motion rely on specific brain regions? Manuscript under review.

Hamer, D. H. 1993. A linkage between DNA markers on the X chromosome and male sexual orientation. *Science, 261,* 321–327.

Johannson, G. 1975. Visual motion perception. *Sci. Amer., 232,* 76–88.

——— 1976. Spatio-temporal differentiation and integration in visual motion. *Psychol. Res., 38,* 379–383.

Kozlowski, L. T., and Cutting, J. E. 1977. Recognizing the sex of a walker from a dynamic point-light display. *Percep. and Psychophys., 21,* 575–580.

LeVay, S. 1993. *The sexual brain.* Cambridge: MIT Press.

Linville, S. E. 1998. Acoustic correlates of perceived sexual orientation versus actual sexual orientation in men's speech. *Folia Phoniatrica et Logopaedica, 50,* 35–48.

McArthur, L. Z., and Baron, R. M. 1983. Toward an ecological theory of social perception. *Psychol. Rev., 90,* 215–238.

Mather, G., and West, S. 1993. Recognition of animal locomotion from dynamic point-light displays. *Perception, 22,* 759–766.

Pattatucci, A. M. L., and Hamer, D. H. 1995. The genetics of sexual orientation: From fruit flies to human. In *Sexual nature, sexual culture,* ed. P. R. Abramson and S. D. Pinkerson. Chicago: University of Chicago Press.

Runeson, S., and Frykholm, G. 1983. Kinematic specification of dynamics as an informal basis for person and action perception: Expectation, gender recognition, and deceptive intention. *J. Exp. Psychol. Gen., 112,* 580–610.

Sahgir, M., and Robins, E. 1973. *Male and female homosexuality.* Baltimore: Williams and Wilkins.

Shiffrar, M., Lichtey, L., and Chaterjee, S. H. 1997. The perception of biological motion across apertures. *Percep. and Psychophys., 59,* 51.

Travis, N. J. C. 1981. A study of the relationship of certain variables to sex characteristic identification from the speech of heterosexual and homosexual individuals. *Dissert. Abs. Int., 42* (6-B), 2323B.

Valenti, S. S., and Costall, A. 1997. Visual perception of lifted weight from kinematic and static (photographic) displays. *J. Exp. Psychol.: Hum. Percep. and Perf., 23,* 181–198.

Whalen, P. J., Rauch, S. L., Etcoff, N. L., McInterney, S. C., Lee, M. B., and Jenike, M. A. 1998. Masked presentations of emotional facial expressions modulate amygdala activity without explicit knowledge. *J. of Neurosci., 18* (1), 411–418.

Zebrowitz, L. A., and Collins, M. A. 1997. Accurate social perception at zero acquaintance: The affordances of a Gibsonian approach. *Pers. Social Psychol. Bull., 3,* 204–223.

Discussion: Section 5

ALFONSO CARAMAZZA: A question for Stephen: People who talk about modules, talk about them in both neural and functional terms as kinds of objects that are dedicated to a particular purpose with a particular functional consequence. You used this term loosely, I think, to simply refer to areas that light up in your experiments. How do you distinguish between data that disconfirm a theory like yours from data that indicate this kind of variability you're observing?

STEPHEN KOSSLYN: It is crucial to distinguish between the theory of how function is organized versus the theory of how function is implemented in neural tissue. There are convergent sources of evidence, from response times, error rates, judgments, effects of brain damage, and so on, that can buttress the theory of function. These, as you of all people know, can be quite independent of any facts about the brain. If you get variability in the areas activated by a function that has been well characterized by independent sources of evidence, this strikes me as good evidence that the implementation is variable. My own view is that many "high-level" processes (not elementary perceptual or motor processes) are constructed as they are needed, and thus the same function need not be implemented in precisely the same tissue from instance to instance—this view is inconvenient, but seems to make sense of the enormous variability I see in the neuroimaging literature.

ALBERT GALABURDA: Is there any evidence that we also image the shape of objects in terms of motor activity affecting a very different group of muscles, more distal muscles, manipulative muscles? Affecting perhaps a very different part of the brain, of course.

ALAIN BERTHOZ: It could be proposed as a general contention that the cognitive foundations of the perception of geometry in general do include a perception of action, of manipulation. And if I may answer not in a neurophysiological fashion, but in a philosophical way, Merleau-Ponty was saying vision is palpation by a gaze.

RHONDA SHEARER: Are you contrasting what you're doing with what Poincaré discussed? Because for Poincaré, the three forms of geometry are visual, tactile and motor. So specifically, he, which was so brilliant at the time, used those three geometries to illustrate the complexity of the integration that we experience at a conscious level as being seamless.

BERTHOZ: Poincaré, as you noted, said two things. First of all, he said the representation by the brain of the world cannot have anything to do with the geometrical space of mathematicians because, as you know, he said that vision is extremely nonlinear; it has many distortions. The muscular sense is an extremely complicated space that has nothing to do with Euclidian space. Even depth perception, as we know now from neurophysiology, is not only a visual property but a combination of visual cues together with efferent copy from motor commands. So, therefore, as he said, there is a difference between representational space and geometry. And then second, as you also point out, he said that we therefore have to propose the idea that action is at the basis of geometry. So I am in accordance with him.

CARAMAZZA: Marc [Jeannerod], it's a very interesting claim that the same areas seem to be activated when a person imagines performing an action and when the person actually performs an action. Now, what are the mechanisms that allow the execution or the blockage of the execution of the action? And have those mechanisms been identified? And how does one go about identifying them?

MARC JEANNEROD: We have looked at the reflexology of the spinal cord during mental activity, with Jean Ricker, in Marseilles, and we found that the H reflexes and the T reflexes are sharply increased during mental imagination of a movement that you make with that limb, a leg for example. And not with the opposite limb. So my claim is that all of the motor system is activated by mental imagery, starting from the motor cortex, going through the cerebellum, and down to the motor neurons. But at the lowest levels, there is a block. It is now commonly claimed that high-level athletes rehearse mentally. And in fact if they improve their performance, it is because they activate all the motor system. So that's one rationale to explain this mental rehearsal.

BERTHOZ: I'd like to make a comment on the question of Caramazza. First of all, I think that the brain is all about anticipation, anticipating the consequences of future actions in order to gain time and allow one to survive. And therefore it projects on the world. There is no duality between imagination and execution of movement. Regarding the similarity between structures in the brain that are involved in execution and imagination of action, there is one experiment that maybe could also shed some light. With Bernard Mazoyer and Lauren Petit, some years ago, and published in *NeuroReport,* we demonstrated that the three canonic structures that are involved in gaze control (SMA, frontal eye fields, and the cingulate gyrus) are activated during both executed and imagined movement. We know the organization of the eye movement system rather well now and we know that there are some neurons in the brain stem, which are called the pulse neurons, that are inhibitory. And therefore the whole brain can perform a saccade, in a sense. But if the pulse neurons of the brain stem do not stop firing, the saccade is not executed. So, in agreement with what Marc says, the whole system can be activated but action is blocked at the local level. But my belief is that there is actually a whole range of possibilities between this local blockage of the periphery and eventually higher level blockage. The blockage of motor output during mental imagery is a case for parallel pathways in the motor system. There is a discerning pathway for activity in the motor neuron and there is a pathway for inhibiting it, probably at the motor neuron level. And this is a challenge for the motor people to find this pathway.

ANNE HARRINGTON: I'm not sure if this is a kind of a ghost-in-the-machine sort of question, but I've been struck by the way in which in the last several papers we've been presented with a set of very intentional kinds of brains. Berthoz said something like, at the beginning is action. Steve, you talked about, what was your quote, you said the brain is constructing the mind as it needs it for its own purposes. And so we've got brains that are looking things up, that are strategizing, that are navigating around on maps. And the introduction of motor imagery really does push the question, or take us right up to the door of the question of what an intentional brain would be all about. And is there some kind of a representational substrate for intentionality that is distinct from and needs to be thought about as we think about the languages of the brain?

FRANÇOIS RECANATI: I would like to underline just the remark on intentionality. There is a spontaneous convergence of the contributions in the first section, which I see as the priority or primacy of motricity. I think this is very well known by the phenomenologists and philosophers. There is a link to be made between the contribution of Berthoz and [Stanislas] Dehaene yesterday. I think number is understood by Edmund Husserl at the beginning of the century, as collection activity. So it could enlighten our view of what Dehaene presented yesterday as a preverbal number understanding. And it's the same geometry of movement that is implied in the action. Husserl named this collection the intentional action of collecting things—that's the route of number understanding. Berger, a phenomenologist of the second generation, wrote a phenomenology of mathematics that also underlined this primacy of motricity. Ponty also spoke of palpating space with the eyes, and one century earlier, others spoke of seeing and took the metaphor that seeing is drawing, and so on.

JEAN-PIERRE CHANGEUX: I have a question for Marc that is related to what in French we call "going to action." I don't know what the translation is in English. You said that prefrontal areas in the middle and inferior frontal gyrus are activated during simulation and observation but not during execution. So does this mean that the prefrontal cortex, which of course is involved in intentionality, inhibits going into action? And then you release the inhibitory activity of the prefrontal cortex, then the action goes on.

JEANNEROD: It's a good question whether there is, in the brain, one area that will inhibit behavior. But just recently there was in *Cognition* a very nice paper on hysterical paralysis in a patient who was scanned in PET by John Marshall. This patient had enormous activity in the dorsal lateral prefrontal cortex, including in the orbital gyrus and so on. These could have been areas that were permanently activated and blocked the motor output from the hysterical site. I think there are several arguments showing that action can be blocked either centrally or at a threshold level depending on the situation.

KEVIN O'REGAN: I have a question for Dr. Ambady on the inhibition, or lack thereof, of certain movements: you might argue that one purpose of making gestures is to transmit our sexuality. In which case it's normal that other people should be able to perceive these. If so, then if people didn't perceive the gestures, we would make bigger and more obvious gestures.

NALINI AMBADY: You're talking about a very marked, very stereotyped category of people who may not want you to perceive their orientation. We do develop gestures to indicate our sex, but not necessarily our sexual orientation, particularly when it is stigmatized and a mocked category. Which is why it is interesting that even when we explicitly asked people to conceal their orientation, they weren't able to do so. Observers were just as accurate. In general, I agree with your point, but this might be a particular category where that might not be the case.

O'REGAN: My real point was that you seem to be surprised that human beings can detect or can perceive sexual orientation via gestures. And seen from my point of view, it's totally obvious. It's a necessity.

AMBADY: The myth is that people can conceal their sexual orientation, and that's why we have policies like "don't ask, don't tell." Or the whole notion of "gaydar," that only certain groups of people who are privileged, in a sense, can detect it. But your point is well taken, and I think your point speaks to what we found. It might seem obvious in hindsight but I don't think it was quite that clear.

HARRINGTON: How universal do you want your argument to be? I gather that you've brought the films to India and showed that the girls in the convent could correctly decode, which seems to imply that this sort of information can be cross-culturally decoded. But you know, if you think about the stylizations of homosexuality in the Western world, it feels to me very historically conditioned and relatively recent. Homosexuality didn't look the same back in ancient Greece as it would in New York City in the 1970s, and so on.

AMBADY: I think the display rules are different, but I think that the observers in our studies were picking on some type of asynchrony in the gestures. They weren't picking any explicit display signals, which of course could vary cross-culturally. But I am not sure how universal I want to make this argument at this point. I just think the data are too preliminary right now.

JACQUES MEHLER: I would like to take a step back. We were asked to focus on the languages of the brain, and in this section there was a clear barrage: everybody was trying to say well, the languages of the brain rely on representations of movement and images. But notice that we share these properties with other higher vertebrates, even very low vertebrates, such as a dog; if I had a dog, my dog would have all of those properties. Yet the dogs do not do what we do. As Liz [Spelke] will agree, even in development you see how perceptual and motoric modules are rather poor when they're not driven by a language with a grammar, like the language of the mind or whatever language you want.

MARK WEXLER: One thing that your dog couldn't do would be to manipulate objects in the very precise way that we can.

MEHLER: Of course a dog is a bad example. It's a quadruped. So take the most evolved of our ancestors and you'd see the same thing. Our linguistic abilities, logical abilities, and so forth, the representations which we have, the productivity which we have in these systems, don't seem to be attainable by other species. And probably one of the explanations that I would favor is that there is an emergent capacity, an evolved capacity of the mind for a linguistic system. We have it, and the other animals who have a module for movement, a module for whatever else, don't have it, period. And this is an empirical question that can be addressed.

KOSSLYN: It seems clear that no module is an island. The brain is a system, and the various components must work together. Which one or ones have priority—if any really do—appears to be an unresolved question, which I hope is an empirical question. Perhaps by studying nonhuman animals we can get a handle on the role of language and its conceptual underpinnings. But of course animals differ from us in more ways than in their lack of language, so this is a tricky method.

Section 6
Representations in the World

Language is used in many ways, but two stand out: communication and mental representation. We so far have focused on the latter, but most language arguably is used for the former purpose. In contrast, most nonverbal representation is used in thinking. Nevertheless, it is also used in the service of communication. In this section we consider what practitioners in the art of communicating nonverbally have learned about nonverbal representation. The act of creating a visual communication requires certain assumptions about the minds of the readers, those who will decode the work. The first three chapters of the section are of great interest in part because their authors are informed about the results of relevant research, and have incorporated such findings into their theories how to communicate effectively—and the fourth paper touches on perhaps the most fundamental question about nonverbal communication, how it (particularly art) is created. Nigel Holmes, long the head of the art department at *Time* magazine and inventor of what is now called "infographics," shows in Chapter 20 how simple patterns of lines can effectively convey information. Holmes draws on findings about the nature of perception to explain why certain patterns are so effective, and notes the key role of prior beliefs and expectations in visual communication. An artist is not simply a channel through which the world passes on its way to the visual communication; rather, what one sees must be organized and filtered, and the final product is a result of the way the artist "manipulates the visual language." Holmes draws a strong parallel to verbal language here, by focusing on units and how they are combined according to rules.

In Chapter 21 the New York artist Rhonda Roland Shearer has developed the idea that the neural machinery used in navigating and organizing the environment is also recruited to organize nonspatial materials. Many linguists have previously noticed the pervasive role of spatial metaphors in language (for example, when asking about time in English, we say, "How long will it take"?). Shearer goes several steps further: she argues that geometry is used as an organizational device in memory and thought. In this case, the type of mental geometry one is using is crucial, because the geometry defines the sorts of spatial relations and organizations that are possible. Some systems of geometry lend themselves to hierarchical organization, and we often use such organization when trying to make sense of the world. But these are not the only possible geometries, and Shearer shows that we can learn much by contemplating features of other sorts of geometries and their implications for how thoughts are organized. Moreover, as new geometries are discovered and developed (for example, fractal geometry), these can provide additional insights into how thought proceeds.

In Chapter 22, Gerald Zaltman describes a procedure for using visual forms to allow people to externalize complex meanings. His technique depends in part on projective tests, in some ways reminiscent of Rorschach ink blots and the like, but also includes sophisticated analyses of protocols developed as people construct visual forms to communicate a message. Zaltman's work explores the conceptual intersection between emotion-laden meanings of metaphors in language and the meaning of specific pictures. Zaltman develops methods for laying bare the "mental models" people have of specific concepts, and in so doing shows how multimodal and multifaceted these internal models are.

Finally, in Chapter 23 Jean-Pierre Changeux addresses one of the oldest systems of social representation—art. This system is older than writing, as is evident in the caves at Lascaux, for example. In keeping with Denis Diderot, who said that one picture is worth a thousand words, Changeux tells us that creation is a remarkably complex activity that draws on much of the brain. He believes that we can interpret perception, creation, and the history of art on the basis of evolutionary thinking. His analysis is predicated on the ideas that (1) there is a universal predisposition in the human brain for aesthetic pleasure; (2) creation can be viewed as a trial-and-error process, with internal rewards resulting in a selection process; and (3) art is an internalization of pictorial representation, with the process of externalizing the image depending on a rich set of factors, including the personal history of the artist.

The Gap between Seeing and Drawing 20

Nigel Holmes

My job is to explain statistics and processes to a particular set of readers in the clearest possible way. Over the years, I have come to realize the obvious—that the best way to do this, the best language to use, is a combination of words and pictures, where the two are inseparable and must be read together. Pictures by themselves seldom complete the job of explaining something; and whereas words by themselves might be able to describe a problem, they very often need pictures for accurate and total understanding. I say that this is obvious, but in the publishing world, editors actually think of the two activities—that is, making words and making pictures—as separate. In fact the whole editorial process conspires to keep the two separate. And while we are generally well trained as writers and readers of words, we are generally badly trained in graphics and in what constitutes understandable graphics.

Since we are a species that has sight as its predominant sense, pictures are among the most effective ways to transmit information. I am convinced that the ability to draw pictures is a vital part of creating good, meaningful graphics.

The act of drawing involves looking at something, then looking in a different direction to actually make the drawing. Thus at the moment the artist tries to represent an object by drawing it, he is looking not at the object, but rather at a blank sheet of paper.

When a picture is "taken" with a camera, there is a straight line between the object to be photographed and the film on which the object is recorded as a picture. But drawing is different. The artist first looks at the object, and then looks away from it to "make" a picture.

The gap between seeing and drawing can be short: those momentary glances up and down from object to paper—what we call "drawing from life." Or the gap can be long: an hour, a week, a decade—what we call "drawing from memory."

Some artists have tried to erase the gap between seeing and drawing—making a picture without looking away from the object. By not looking down at the surface they were working on, they tried to fuse the act of seeing with the act of drawing. Rodin is the most famous example of someone who tried this. Many of his drawings were made without taking his eyes off the object, or in his case more usually, the model.

I tried it, too. Using a pair of scissors as my object, I covered my right hand on the drawing paper and looked only at the scissors, while drawing them. The result showed how hard it was to do this, however interestingly quirky the sketch might look. A minute later I did a second drawing—slightly worse! Just to check that I hadn't lost the ability to draw at all, I removed the cover on the drawing surface, and did a straightforward rendering. I wondered if by drawing the scissors normally, I would somehow train my hand to make marks on the paper in a way that when I returned to drawing "blind," there would be some "memory" of how to draw the scissors. Indeed, the next "blind" drawing was a little better. But a minute or so later, it was more disconnected than ever. If Rodin were alive, I'd ask him what the trick was, because for me, this was an exercise that showed that I cannot do a convincing drawing without looking away from the object being drawn. I cannot be a camera, with the object going straight through me to the paper.

But "making" a drawing is not like "taking a picture." A drawing of an object or a landscape does not look like a photograph of the same scene, taken at the same time, from the same position.

Many elements rush into the enforced, and as we have seen, necessary, gap between seeing and drawing, and an interesting result of not looking at the object at the very time the act of drawing takes place is that no two artists will ever make the same drawing of an object. This is because what artists usually do when they draw is to manipulate elements of a visual language. I will deal with two of these elements: the first is the use of a set of basic shapes, or geons, the second, perspective. Drawing involves much more than the use of geons and perspective, of course. A major part of drawing for any artist is how to make use of all the elements to arrive at a personal style.

First, I will consider the building of an image from universal shapes. It is very interesting for me to read about what's going on in our minds when we look at things. For instance I now understand that David Marr's theories, and subsequently Irv Biederman's set of geons, might start to explain how we recognize objects. A long time ago, at art school in England, I was taught to break down objects into their component parts, first, so as to be able to understand their structure and, second, so that I could reconstruct the objects on paper in the form of a drawing. To know that a bottle was a small upright cylinder, then a hemisphere, and below that a fatter, longer cylinder was interesting, but not the kind of activity, intellectual or otherwise, that I was looking forward to in London in the 1960s. And of course the bottle on the still life table didn't look anything like a cylinder, a hemisphere, and a bigger cylinder. For a start, I was not sitting directly opposite it. It felt much more natural to draw around the bottle, tracing the outline, trying to put down on paper what it looked like—and from my particular angle of view.

And some days more complex objects were put in front of us. "Taking a line for a walk" is how Paul Klee described the act of drawing, and that is what this image of a microscope is. The tip of the pen has walked around the object, leaving a trail.

But graphic artists are seldom making records of a still life—in fact they are seldom involved with that very short gap between seeing and drawing, and that is why the building blocks are so important in commercial, as opposed to fine, art.

By thinking in masses, in shapes, in geons, instead of drawing "around" an object, you are thinking about what the object is, rather than what it looks like. At this moment, instead of drawing what you see (either in front of you, or in your memory), you are drawing what you know about an object. It follows that the object does not have to be there for you to draw it. Thus the microscope can be thought of as being composed of shapes that can be fitted together. The resulting image is better for having been constructed this way, as opposed to being made by taking a line for a walk around it.

There is another way to express the difference between these two forms of drawing: when we first look at something and start to draw it, the act of looking is more important than the act of drawing. However, as the artist proceeds with the drawing, his responsibility shifts away from the object to what he is creating—that is, what's left on the paper. Notwithstanding those art historian photographers who are interested in comparing a drawn landscape to a photo taken from the place where the artist sat and drew it—there are examples of this, for instance, comparing Cézanne's paintings of Mont St. Victoire to photos of the place—the artist generally knows that he will be judged by his representation of a scene, or an object, not by his ability to mimic the photographic look of a place or a thing.

In the graphic arts, geons, or pictorial building blocks, can be used with great efficiency to make symbols that are understood quickly, and that can reproduce easily and in multiples for use in statistical charts. The master of this was Otto Neurath, whose ISOTYPE system was developed in the 1920s with the help of the very gifted artist Gerd Arntz. Neurath never expected his visual vocabulary to stand alone as a communications tool; rather, he called his system a "helping language," one that worked together with words. The work of Neurath and Arntz gives a clear answer to those who say that drawing from a kit of parts can result in a cold, inhuman art form. In fact, in his efforts to be both pictorial and statistically accountable in his charts, Neurath did want his images to be neutral, or deadpan, but it is hard not to have real feelings of sympathy for this man, who is so obviously cold and out of work, or to recognize that this man is clearly at the other end of the financial scale. The reason these images are effective is that they are well observed. However simply executed, they are very good drawings.

The speed of transmission of understanding is faster now than in Neurath's time. This simple manipulation of three circles is all we need to recognize one of the prime movers of our entertainment-mad world. Following the example of Mickey Mouse, toy makers often use circles, or parts of circles, for cuddly characters: this one is Elmo from Sesame Street. And I think I disagree with Steven Pinker's passage in

How the Mind Works, about geons being "not good for everything . . . it is almost impossible to build model of a particular face"—there is a whole school of caricature that employs basic geons to create perfectly recognizable faces. In the 1920s and 1930s Paolo Garretto did wonderful "geon" faces, which showed how simple shapes, when cleverly arranged, can be very powerful, not to mention instantly recognizable. Of course some celebrities have deliberately made their faces into icons: Charlie Chaplin is an example. And with what little graphic effort can Chaplin become a monster! Remember this about drawing: artists are often having a secret kind of fun. It becomes a game to see how few marks one can make and still hold an image. There is pleasure, for the viewer and the artist, in recognizing both the geon structure in a drawing and the face the geons make. Thus the formulas and marks that artists use become interesting in their own right, as well as being a means for portraying something. And just as a passage in a jazz solo or a book might quote or allude to another tune or another author, so do graphic artists in their work. David Suter is an artist whose drawings often use optical illusions, some quoting Edgar Rubin's 1915 face and vase. Using the same play between object and ground, the designers of the current Fedex logo have hidden an arrow between the last E and the X in the name. (Maybe they were a little too clever. Who noticed this nice bit of fun? A press release from the designers pointing it out alerted me to its presence.)

I do not want to suggest that using geons is the only way to draw. The gap between seeing and drawing can also be filled by what I might call a "scribble-up" technique. Here, images are built up in much the same way that a sculptor adds clay to an armature, piece by piece, from the inside out. But this is really just another way of arriving at the outside shape, the form of an object. Neurath suggested that the best way to keep an image simple was to cut it out of black paper, the action of the scissors limiting the artist's choice of shapes.

After geons—the building blocks of images—the second major element in the language of drawing that I briefly want to discuss is perspective, that is, the understanding that some objects, or parts of objects, are in front of others in a picture.

When we look at this image we can read that it says "tall" and "short," but it's pretty hard to see it that way. Despite the accompanying words, we see this as a picture of one person near to us and one person further away. The power of perspective is enormous. It is a set of rules that tells us how to read pictures. Only with considerable mental effort can we see this as a tall person walking next to a short person. Now consider this image: it's Billy Crystal and Gheorghe Muresan, the costar of his movie *My Giant.* This picture consists of the same arrangement of people, one tall, one short. But here both sets of feet are clearly on the same line, and there's even a helpful mark on the pedestrian crossing. These people are anchored in space. Now we can concentrate on just how small Billy Crystal really is, compared to the 7′ 7″ giant next to him, instead of wondering how far behind the giant he is walking.

Why is it important for graphic artists to understand the power of perspective? Here is an example. The problem was to chart the length of a number of ships in the U.S. Navy. Since it is my firm belief that readers respond more quickly and favorably to pictures rather than abstract bars, my first step was to make the bars into drawings of the ships. Two interesting things happened. First you could see that a patrol boat is not only shorter, is also altogether very much smaller than a frigate, a fact that you did not understand from looking at the bar chart, where it is actually shown to be taller than it is long! The second effect of substituting images of ships for bars is that a total picture is created here, one that has the power of perspective in it. And that is misleading, for inevitably one views this picture as a whole, not as a set of individual bars. The picture that we see is of a fleet of ships that recedes from the viewer into the distance. If the graphic artist understands the power of perspective, he will reverse the order of the ships, and put the largest one at the top, so that the viewer is forced to see it now as a flat image, with all the information up against the front picture plane, and not as an impression of a naval shipyard.

Every day an increasing amount of data rushes past us. The use of clear, geon-based drawings together with the power of perspective will help us to understand more of the data. All we need are well-drawn pictures of the information.

Rethinking Images and Metaphors: New Geometries as Key to Artistic and Scientific Revolutions

21

Rhonda Roland Shearer

The daily grind of repeating experiments that meet our expectations and reinforce rather than revolutionize our fields is the gristmill of convention in both art and science. However, history has recorded rare leaps of change, and the resulting novelty in approaches, thought, and perceptions that occurs in both fields correlates with major, but infrequent, new developments in geometry. If the brain's evolution in operating a body in space involves representations or maps and these same maps are extended for use in abstract thought, then the organization of knowledge and perception can be usefully conceptualized in terms of geometry and part-whole relations in space. Revolutions in both art and science serve as evidence for my claim that the brain's utilization of space indicates a fundamental role for order and change in part-whole relationships not only in these special large-scale cases but also as a general rule in everyday perception and cognition.

Whenever we perceive or conceptualize—whether it involves a process of recognizing large/small, up/down, near/far relations or of utilizing Newtonian space or Darwinian taxonomies—order is the only conduit to understanding and perception. Once an order is established, it must be replaced with a new order before we can understand or perceive something anew. Therefore conscious manipulation of established, fixed order is a direct, experimental means for provoking innovation. The issue is not a "chicken or egg" problem. If we "turn the tables," "go to the top of the mountain" and *then* see something new, is the creative act what we see or the geometric act that made such seeing possible? The second, or geometric step, must always come first.

For example, when we examine the history of art, the two largest-scale developments consistently noted by scholars are Renaissance perspective and the early twentieth-century birth of modern art. Perspective geometry transformed the painter's surface from a convention of two-dimensional symbolic space (where Jesus' left and right hands symbolically pointed to people who were bad and good respectively) to a new set of geometric relations that emphasized one set of retinal rules (for example, that a close object is large and the same object far away is small) against our more rational sense of constancy, which ignores or filters out perspective distortions.

By the early twentieth century, early modernist artists were thinking within the new geometries of Riemann and *n*-dimensions (popularly known as curved space and the fourth dimension), which inspired a radical break with the artistic convention of representations as limited to three Euclidean dimensions (Henderson, 1983).

The geometry that was fodder for radical change in thought and spatial application in art was the same Riemannian geometry of curved space that Einstein claimed as his inspiration for general relativity, a dramatic break in science on a similar scale to the birth of modernism in art. Newton's vision of the perfect, smooth regularity of space was radically altered when Einstein applied Riemannian geometry to nature. Einstein envisioned space as deformed by gravity and curved.

Copernicus' discovery remapped the earth from the center of the universe to a peripheral position—a geometric change involving a literal alteration both in spatial mapping and in mental space, as we reverse the relational bins of conventional categorization schemes to place the sun in the center and the earth as one of many revolving planets.

Darwin's theory of evolution was also a change in conceptual space (taxonomic part-whole relations). For many, he uncomfortably recategorized humans as genealogical relatives of monkeys and apes rather than a separate order of creation. These examples from the history of art and science indicate that we can usefully conceive revolutionary change, not only as shifting images and ideas, but also as alterations in the fundamental geometries of our spatial maps, whether literal or conceptual.

It is not only the largest-scale revolutions in art and science that allow us to experience a new sense of reality created by geometric change. We can experience this geometric effect on a smaller scale, and thus in a similar way. That is, by smaller but similar construction we may be able to think in new ways. My first example involves the smaller-scale effects of geometric change in perception. Figure 21.1's upside-down image is not a printer's error. Rather it represents a conventional technique for training artists to draw. Rotated 180 degrees, photographs are easier for budding artists to draw in this unexpected, unfamiliar spatial orientation. It is as if we were suddenly able to see the shapes of human footprints in sand as pure form disassociated from the baggage of any context, story, or meaning. Novel orientations of objects enable artists not only to psychologically unlink form from meaning, but also to mentally focus on lines, shading, and shape alone. With novel rotation, the operation of drawing then becomes "These are lines, shades, and shapes to reproduce"—not as complex a mental task for young artists as "lines, shades and shapes, forming a reclining human female, known as Sappho, exposed breast, complex draping cloth," and so on, as would be found in an upright Figure 21.1. My second example, in contrast to the first, suggests the significance of change in conceptual maps that link form to meaning, instead of the removal of meaning from form (with novel orientation) to enhance perception.

Consider the old joke about a man who, while in a foreign country, always inquired about the meat included in any menu fare. In a restaurant, this man asks a waiter, "What meat is in the Rabbit Stew?" The waiter answers, "Rabbit and horse." "How much rabbit and how much horse?" asks the man. "About half rabbit and half horse," answers the waiter. "Half and half?" asks the man. "Yes," answers the waiter, "one rabbit and one horse."

Figure 21.2 maps the running account of part-whole relationships as they change within this Rabbit Stew joke. We realize, in the punch line, when we finally determine the most accurate part-whole relationship, that the rabbit stew was really horse stew all along. This joke provides a good example of how spatial changes don't have to be Copernican in scale to have a significant impact upon our perception and cognition. Forms in space create meaning.

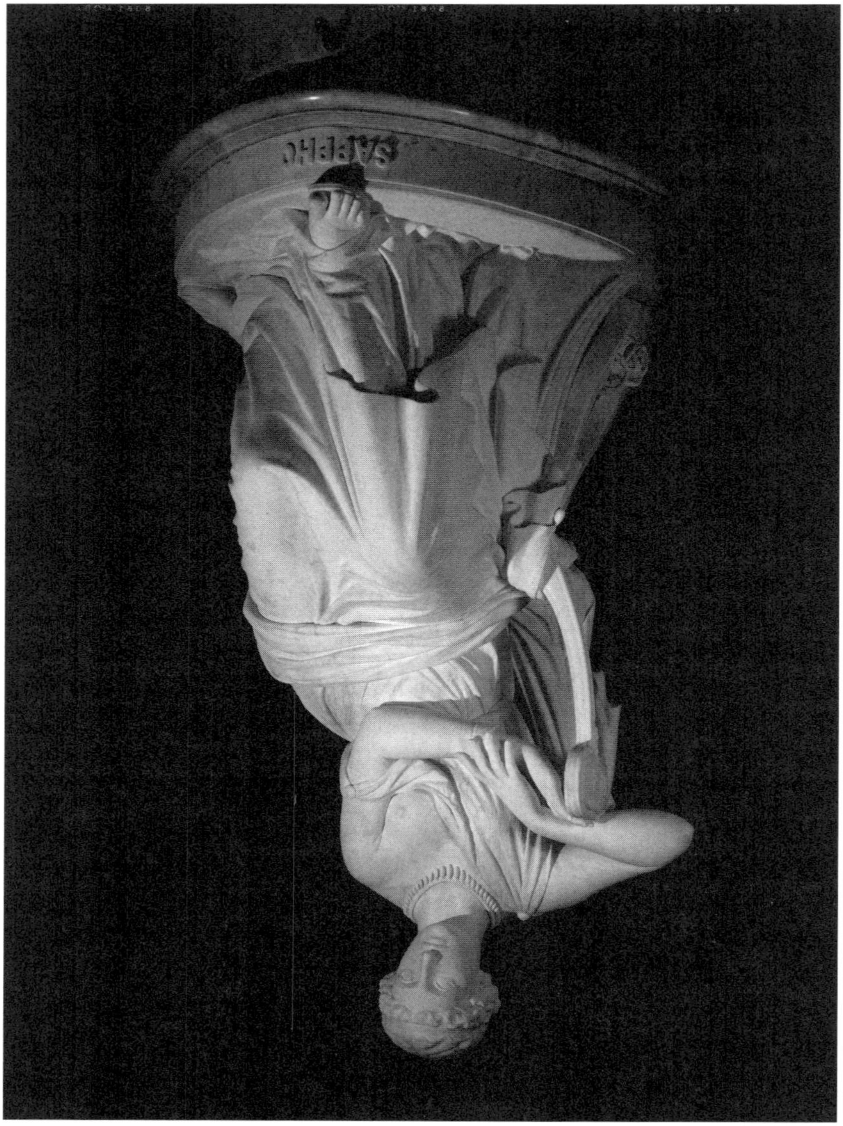

Figure 21.1. Rotating a photograph of a figure by 180 degrees is a conventional technique for teaching drawing. Nineteenth-century marble figure courtesy of Berry Hill Gallery.

Reality Is Horse Stew
Geometric analysis
1.
Rabbit stew
2.
Rabbit stew with a little horse
3.
rabbit, horse
4.
Entire rabbit, entire horse,
make it really horse stew

Figure 21.2. Progressive part-whole relationship changes in "Rabbit Stew" joke.

With New Geometries, Innovations Follow

New geometries, like revolutions in art and science, are rare historical occurrences (see Figure 21.3). Since new geometries have acted as significant conceptual provocations linked to major innovations in art and science, examination of the conceptual and perceptual differences between classical geometries and the new geometry of fractals could be an important means for predicting and/or creating innovations. Fractals, devised by Benoit Mandelbrot in 1965, are the most recent and largest-scale change in the history of new developments in geometry. Like Russian stacking dolls, ranging from small to large in size, fractals are defined as similar shapes that occur across various sizes or scales (also referred to as fractal self-similarity). Nature expresses nu-

Euclidean geometry	Euclid 300 B.C.
Perspective	Artists in Renaissance 15th century
Non-Euclidean geometries *N*-dimensional geometry	Several geometers Mid-19th century
Fractal geometry	Mandelbrot 1965

Figure 21.3. Large-scale developments in geometry: new geometries are rare historical occurrences.

merous examples of fractal forms—clouds, fire, trees, mountains, rivers, erosion patterns, chemical reactions, snowflakes, and so on. In fact, it has been argued by Mandelbrot and others that nature is much better described as fractal—for Euclidean lines, circles, and cubes occur only as the exception rather than as the rule.

The other new and related aspect of Mandelbrot's fractal geometry has been defined as fractal dimension (Mandelbrot, 1983). When fractals are evident, numerous scales or sizes (and in the case of computer-generated fractals, infinite scales) of similar forms irregularly pack themselves within a finite boundary—for example, Russian dolls fractally increasing on a line confined between two points. As the fractal forms iterate in time and continue to subdivide into smaller and smaller partitions of space, a reduction in scale occurs, with a simultaneously increasing volume of the totality of dolls. More and smaller dolls are generated, but subdivisions of space can infinitely continue and never fill beyond the one-dimensional line into two complete dimensions. Therefore the line in between the two points of fractal dolls will express a fractal dimension somewhere between one and two (either closer to one dimension with fewer iterations of dolls, 1.3 for example; or closer to two dimensions with more iterations, as in a 1.7 fractal dimension). With fractals, we experience a new reality in comparison to the convention of mapping and embedding forms within a whole integer dimensional reality of zero, one, two, or three dimensions, and so on.

Like the spatial changes that we experienced in the Rabbit Stew joke, moving from Ptolemy's to Copernicus' cosmic map, or from a smooth Newtonian space to the irregular curves of Einsteinian spaces, fractal geometry gives us a new way to perceive space and its part-whole relations. Instead of envisioning nature through classical geometric descriptions—which includes a built-in bias for viewing irregular forms as dirty, noisy shapes with Platonic, Euclidean ideals hidden inside (for example, a lumpy grapefruit surface disguised as Plato's perfect sphere)—fractals offer a radical alternative to the historical bias that "irregular" equals "disorder" and the absence of geometry.

Fractal Geometry and the Earmarks of Scientific Revolutions

In Figure 21.4, I present a list of eight traits that historians of science have identified as earmarks of scientific revolutions (Cohen 1985; Hanson 1965, 1969; Holton 1988; Kuhn 1972; Thagard 1992). Here I will focus on category change and new language.

Figure 21.5a demonstrates that genealogical taxonomies, which map relations of influence by generations and time, exist not only in the domain of science but also in art. Alfred Barr, curator and histo-

1. New ideas
2. New language and metaphors
3. New kind/hierarchies and categories (taxonomies)
4. New part/whole relationships
5. New icons (visual symbols)
6. Sense of "conversion" or Gestalt switching (new thinking, seeing values, "reality")
7. Many revolutions have an "ideological component"
8. History needs to be rewritten for logical and factual congruence

Figure 21.4. Traits of scientific revolutions cited by historians of science. (Sources: Kuhn, I. B. Cohen, Popper, Thagard.)

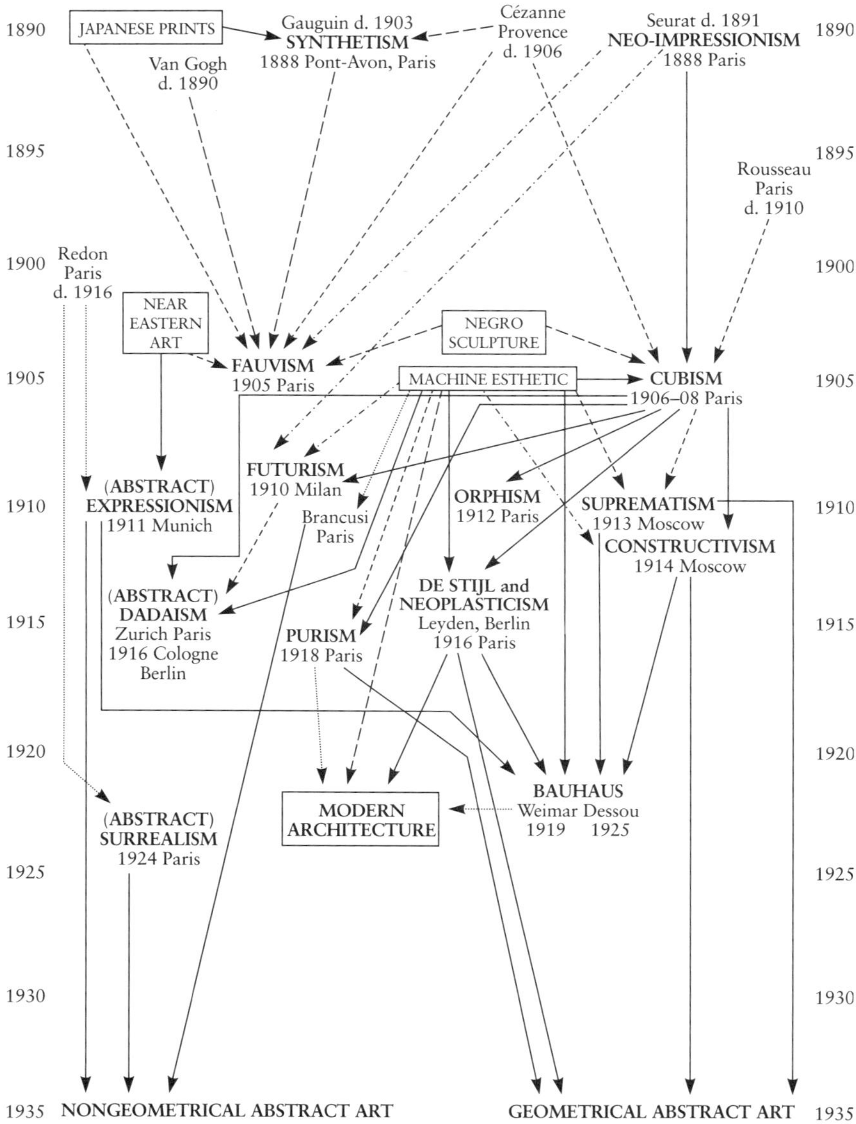

Figure 21.5a. Alfred Barr's taxonomic chart of modern art's genealogical evolution through time. (© Art Science Research Laboratory; original in Museum of Modern Art, New York.)

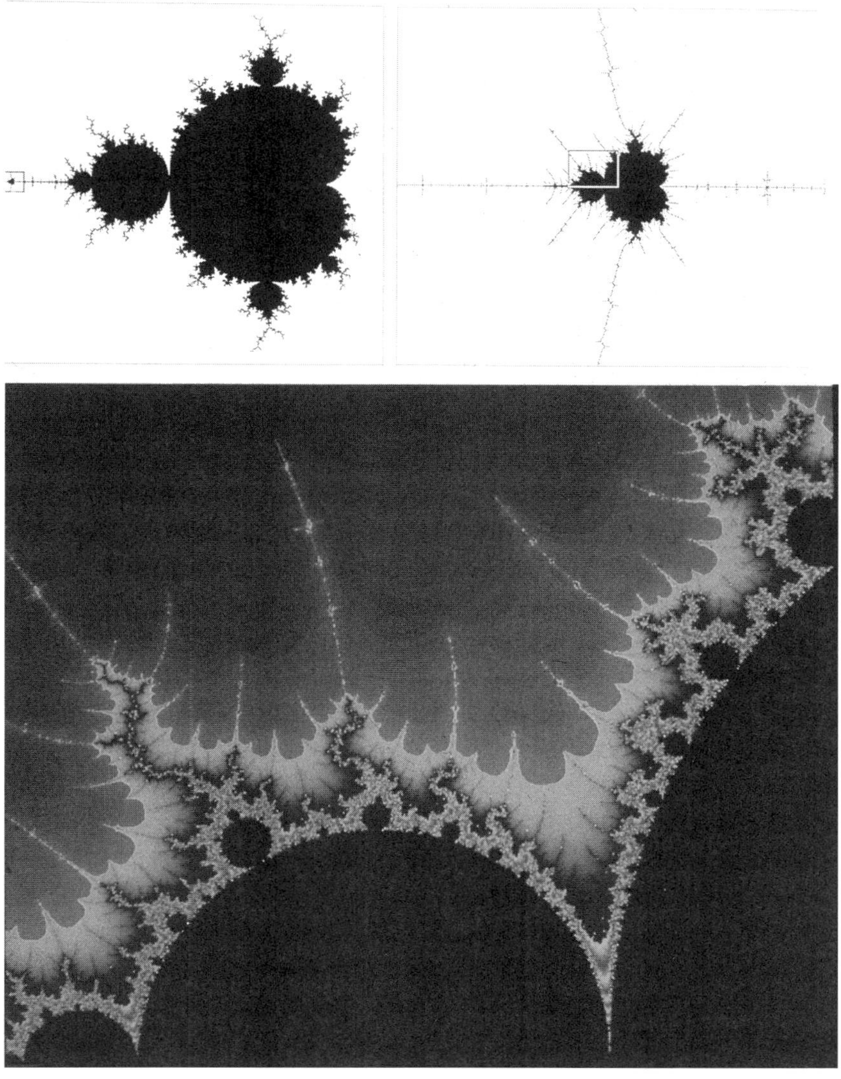

Figure 21.5b. Computer-generated fractal. Mandelbrot set by Richard Voss.

rian of art in the mid-twentieth century, drew up a strict taxonomy of the evolution of modern art. It culminated in a bifurcating split between geometric and organic abstraction. But what about the fractal in Figure 21.5b? Surely under Barr's conventional scheme, this fractal is both organic and geometric by definition and appearance.

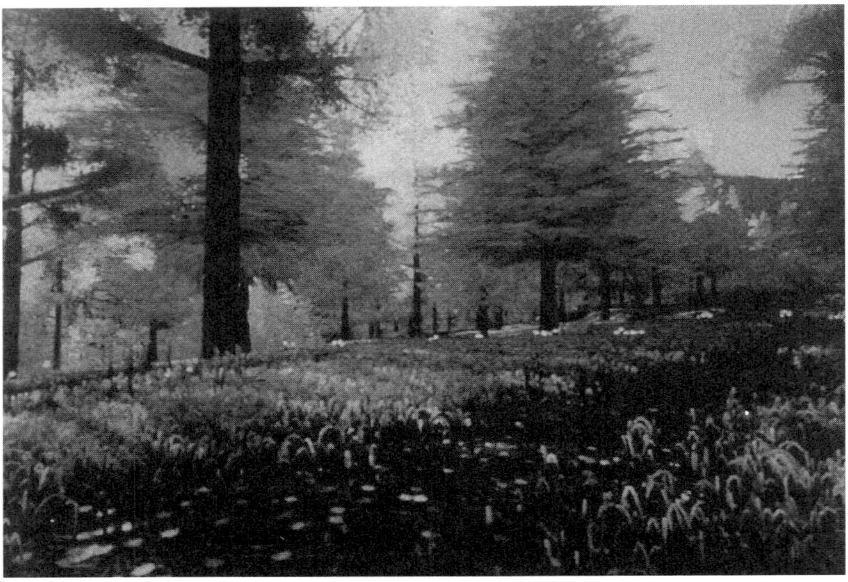

Figure 21.6a. Computer-generated fractal landscape by Przemyslaw Prusinkiewicz.

A comparison of a fractal geometric landscape and a photograph of an actual landscape further indicates how dramatically we must alter our conventional categories and the fundamental operating taxonomy of our beliefs and definitions in art history (Figure 21.6a,b). The fractal landscape, generated as pure geometric form in a computer, is a mathematical object and therefore qualifies for residence in the category of geometric abstraction. Yet the fractal shapes, as organic or biomorphic forms, simultaneously exist in the other, formerly opposite and separate category of organic abstraction. In the fractal landscape, moreover, the categories of abstract and real, long considered objectively to be opposite and separate in definitions of nature and reality, can now for the first time describe the same geometric forms.

Not only must the dualisms of organic and geometric, or abstract and real, now be mapped as connected, but the hidden, hierarchical preference for, and supposed superiority of, one side of the dualism (abstract and geometric) over the other, devalued side (organic, real) is exposed as a false conclusion based upon the false premise that "irregular" is opposite to geometry. When we only had classical

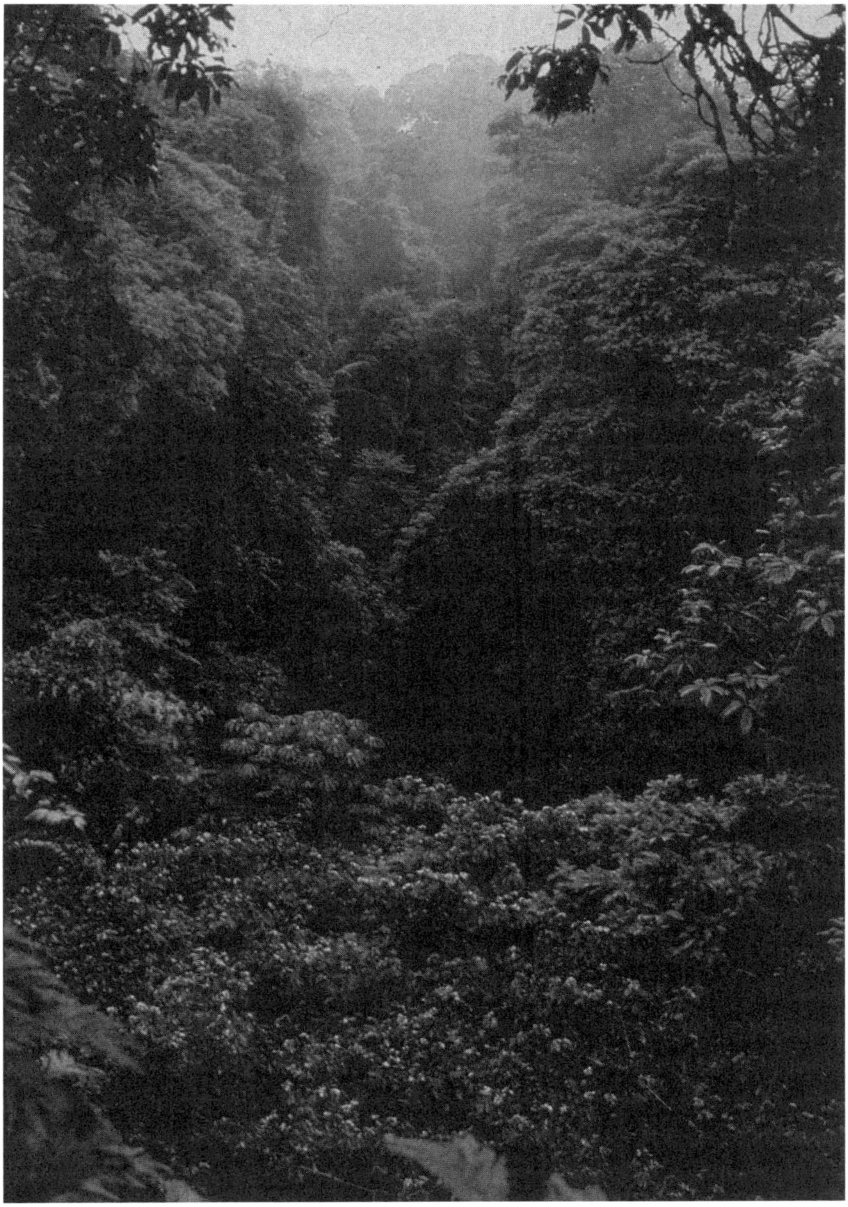

Figure 21.6b. Photo of actual landscape.

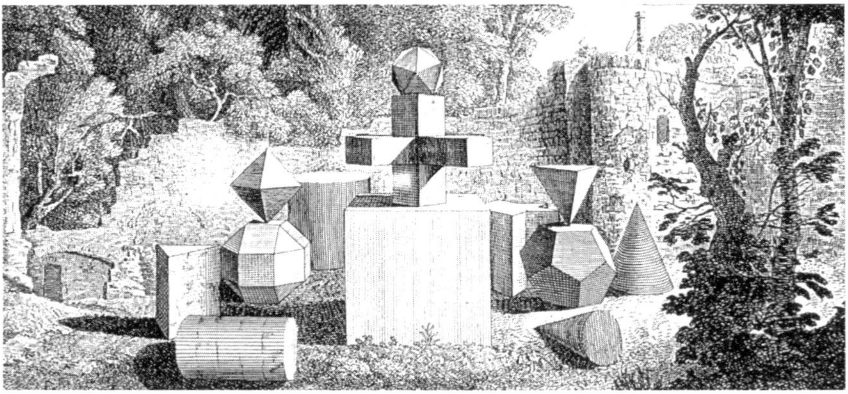

Figure 21.7. Illustration from eighteenth-century book on perspective by Joshua Kirby. (Joshua Kirby, *Dr. Brook Taylor's Method of Perspective Made Easy; Both in Theory and Practice: In Two Books,* Book One, London: Francklin & Bunce, 1765.)

geometries to define nature, we faced an unmistakable discordance. Consider the scene shown in Figure 21.7 from an eighteenth-century book on perspective, in which the Euclidean polyhedra look like foreign vessels sitting uncomfortably in the surround of nature's unruly abundance (Kirby, 1765). Since only certain regularities could be mathematically described, the rest of nature (which mathematics could not define, control, or allow us to understand) was dismissed as noise and regarded as irrational, disordered, and even feminine. Hence Bacon's statement, which is part of a continuum that has equated women and the feminine with the irrationality of nature: "Woman is nature and hence detestable." In this vein we find a recent cartoon (Figure 21.8), in which two men in suits leave the office of a woman executive who is wearing a dress covered with flowers. One man says to the other, "Her flowered prints fooled me too . . . She's tough as nails!" Here a belief in flowers and nature is categorized as essentially feminine in opposition to the masculine, a conviction found not only in high art but in popular culture. This perspective influences not only artists' selection of subject matter but what people choose to wear and even the image they wish to project (Shearer, 1996).

The choice of subject matter preferred by artists and art historians has always been based upon the belief of prefractal dualism and hierarchy that the abstract and geometric were, a priori, intellectually superior to any representation of the organic and real (Bryson, 1990).

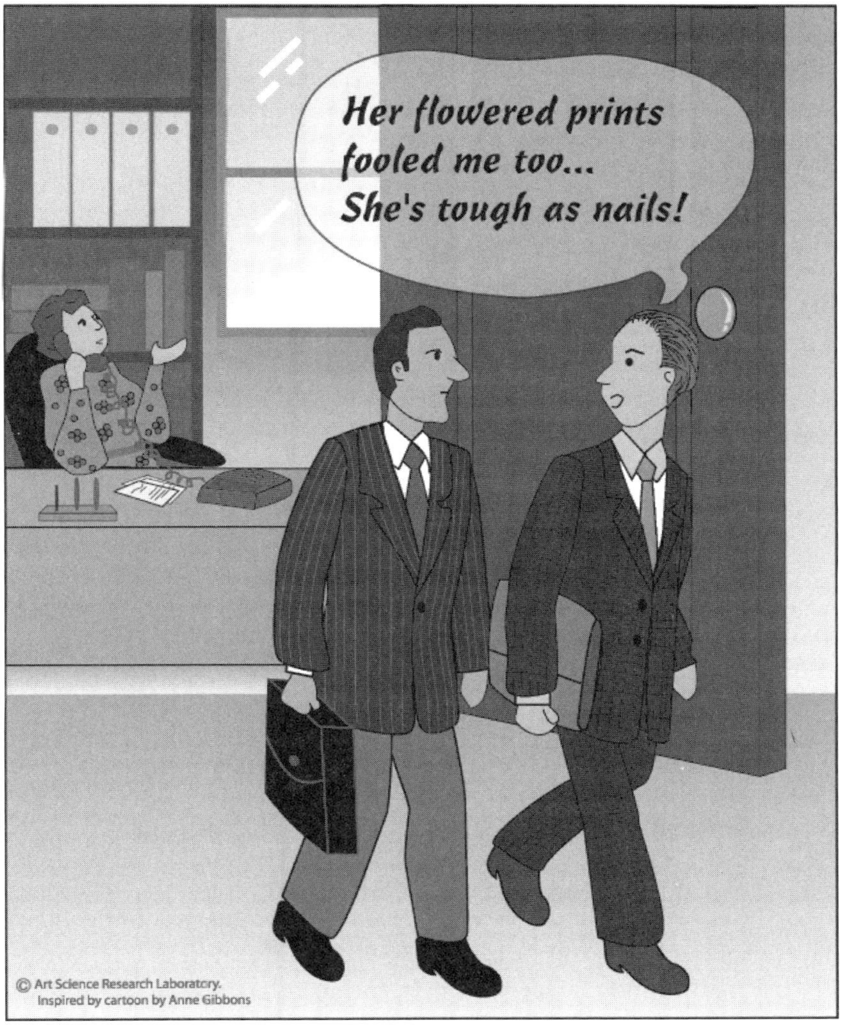

Figure 21.8. Cartoon refers to the conventional belief that flowers and nature represent the feminine and female in popular culture, clothing, and high art. (Inspired by a cartoon by Anne Gibbons. © Art Science Research Laboratory.)

When old categorization schemes can't consistently contain or map new relations, they must be changed, thus creating not only a new taxonomy but a belief system that alters our sense of the world, as in pre- and post-Darwinian biology. In addition to changes in categories, change in language is another earmark of scientific revolutions. The geometric description of a cloud serves as an example. Before fractal geometry, it could only be said that clouds were irregular or cloud-shaped. Language or classical geometric conventions allowed little else—ovals and circles would never do as descriptions of clouds.

Fractal relations always surrounded us. But we could not see, understand, utilize, or even talk about their structures without the language of the new formal geometry—just as we believed that the man was getting rabbit stew until the changing part-whole description revealed his meal to be better labeled as horse stew.

Conclusion

My argument for the significance of new geometries is itself fractal. Examples I have given range, like Russian nesting dolls, from large-scale revolutions of beliefs (like those of Copernicus and Einstein) to single jokes (Horse Stew). The invariance in the importance of new geometries across all scales demonstrates the structural similarity between the role of changes in part-whole spatial relations in large leaps of knowledge and the brain's everyday, smaller-scale operations.

We map the world in part-whole relations. As Giordano Bruno said of symbols, these maps are simultaneously vehicles (routing our thinking and perceptions) and chains (for once we think within these fixed maps, we are limited or chained because we cannot think outside of them until a shift to an alternative map is made).

For discovery, we must literally reorder the conceptual and literal spaces represented in our heads to allow new information into our beliefs and perceptions. Since we can relate prior success in art and science to such remappings, we can now directly choose to work with literal and conceptual part-whole relations in our minds as a more conscious means for creating innovation.

Fractals, as our most recent geometric development, become an obvious choice for such application if we consider how effective new geometries have been for past creativity in art and science. We have usually considered universality and individuality, for example, to be entirely disconnected and opposite. But if we think within fractal structures, we will be able to see how they can be linked. A given tree branch, with its individual irregularities, is like no other—and yet, as a fractal, it is (despite this full individuality) completely and universally related to all tree branches; on a greater scale, all human vascular systems, and river systems as well, are fractal branching structures. Similarly, with fractal geometry as our mental eyeglasses, we can see an intriguing linkage between ourselves as organic structures and inorganic forms found within nature. Science has experienced a long-standing separation between the organic and living and the inorganic and dead—all as a reaction to the once believable, and now irrational, taxonomy of premodern science that categorized rocks as alive.

Just as many years had to elapse from the first development of non-Euclidean geometry in the mid-nineteenth century until its significance could be validated through early twentieth-century success when applied in science (Einstein) and art (birth of modern art), we should note that only a short time has elapsed since fractal geometry's discovery in the mid-1960s.

Throughout the history of mathematics, what initially appeared as theoretical has often later been found to have practical application as a discovery in nature. The discovery of the Buckminsterfullerenes, or Bucky Balls, having moved from only theoretical status to being observable in nature, is a good example (Baggott, 1996). Pharmaceutical companies are currently manipulating the geometric relations of molecules in computers and *then* testing them as a novel means for drug discoveries. This new, direct geometric approach is rapidly replacing and reversing the old experimental method of direct testing of substances and compounds, and only then resolving the molecular geometry.

Universal structures exist in nature and we, over time, have accessed them with various and improving descriptions. It is within these very descriptions (which we embed in conceptions of time and of part-whole relations in space) that our creative limits and potential for innovations simultaneously lie. We therefore find a distinct advantage in the direct procedure that I have called the Flatland Hypothesis: first, map the part-whole relations of your thoughts and feelings and of the conventional idea or order to clearly identify and become consciously aware of its structure; second, consciously alter these structures into novel relationships and spacial orientations or apply to them the newest development in geometry. With novel or unexpected geometric relations you will be able to see and think anew (Shearer, 1996).

References

Baggott, Jim. 1996. *Perfect symmetry: The accidental discovery of Buckminsterfullerene.* New York: Oxford University Press.

Bryson, Norman. 1990. *Looking at the overlooked: Four essays on still life painting.* Cambridge: Harvard University Press.

Cohen, I. Bernard. 1985. *Revolution in science.* Cambridge: Harvard University Press.

Hanson, Norwood R. 1965. *Patterns of discovery: An inquiry into the conceptual foundations of science.* Cambridge: Harvard University Press.

——— 1969. *Perception and discovery: An introduction to scientific inquiry.* San Francisco: Freeman, Cooper and Company.

Henderson, Linda Dalrymple. 1983. *The fourth dimension and non-Euclidean geometry in modern art.* Princeton: Princeton University Press.

Holton, Gerald. 1988. *Thematic origins of scientific thought: Kepler to Einstein.* Rev. ed. Cambridge: Harvard University Press.

Kirby, Joshua. 1765. *Dr. Brook Taylor's method of perspective made easy; both in theory and practice: in two books.* Book 1. London: Francklin & Bunce.

Kuhn, Thomas S. 1972. The structure of scientific revolutions. Chicago: University of Chicago Press.

Mandelbrot, Benoit, B. 1983. *The fractal geometry of nature.* New York: W. H. Freeman.

Shearer, Rhonda Roland. 1996. Real or ideal? DNA iconography in a new fractal era. *Art Journal 55,* no. 1 (Spring): 64–69.

Thagard, Paul. 1992. *Conceptual revolutions.* Princeton: Princeton University Press.

Eliciting Mental Models through Imagery **22**

Gerald Zaltman

Knowledge is treated broadly here as the tacit and explicit beliefs people hold, often expressed as feelings, thoughts, and assumptions. Together, tacit and explicit knowledge form topic- or issue-oriented systems called mental models. Trying to understand a mental model, the orienting template people use to address particular situations, without addressing its tacit elements is like anticipating the picture of a fully completed jigsaw puzzle when many of it most important pieces are unavailable as clues (and no puzzle box cover is present, of course).

This chapter is particularly concerned with tacit knowledge, or what people don't know they know. This hidden knowledge is quite substantial and surfacing it is a major challenge. It is also important, for several reasons. For instance, tacit knowledge:

- constitutes most of what we know;
- has a significant impact on thought and action;
- is often acquired without awareness;
- even when acquired formally, frequently drops from "sight";
- may be used inappropriately;
- may be wrong; and
- whatever its merits, may be inconsistent with explicit knowledge.

Perhaps more important, tacit assumptions, decision rules, and expectations, feelings, and other thoughts co-mingle with explicit or formal knowledge. Tacit knowledge likes to play hide and seek, often hiding behind explicit knowledge.

Using Metaphors to Surface Mental Models

One approach to surfacing mental models is to use metaphors. Viewed broadly, metaphors are the representation of one thing in terms of another. They are central to the process of categorization and hence essential for thought. Metaphors are powerful not only because of what they reveal but also because of what they hide. One estimate is that we use about 5.7 metaphors per minute of spoken language (Gibbs, 1992).

Many metaphors reflect embodied cognition (Danesi, 1990; Johnson, 1987). The central idea of embodied cognition is that our sensory and motor systems—how we understand and react to our world—provide important tools for expressing abstract thought. Because of the centrality of our sensory and motor systems to everyday existence, it is not surprising that we often exploit their properties in the form of metaphor to represent thought. These metaphors are so prevalent that we are often unaware of their use (Goatly, 1997). I hope you *see* what I mean, *grasp the central points,* that I am not getting too *far ahead* of myself, *in over my head,* this presentation does not *put you off* by being *beneath* you, is *balanced, sounds* good, *reaches* people with different *viewpoints,* and that important points are not *left out.*

Metaphors are useful devices for helping people open internal windows to tacit knowledge, look in, and then share what they see. In the process, there is considerable discovery of tacit knowledge as it comingles with more explicit knowledge. "[M]etaphor straddles the worlds of cognition and affect, it expedites thought process in the world of feeling," where much tacit knowledge lives (Pearce, 1996, p. 3). Understanding both types of knowledge enables a researcher to build mental models that reflect the guidance systems people possess that influence what data they attend to and how they process and respond to these data.

This chapter describes a way of using metaphor to elicit the tacit and explicit knowledge a group of people share about a topic of common interest.[1] Important issues of validity and reliability and the interpretation of the data obtained using this approach are discussed in detail elsewhere (Zaltman and Coulter, 1995; Zaltman, 1997).

In as much as the mind is what the brain does (Kosslyn and Koenig, 1992), and the mind/brain does many things, it is important to integrate many perspectives to understand its operation. The method described here bundles ideas from several areas to help elicit most constructs shared by most people most of the time about a topic of relevance to them. Here a brief and admittedly oversimplified excursus on thought might be useful.

A Short Excursus on Thought

Thought often occurs as neural representations or "images." These images are topographical displays of neural activity. The processing or manipulation of these representations gives rise to thought processes (Damasio, 1994, pp. 89–90; Kosslyn, 1994, p. 3). Basically, to use a metaphor, some neurons cluster together to form discussion groups or chat rooms. These clusters are what I will call "constructs." For instance, one neuronal cluster might represent trust, and others represent escape, risk, patriotism, and so on.

Neural clusters (or constructs) by themselves do not have particularly interesting conversations, so they like to exchange information or gossip with other neuronal groups. They may choose to avoid certain groups and may or may not show good judgment in those they do select. This creates a complicated but more interesting pattern. A construct, that is, a cluster of neurons, by itself has little meaning; constructs take on meaning largely by virtue of other constructs they associate with in excitatory or inhibitory ways. Trust, for example, means somewhat different things when seeking medical assistance, falling asleep in someone's arms, voting for a candidate for public office, or telling a close friend a personal secret. Each context has other constructs that are linked with trust and which give it different shades of meaning. Trust, in turn, gives meaning to these other constructs.

Thought becomes more interesting still, because relationships among constructs are not static. The special property that emerges from the interaction of trust and, say, commitment, may react back upon these two constructs and subsequently alter them. These alterations, in turn, cause something new to emerge as the two (now somewhat changed) constructs continue to interact, which further alters trust and commitment, and so on (Stewart and Cohen, 1997).

While trust retains common qualities across contexts, it also takes on distinctive qualities in each context as well. It matters, then, what other groupings a particular set of neurons link with. Edelman's notions of reentry and neuronal grouping suggest that the nature of trust in one mental model (about the workplace, for instance) may affect its operation in another mental model (voting for a government official) and the likelihood of both mental models becoming co-active and mutually influential.

Linkages or activity patterns among neuronal groups are what researchers try to surface and represent as a mental model. Each construct in a mental model is a researcher's metaphor for what a single neuronal group is believed to represent. The overall model researchers create is their representation of or metaphors for how multiple neuronal groups interact.

However important verbal language may be for accessing and expressing thought, the thought patterns mental models represent are nonverbal (Donald, 1991). A thought may be triggered by sensory input or by other thoughts. In either case, it occurs in silence, no matter how powerful or "noisy" the initial stimulus or subsequent actions in response to thinking. Even the content of conversations we carry on with ourselves is the product of a less silent prior thought process. These inner conversations (even if mumbled out loud) become stimuli to further thought.

Thoughts are silent in the sense that, if we are aware of them at all, it is after they occur, and they "occur" to the "aware" us only if sufficiently activated. Herein lies another challenge in surfacing mental models: not all important thoughts ever reach this level of activation. They remain tacit or hidden. This is where metaphors, particularly those involving visual images, can help people inspect their tacit and explicit knowledge and then share with us what they see. In doing this, we face the added challenge of minimizing our presence in their line of sight. How, then, can we elicit the organized tacit and explicit knowledge people have while limiting our presence?

Eliciting Mental Models through Metaphors

This section outlines a method for surfacing mental models that is gaining acceptance in diverse settings. An illustration of just one element of the method is provided at the end. The method involves a two-hour, one-on-one personal interview, in which the interviewer engages the participant in a process of metaphor exploration. The process is best described as a series of steps, although the interview or guided conversation does not have the linearity the word *steps* implies.

After being recruited for a study, participants receive a letter of instruction asking them to bring to their interview twelve pictures that represent their thoughts and feelings about the chosen topic. (Examples of topics include how women picture their day, what feeling good means, the meaning of personal safety and security, the importance of skin, the meaning of cholesterol, how executives approach ill-structured problems, the use of computer-mediated communication, and innovation processes within an organization.) It is very important that images be collected by the participant in advance of the interview, and approximately seven to ten days are allowed for this activity. Participants are told their pictures may come from any source, such as magazines, newspapers, or family albums, or may be photographs they take specifically for this interview (a single-use camera is offered). Other instructions indicate that the pictures need be meaningful only to them. People typically report spending four or more hours thinking about the topic and finding pictures. Thus they arrive for their interview already engaged with the topic and with many thoughts represented by pictures.

Step 1. Storytelling

In this step the participant describes how each picture relates to the topic. The interviewer uses various questions or probes to explore these relationships further. After discussing each picture the participant is asked to assign it a title.

Step 2. Missed Pictures

Interviewees are asked if there was an idea they wanted to express but could not find a picture for or if they had sought a certain picture but could not find it. If the answer is yes, the missing picture is drawn on a card, its story told, and included along with the other images.

Step 3. The Kelly Repertory Grid

Here, three images are selected at random from the set of twelve and the participant is asked how any two are similar to one another and yet different from the third. This typically yields two basic constructs, which are then probed with various questions. This probing surfaces the thoughts and feelings leading to or activating the construct and others it activates. The random selection of three pictures and questioning is usually repeated three times.

Step 4. Altering the Picture

Techniques adapted from art therapy are used here with images selected purposefully by the interviewer. There are many ways of implementing this step. For instance, participants may be invited to widen the frame of the picture in any direction, including extending its foreground and background, and then asked what would enter the picture that would reinforce (or contradict) its meaning. If they do not automatically place themselves in the picture, they are asked if they might be in it and, if so, where. Sometimes they are invited to place a product or service provider in the picture and asked about the reasons for its placement. Another option is to select two of the pictures and ask interviewees to create a third picture in their mind's eye which, together with the other two pictures, tells a story about their thoughts and feelings on the topic. Participants describe the "missing" picture, its linkage to the other two, and describe the overall story. This step is usually repeated two or three times.

Step 5. Preparation for Digital Imaging

At this point participants are asked to consider some of the important ideas they've shared and to select five or six pictures that together might reflect these thoughts. A digital imaging expert is present at this point and provides a short explanation of that step (see below). These images are scanned into a computer in another room while the interview continues.

Step 6. Other Sensory Images

Next, the participants are asked about other sensory images that would reflect their thoughts and feelings about the topic or a specific aspect of it. For example, they might be asked what sound would represent their thoughts and feelings about the role of exercise in their lives. What would not be the sound? Answers are then probed for the more abstract ideas a particular sound represents. Each of the major senses is explored this way. Again, there are alternative ways of introducing and exploring this step.

Step 7. Vignette

This step emphasizes the creation, in the mind's eye, of a short home movie, video, or one-act play to elicit thoughts and feelings. Prompts are used to encourage descriptions of actors, settings, actions, conversations, background sounds, and so on. Sometimes specific characters will be specified for inclusion. These characters may include people or things and constructs that are imagined to be able to have and express thoughts and feelings.

Step 8. The Digital Image

At this point the pictures selected in Step 5 have been scanned into a computer and an expert in digital imaging serves as the participant's hands while the participant directs the creation of a collage. Participants understand that the original images can be altered in virtually any way they can imagine. Each time the participant requests a manipulation the digital imager asks what that manipulation helps express. Examples of manipulations for which explanations may be sought include: having a person or object in an image face in the opposite direction; changing the time shown on a clock; altering the color of an object; having something be transparent and placed over something else or having it magnified/shrunk in size or distorted; placing one image within another, for example, placing a picture of the Eiffel Tower in a pair of hands, and so on. At the end of this step, the participant tells the overall story the final image represents. The narrative story accompanying a digital image about coping with cholesterol is presented in Box 22.1.

Box 22.1 Visual summary explanation: Cholesterol level

Well we are looking at a picture and the central figure is a woman in a body suit, she is on her hands and her knees, she is balancing several objects, a lamp and a tea set or a coffee set on her back. She has a very perplexed look on her face, a little bit angry, a little bit puzzled. This represents how I feel about my high cholesterol. I feel like I am balancing a lot on my back. I don't quite know what to do about it. She looks like she is afraid to move and that's how I feel about eating different foods and trying to watch what I am doing. In the crook of her leg there is a magazine with a picture of man and he also has a very angry but yet kind of defiant yet hurt look in his eyes if you look very carefully, just kind of mixed up and mad and just everything, all kinds of emotions and that also represents how I feel. Down in-between the legs and the arms of the woman, there are some space-type-clad people with silvery gold space suits with one figure in the middle standing on his hands and that person is in the purple outfit and that represents myself of being just a little bit different from people who do not have high cholesterol. The others look normal where I look very out of place like I don't belong there and of course I am standing on my head and the rest of them are not. Up in the lefthand corner there is an abstract painting and this totally describes how I feel about this whole condition with cholesterol. It's confusing in my mind, the physician is not addressing it and it is very abstract, it's just confusion. The lamp has a shade on it and on that shade there is a land rover—type vehicle and there are some mazes with high steep sides and this indicates to me that this again, the land rover represents myself and I am down in this abyss, this place where I really can't get out of it and that the rocks and the shale are crumbling in and that also is like the cholesterol, it's invasive. And then we have a little bit beneath that there is a small insert of a merry-go-round and this represents the merry-go-round I am on with the high cholesterol. I feel like I am going round and round. I really don't have answers or things that will help me with this situation and you will notice that there is a fence on around the merry-go-round and you can not see there is no exit, you can't get out of it

Box 22.1 *(continued)*

and that represents how I feel about my condition also. Lastly, there is a small insert of a child sitting in a very pastoral like setting reading a magazine completely at peace with himself and the world obviously without problems and this represents how I would like to be regarding this cholesterol problem. I would like to be like that child. I would like to be free of this problem and I would like to know that it is all right and I have done something about it. I think the composition is very interesting and it's certainly in a very small space it encompasses all of the things and feelings that I have about my condition and in my mind it illustrates it very well.

Using the Data

Between fifteen and twenty people are typically interviewed for a research project. For instance, in a project seeking to understand the experiences of patients participating in trials involving a rheumatoid arthritis treatment, Enbrel, twenty-one patients across the United States and fourteen physicians treating these patients were interviewed. Each interview is tape recorded and transcribed. A special computer program, Metaphoria, helps the overall analysis considerably.[2] Generally three people code the data. Typically this involves two of the interviewers and one person not involved in the interviewing. This team must reaching agreement about what constructs are being elicited as participants describe their metaphors and respond to the interviewers' questions. A list of constructs is prepared and the coders return to the transcripts and note construct pairs. For instance, in the Enbrel example the construct of freedom may be connected to giving more attention to family. Giving more attention to family may be connected with lessened guilt. In this case, freedom and attention to family are noted as a construct pair as are attention to family and lessened guilt.

The mental model is built using constructs that (1) are mentioned at least once by half of all participants and (2) are directly linked to another such construct by at least one-third of the participants. (More or less constrictive guidelines can be used.) This produces a mental model or map involving between twenty and thirty constructs that usually represents 85 percent or more of all constructs mentioned by any one interviewee. Moreover, we find that it generally requires no more than three or four interviewees selected at random to generate all constructs represented in the map. This is consistent with the position that the mind is not the possession of the individual, that meaning arises from associations and interactions with others. (See Brothers, 1997, and Zerubavel, 1997.) Because the resulting mental model captures so much shared knowledge, we also call it a consensus map.

An example of a mental model for a consumer product is shown in Figure 22.1. The mental model shown is the researcher's understanding and representation of the constructs and their connections he or she believes are being expressed by participants in a study. In effect, it is the researcher's metaphor for the pattern of thoughts believed to be shared by study participants. This belief is based on the use of metaphors to elicit these thoughts (constructs) and their associations with one another.

The connections between constructs are particularly important, as noted earlier. These connections represent reasoning processes that give definition to the constructs. An analogy is provided by social network research, where the unit of analysis is the connection or relationship between people rather than the individuals themselves.

Mental models have varied uses. For instance, one organization used this method to elicit a model describing how its senior management viewed the process of introducing new ideas into the company. The resulting mental model consisted of both explicit and tacit knowledge and was accepted by the managers as an accurate and rich description of the issue as they experienced it. The model produced a healthy mixture of surprising and expected results. The managers were then asked to redraw the model to reflect how they would like it to look a year later. This resulted in their identifying constructs and associations that should be reinforced, deleted, and added. They were also able to identify how altering certain constructs and relationships among constructs might have unexpected effects on other relevant constructs that would facilitate or inhibit the introduction of new ideas. For example, it became evident that by strengthening certain reward structures, the incidence of new ideas of immediate value would increase, but quite possibly at the

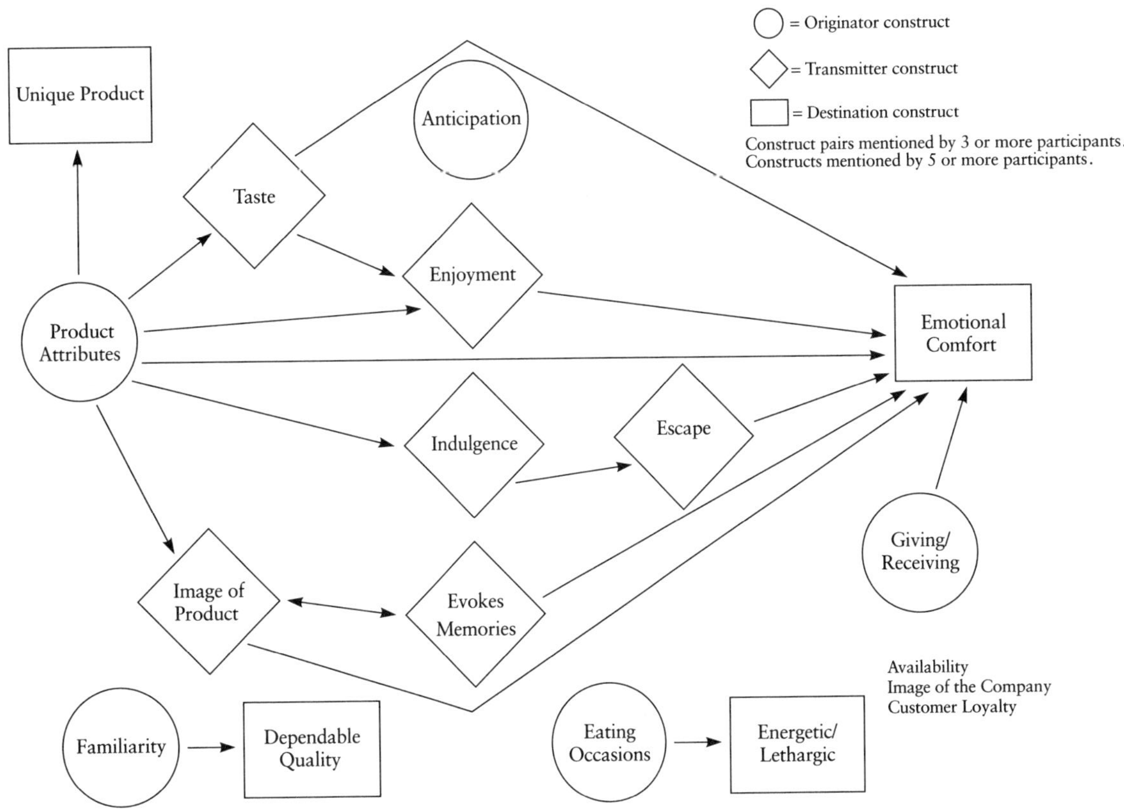

Figure 22.1. Snack food consensus map.

expense of ideas that would have potentially far greater benefit in the long run. The mental model also showed that the company had a sense of confidence in the process of introducing new ideas that was unwarranted; the model suggested ways of altering several aspects of the company's organizational learning experience.

Conclusion

A research method has been described in which people are asked to select visual and other sensory representations of their thoughts and feelings about a topic. Time is allowed to enable them to think carefully and find appropriate images on their own. These images are initial metaphors whose descriptions give rise to yet other metaphors. The interviewer's method of probing these metaphors along with nonmetaphoric expressions of thought brings to the surface considerable tacit as well as explicit knowledge. This is done in a way that focuses on the relationships among constructs, so that a mental model can be created that captures the shared thinking of otherwise different people. It is believed that the use of sensory and other images, when explored appropriately, activates the neuronal groupings that represent thought. Moreover, the "mental model" these patterns create provides the initial bases for the more conscious selection of relevant images. The mind/brain directs the selection of visual and other imagery, which in turn is used to reveal the tacit and explicit mental model actually in use.

Notes

1. The method described here is called the Zaltman Metaphor Elicitation Technique and is patented as U.S. Patent no. 5436830.
2. Information about Metaphoria may be obtained from Professor Jerry Olson at Pennylvania State University.

References

Brothers, Leslie. 1997. *Friday's footprint: How society shapes the human mind.* New York: Oxford University Press.

Damasio, Antonio R. 1994. *Descartes' error: Emotion, reason, and the human brain.* New York: G. P. Putnam's Sons.

Danesi, Marcel, 1990. Thinking is seeing: Visual metaphors and the nature of abstract thought. *Semiotica, 80* (3/4), 221–237.

Donald, Merlin. 1991. *Origins of the modern mind: Three stages in the evolution of culture and cognition.* Cambridge: Harvard University Press.

Gibbs, Raymond W., Jr. 1992. Categorization and metaphor understanding. *Psychological Review, 99* (3), 572–577.

Goatly, Andrew. 1997. *The language of metaphors.* New York: Routledge.

Johnson, Mark. 1987. *The body in the mind: The bodily basis of meaning, imagination, and reason.* Chicago: University of Chicago Press.

Kosslyn, Stephen. 1994. *Image and brain: The resolution of the imagery debate.* Cambridge: MIT Press.

Kosslyn, Stephen, and Olivier Koenig. 1992. *Wet mind: The new cognitive neuroscience.* New York: Free Press.

Marks, Lawrence E. 1978. *The unity of the senses: Interrelations among the modalities.* New York: Academic Press.

Pearce, Stephen S. 1996. *Flash of insight: Metaphor and narrative in therapy.* Boston: Allyn and Bacon.

Stewart, Ian, and Jack Cohen. 1997. *Figments of reality: The evolution of the curious mind.* Cambridge: Cambridge University Press.

Zaltman, Gerald. 1997. Rethinking market research: Putting people back in. *Journal of Marketing Research, 34* (November 1997), 424–437.

Zaltman, Gerald, and R. Coulter. 1995. Seeing the voice of the customer: Metaphor-based advertising research. *Journal of Advertising Research, 35* (4), 35–51.

Zerubavel, Eviatar. 1997. *Social mindscapes: An invitation to cognitive sociology.* Cambridge: Harvard University Press.

Creation, Art, and the Brain

23

Jean-Pierre Changeux

Visitors to the Imperial Collections at the National Museum of Taipei are struck upon entering the exhibit by a peculiar set of objects: oracle bones from the Shang Dynasty. These fragments of tortoise shell feature unusual fractures, mostly randomly distributed, and resulting from the insertion of white-hot firebrands into cavities that are pierced along the internal wall of the bone. With respect to these fissures, texts written in the oldest-known Chinese characters attribute meaning to each fracture line: the answer (auspicious or ominous) to a set of questions asked by a fortune-teller (military success, harvest, illness, dreams, and so on) and, by logical extension, the supposed "verification" of the prediction.

These first written traces testify to an activity that is fundamental to the human brain: that of giving meaning to a physical makeup (in this case, randomly distributed line patterns) with the goal of mastering the evolution of time in a world that escapes us. The human brain proceeds in a direction opposite to the "input-output" mode long proposed by cybernetics. It always projects onto the world, in a spontaneous and internally generated fashion, "mental representations" that it tries to test against an external reality that is intrinsically devoid of meaning. This projection, as a generator of mental form, represents an essential predisposition of the human brain toward creation (Changeux, 1994).

Scientists are cautious in discussing a subject as difficult as "creation." Experimental data available to the neurobiologist remain fragmentary and limited. In the absence of human data, animal models are useful, but insufficient. In addition, current scientific methods do not yet allow us objectively to reconstruct the life experience of the creator and his imaginary world. My discussion must remain hypothetical.

The Human Brain's Predisposition toward Creation

Is it plausible that a group of nerve cells and their axonal and dendritic extensions, in which electrical and chemical signals travel, could be at the origin of a function as seemingly elusive as creation? At this stage, I would only say that there is no physical reason why not (Changeux, 1983, 1994; Edelman, 1992). The human brain is made up of approximately 100 billion neurons, and each neuron has an average of 10,000 discontinuous contacts (or synapses), with its multiple connections. Thus there are on the order of 10^{15} synapses in the human encephalus, or approximately 600 million synapses/mm^3. The number of possible combinations between neurons reaches astronomic powers of 10, followed by millions of zeros, on the same order of magnitude as the number of positively charged particles in the universe. In addition, the efficiency of these synaptic contacts varies as a function of experience. No numerical limit can legitimately be placed on the functional combinations of the neuronal network.

Moreover, connections in the neuronal network are neither totally random, like a gas, nor completely regular, like a crystal. They are organized. Relationships of convergence—of many axons on one neuron—and of divergence—of the same axon on several neurons—succeed in bringing together local specialization and global integration within the cerebral network. Finally, the brain's organizational pattern, stable from one generation to the next, results from an essentially genetic, biological evolution that is several hundred million years old. During this evolution, according to Herbert Spencer's description, "coordination between sensory and motor groups developed and were made even more complex by the introduction of new elements combined in various ways to make up spheres of increasingly vast extent that could become mentally present" with, continues Hughlings Jackson, "passage from the simplest toward the most complex, that is from the well-organized, inferior center, to the superior, less-organized centers . . . that continue to gain structure *throughout one's life.*" In other words, the higher one goes in the hierarchy of the nervous system, the more self-organization and, by extension, the capacity to create can be seen to emerge, as long as the system remains "open" to its environment.

Within the Darwinian model of evolution, that condition of openness to the environment is fulfilled by the process of "variation-selection-amplification." This model explains (even if many uncertainties remain) the successive hierarchical nesting of organizational levels that are internal to the organism, and specifically to the brain, through random and spontaneous variations of specific genetic determinants. These developmental genes (or homogenes) (Lawrence, 1992), which express themselves in a sequential and combinatory manner in the course of development, must have contributed to this evolution, from flies to mammals, from the Australopithecus to *Homo sapiens* (Changeux and Chavaillon, 1995). Within a few million years, we witness an increase in the relative surface of temporo-parietal, and especially prefrontal, cortices and at the same time hemispheric dominance becomes more pronounced. Correlated with these changes in brain morphology are the development of language, higher cognitive functions, and social life. The first tools were invented approximately two million years ago. The first paintings appeared on cave walls about 30,000 years ago. The conscious creative activity of the human brain thus takes over from the "blind" morphogenetic activity of biological evolution.

At the same time, new, nongenetic types of evolution, with much shorter time scales, take root in the human brain. Neurons and synapses are not assembled from prewired microprocessors as if they were ready-made by an engineer. Cerebral connectivity takes shape in a progressive manner, with a margin of random variability. Phases of runaway connective development are followed by prunings and eliminations, under the control of the spontaneous and evoked activities of the network (Changeux and Danchin, 1976). At sensitive periods in the extra-long postnatal development that characterizes humans, the neurons acquire their functional singularity (Wiesel and Hubel, 1965). For example, when a newborn cat is exposed to an environment where all the bars are vertical, the orientation of its visuo-cortical neurons is drastically reduced to all but vertical lines (Movshon and

Blakemore 1974). In the same manner, the human child experiments at an early age with his physical and social environment, acquires his mother tongue, and imprints himself with visual images and sounds, with a musical "temperament," and with symbolic systems and rules of conduct proper to his cultural reference group. This epigenesis by selective stabilization of synapses frees human beings from "genetic automatism." It makes cultural evolution possible, and it makes the human brain a key player in the story of creation.

Mental Representations and Creation

Commenting on her activities as a sculptor, Louise Bourgeois (1995) writes: "I am bombarded by so many images when I think that my thoughts are not convincing metaphors. I see these images all one next to the other." Similarly, "through focusing his attention on imaginary experience," Jacques Monod (1970, p. 170) finds himself "taking on the identity of a protein molecule."

The most widely accepted model of visual representation, proposed in 1949 by the Canadian psychologist Hebb (1949), is that these "images"—or rather, mental objects (Changeux, 1983)—result from an internal, private physical state of the cerebral network. This physical state occurs when basic electrical and chemical neural activities are dispatched over time to affect a specific topologically defined group of neurons. This produces discrete and autonomous "neural forms" that are made up of neurons distributed across multiple brain regions, themselves connected in different ways. The connection mechanisms that ensure their coherence may rely on changes in efficiency in the transmission of signals from one neuron to another, and these changes may depend on molecular—or "allosteric"—transitions of neurotransmitter receptors (Changeux, 1983). The "indication function" (Dretske, 1995) connecting this physical state of the brain to its meaning must depend, under these conditions, on the geography of brain maps, which, as noted, took shape in the course of evolution, then stabilized and narrowed in on their specific functions in the course of postnatal epigenesis.

On the sensory side, the formation of visual representations is, by far, the best known. In the macaque, Felleman and Van Essen (1991) have inventoried, mainly in the occipital regions, 32 visual areas organized in 14 hierarchical levels, and linked by 305 different types of connections that use only 40 percent of the total potential capacity. The observation of areas V1 and V2 in humans using functional magnetic resonance imaging (fMRI) (Sereno et al., 1995) reveals these regions' perfect symmetry, which corresponds to a geometric projection of the topology of the retina. Functional MRI also reveals the seemingly epigenetic variability of the borders of each of those regions. Moreover, each of these topologically defined areas is linked to a specific functional specialization. Zeki (1993) has shown, for example, that presenting a subject with a montage of colored rectangles (which he somewhat incorrectly calls "Mondrians") results in increased differential activity in area V4, while watching black-and-white squares (in the style of the Belgian painter Pol Bury) in motion selectively stimulates V5. The hierarchically inferior V1 and V2 respond to both types of stimulation. These are examples of mental representations that take shape and are recorded while the observer is in the physical presence of the stimulus. It is remarkable that, when a subject is asked to call up images from memory, stored in latent form, we see reappear on the screen a pattern of activation that much resembles the original pattern observed when the stimulus was physically present (Le Bihan et al., 1993). Calling up a memory trace materially re-creates the brain's past experience.

Moving up the cortical hierarchy, attributes of color, shape, motion, and real-world object depth, first processed independently, progressively come together to build a coherent image of the world. At the level of the inferior temporal cortex (Perrett and Oram, 1993), one can find neurons activated by simple geometric shapes or upside-down "T"s, as featured in certain works by Klee. One can also find there neurons that respond specifically to hands (Perrett and Oram, 1993) or to faces (Perrett, Rolls, and Caan, 1982; Perrett and Oram, 1993), and whose counterparts seemingly must have been active in Philippe de Champagne's brain when he painted the *Magdalene in Ecstasy (Madeleine en extase)* displayed at the Rennes Museum, in the same way that they also become active in our own brains when we contemplate that painting. Other neurons respond to a head, regardless of its orientation, and thus are sensitive simply to the concept of a "head"

(Perrett and Oram, 1993). The abstraction process continues as we "ascend" toward the anterior temporal cortex, where one can identify neurons that, with training, are able to distinguish between ninety-seven individual types of fractal shapes of extraordinary geometric complexity (Miyashita and Chang, 1988). The monkey turns out to be an excellent geometrist.

The musician (MacAdams and Bigand, 1994) must not be made to feel left out of this mostly visual world of the brain. Specialized areas of cortex in the temporal lobe, and especially in the right hemisphere, are separately devoted to processing the frequency of sounds, the localization of sounds with respect to their point of origin, melodic organization (contour, interval, tone), and time-based factors such as rhythm and metrics. There is even a system that specializes in the perception of noises in the environment. And it seems likely that composers like Pierre Schaeffer or John Cage took care to put it to use in their works.

Finally, since the days of Broca, it has been known that language representations selectively occupy specialized areas of the left hemisphere. The images obtained by Posner and Raichle (1994), using a positron emission tomography (PET) camera, illustrate differential activation of temporal areas during hearing, occipital areas during reading, Broca's area during speech, and frontal areas during word generation.

In spite of the progressive rebuilding and restructuring that takes place in climbing up the hierarchical ladder of cortical regions, we are still far removed from that "singing state" evoked by Valéry, that "musical place of words," where images, words, and rhymes meet at the point of creation, specifically poetic creation. But it seems that we are getting closer with an important brain-imaging study by Mazoyer and his colleagues (Mazoyer et al., 1993). These researchers compared the cerebral activity of monolingual French-speaking subjects to whom three types of stimuli were presented aurally: a story in Tamil, which they could not understand; a list of French words that they could understand; and finally, a well-structured story in French. Investigators found that the more comprehensible the stimuli became, the more activation was found in the left hemisphere, with the number and intensity of the activations increasing. Multiple cerebral domains find themselves "stuck together" *cum prehendere,* when the subject comprehends. With complete understanding of the story, a new cortical region comes into play: the prefrontal cortex. It is known that its relative surface increases in size exponentially from the monkey to the human (Furster, 1980). It is also known that damage to this area results in serious behavioral problems, that, according to the specific site of the lesion, affect attention, reasoning, or mental planning. The prefrontal cortex contributes to mental synthesis, to organizing thoughts into intentions. It helps to build mental representations that relate to social interaction. It plays a central role in attributing mental states to others, in the recognition of one's own "singular otherness," to use the term of the French philosopher Emmanuel Lévinas, and thus contributes to one of the central abilities of the brain in the appreciation of aesthetic qualities of artwork and in moral judgment: empathy.

The concept of empathy calls forth an entire domain of the creative brain to which I have not yet alluded: that of the emotions (Damasio, 1995). Ancient and primitive, some would say "animal" (because of its role in vital survival functions), the limbic system plays an essential part in assessing danger as well as pleasure and in shaping the subject's physical and emotional landscape. It is linked to neuronal systems of the brain stem that underlie self-stimulation among rats. Intricately connected to the frontal cortex, the limbic system marks out emotional reference points to guide other systems that act upon the world. Because of the limbic system, reason and pleasure are allowed to live in harmony in the brain of the creator.

Creation and Mental "Darwinism"

In defense of the "genetic critique" of the literary creation process, illustrated in manuscripts by Gustave Flaubert or Francis Ponge, Almuth Grésillon (1992) emphasizes that "against the straight highway, the inexorable march toward resolution and outcome, the teleology of the straight line, we find opposite metaphors that indicate a more winding path: forks, turnoffs, wrong turns, unbeaten paths, detours, crossroads, backtracks, dead ends, accidents, and false starts." According to Claude Simon, "the writer progresses laboriously, gropes around blindly, gets bogged down, and starts up again." Matisse compares the path of his pencil to "the gesture of a man feeling his way forward in the dark." In many respects, the memory of Jacques-Louis Lions's (Franck, 1995) black painting, preserving what Laurent Schwartz, a French mathematician, refers to as the multiple "sharp lines" and "zigzags," is more informative about the mechanisms of mathematical creation than is a report published in the *Proceedings* of the Academy of Sciences. The process of creation proceeds along a slow road of trial and error.

Artists' and scientists' brains have not yet been imaged in the PET scanner to record the creative process in an objective manner. We are restricted to a "diet" of data that confines us to schematic models of theorization. The proposed hypothesis (Changeux, 1983, 1994; Changeux and Dehaene, 1989) is that creation proceeds, in psychological time, according to an evolving process of trial and error. This process encompasses biological evolution and connectional epigenesis within a framework of "mental Darwinism" and according to a projective style (Changeux and Dehaene, 1989). During periods of "preparation" and "incubation"—in the words of Jacques Hadamard, a famous French mathematician—fragmentary images of sketches of mental representations or *prerepresentations* (Changeux and Dehaene, 1989) pop up spontaneously and transiently in the brain. A combinatory function, a kind of "mental handiwork," associates and dissociates objects from memory and current perceptions, until, in this competition, one "recombination" wins out. According to Hadamard, this is enlightenment or, more generally, the selection of a particular representation. This meaningful object will generally serve as a step in the halting, constantly renewed process of mathematical invention, biologic modeling, or in the early design of a work of art. This work of the imagination will sooner or later engage a selection-by-evaluation mechanism that, seemingly, brings into play the limbic system and its outposts, already mentioned in the context of emotion. The limbic system, flooding the synapses of the relevant neuronal group with neurotransmitters, thus modifies their efficiency and, consequently, produces a material trace in long-term memory.

As one might expect, the space in which these mental images "struggle for life," as Taine wrote, is not perfectly identified. The brain analog of Claude Bernard's "interior milieu," this conscious milieu, a "simulation space" of virtual activities, provides a meeting place for current perceptions of the outside world, for representations of "self," and for memories of past experiences, somatically marked with emotional valence. Also contributing to these deliberations are many internalized social rules, as well as innate forces that stem from biological evolution and whose influence is often beyond the scope of the subject's perception. The physical borders of this "conscious milieu" seemingly include the frontal cortex, the limbic system, and the brain stem, among many other brain areas that, through their "reinputs" (Edelman, 1992), create a looping system.

Touchstones of a "chemical" definition of the conscious milieu, psychotropic drugs, such as mescaline, bind selectively with certain categories of receptors and neurotransmitters (in this case catecholamines). The Huichol Indians take mescaline as part of an annual ritual during their pilgrimages to Wirikuta. They then often experience multicolored hallucinations, with strong geometric components of remarkable symmetry. Once they have returned home, they set these fleeting images to wool canvases that are supposed to represent their journey to "the beyond." Could it be that these colored and regular images reflect the neural geometry of the color areas of V4? Do they engage the same receptor, as when similar shapes emerge, albeit in a voluntary way, in the minds of artists such as Kandinsky, Manessier, or Messiaen, who "heard" colors when he was creating?

During the "mental experience" of creative work, multiple evolutions overlie and connect with each other. Beginning with the first "confused shapes" (Leonardo da Vinci), "randomly born bits" on which, according to the French poet and essayist Yves Bonnefoy, "the imaginary rests," one can distinguish the "first idea," a still-crude outline that is nevertheless so importantly connected to the subject's own definition. Then this mental object, sifted through the filter of reason, becomes reality on paper by multiple "external drawings" of the graphic sketch, or *disegno*. Representations from the "internal circuit" give way to precise movements of the hand and fingers (often acquired after a long period of practicing one's art) that finally direct the pen or the paintbrush. A cascade of activity in premotor, then motor areas extends the internal, implicit evolution of mental creation.

The neuroscientist Apostolos Georgopoulos (Georgopoulos, Taira, and Lukashin, 1993) has deciphered, using monkey models, the activity of motor neuron populations responsible for guiding hand movements. The average vector of the recorded neural activities, in frequency and in direction, coincides remarkably well with the orientation vector for finger movement, especially when the animal is drawing a spiral (Schwartz, 1994). An "evolutionary dialog" takes shape between the brain of the creator and the work being created, "adjustments of the eye with reasoning," which accompany corrections, cross-outs, and restarts of the work in progress.

Individual and Cultural Histories of Creation

Artistic and scientific creation are part of an individual history which itself stems from an anterior historical evolution. Thus Hélène Seckel (1988) would place *La vision de saint-Jean* (*Saint John's Vision*) by El Greco at the origins of Picasso's *Demoiselles d'Avignon,* followed by *Les baigneurs* (*The Bathers*) by Cézanne, the *Bain turc* (*Turkish Bath*) by d'Ingres, and, among Picasso's own works, *Le harem de 1906* (*The Harem of 1906*) and *Deux femmes nues* (*Two Nudes*) from the same year, with an obvious influence of African art, and finally several sketches for the painting itself.

In the same way, every scientist, as much as he may think himself a genius, knows what he owes to the cultural environment in which he took his first steps, to the discoveries of his predecessors, to unstructured meetings with colleagues, to accidental observations, to references gleaned here and new techniques borrowed there. In this elusive network of unforeseen interactions, where contingency and rationalization mix, "cognitive crystallizations" take shape. Their eventual validation and final acceptance will occur when universally aimed critical debates are held. Historians of science (Creager and Gaudillière, 1996) have conducted a sophisticated analysis of the inherent difficulties of untangling such a web. To the problem of conceptual content is added that, no less important, of claims of "priority" or "credit" (essential to the psychology of even the most eminent scientists), which mask the processes that are intrinsic to the evolution of knowledge (or even lead us astray on the subject). Thus research on the history of science prefers to count not so much on unreliable written or oral autobiographical accounts, but rather on in-depth examinations of experimental notebooks, on exchanges of correspondence, and on other testimony that is more neutral from the point of view of the personal visibility of the researchers (Creager and Gaudillière, 1996).

The historic evolution of artistic and scientific representations does not, however, follow as obscure and random a path as it may seem. It engages a rather severe selection mechanism following specific rules—mental tools—that creators have imposed on themselves from the beginning of time, and that they themselves have made evolve throughout the course of history. "I love the rule that corrects emotion," notes the French cubist Georges Braques. And Louise Bourgeois (1995) continues: "My sculptures are like algebraic equations with variables. The equations must be tested."

A first, very general, rule is the coherence between the parts and the whole. For the mathematician, the coherence of a new mathematical object with mental objects that already exist in his brain marks a true "invention." In the realm of art, Alberti (1970 [1435]), taking after the Stoics, sets down as an absolute law the principle of *harmonia* or *consensus partium,* which occurs "if all the elements, whether they be dimension, function, type, color, and other similar things, converge upon a single and same beauty." Matisse seems to concur with Alberti when he writes: "I take from Nature what I need, I carefully combine all the effects, I *balance* them in description and in color, and this condensation in which everything harmonizes is never reached on the first attempt." The successive steps, photographed by Matisse himself, that led to the creation of *Grand nu allongé* (*Large Reclining Nude*) (1935), displayed at the Baltimore Museum, testify to this tireless search for "the harmony of the whole" when creating a work intended to become a masterpiece.

The neuronal counterpart to what Diderot calls "the apperception of ratios" still remains very enigmatic. I will first discuss a series of experiments that examine "illusory contours." These occur, for example, when a subject perceives a continuous luminous bar connecting notches cut into two darker elements, distinguishable when the notches remain open on a light-colored background. Peterhans and Von der Heydt (1989) have shown that signature neural activity, in this case in area V2, characterizes the occurrence of the illusory contour of the luminous bar. The brain constructs a coherent representation of the world, even if only virtual. This goes hand in hand with an even more fundamental perception of the invariability of the world that surrounds us. When we voluntarily change the position of our head or the orientation of our gaze, we feel like the outside world is immobile and that we are moving within it. This perception poses a serious problem of reference coordinates for our brain. Droulez and Berthoz (1988) suggest that the brain constructs an internal model of the environment, which it updates continuously by subjecting our sensory representations to the overriding input from motor-based controls responsible for the orientation of our head and gaze. The connections linking temporal and frontal areas may be said to play a role in the synthesis of that mental object, unique and coherent, to which artist and scientist may well refer in their search for harmony.

In this context, several series of experiments refer more specifically to symmetry, a concept dear to the hearts of mathematicians and architects, and one found abundantly in Islamic art and Buddhist mandalas. Among many types of swallows (Moller, 1992) and earwigs, it has been shown that females prefer males who are symmetric. The evolutionarily based reasons that are given, valid for superior vertebrates as well, vary from the "honest ad effect" to the universal necessity to recognize objects whatever their orientation in the outside world. Among humans, the attractiveness of a face does not depend only on its symmetry. Perrett (Perrett, May, and Yoshikawa, 1994), using composite digitized photographs, has shown that, contrary to popular belief, the "average" face is not the most attractive. Japanese, like Caucasians, in fact prefer a composite face constructed from facial features individually recognized as being the most seductive, the exaggeration of shape differences compared with the norm making the composite that much more attractive across cultures. There is a search for "individuality" amid a basic symmetric organization. The ultimate coherence of perfect symmetry yields to the search for quasi-symmetry, for the baroque style that we see reappear throughout the history of art.

One rule on which all agree in science as in art is that of novelty, which excludes the familiar, things already seen or heard before. A powerful brain device comes into play in detecting the novel, the unpredicted, a device essential to the survival of the organism. Pavlov and then Sokolov have shown how an animal subjected to a repetitive stimulus, let's say a sound, ends up no longer responding to that stimulus. A "desensitization" occurs. However, as soon as the stimulus changes, the organism produces an orientation response toward the source, by its gaze and its posture. Thus this important brain device comes into play not only in the detection of novelty but, consequently, in its production as well. Neuroimaging observations by Posner reveal, along these same lines, that when a subject becomes familiar with a list of nouns that he has read several times over, brain activity gradually turns off. But as soon as a new list is presented, the frontal (cognitive) cortex and Wernicke's area (language) light up on the lateral surface, as well as the cingulate cortex (limbic) on the medial surface. No doubt reading a poem by René Char, a melody by Poulenc, or a *Proceedings* paper by Louis Pasteur would maintain a permanent level of high blood flow in the listener, whose brain could be said to "echo" that of the creator.

Coherence and novelty are insufficient to select mental representations that deserve the attributes of "true" or "beautiful." The rule of reality testing *(adéquation au réel)* had united science and art for centuries, until romanticism created an irremediable rift. In the natural sciences, experimentation rules. A very attractive mathematical model can, from one day to the next, be relegated to the throwaways of history because of its incompatibility with external reality. This is what happened to Pauling's triple-helix DNA model after the presentation and subsequent validation of Watson and Crick's double-helix model. In the natural sciences, invention cannot stray from the narrow and demanding path of discovery of a preexisting physical reality and the mastery of the rules that govern it (Changeux and Danchin 1976).

"Mental tools" that are produced by the scientist's brain, theoretic models, as adequate as they may seem, always remain limited and cannot pretend to exhaust the reality of the world; at most, they can only define its "horizons" (Cohen Tannoudji). At the same time, the validation of a model cannot be accomplished by a single human being: it necessitates collective, open, critical debate, an exchange of "representations," as already mentioned, between scientists' brains. Whatever may be said about it, the application of the rule of "reality testing," which makes one accountable to the principles of objectivity and universality in scientific knowledge, leads to indisputable progress in the field of human knowledge.

The idea of progress in art appears, to the contrary, to be absurd. Certainly, from the beginning of time, the artist has referred to the natural world. For example, the composer André Jolivet, in his work, uses the natural rhythms of the heart, of breathing, and of sex. The painter Mondrian uses lines, basic shapes, and colors that, as we have seen, are underpinned by fundamental neural mechanisms of visual perception. However, is Stravinsky's *Le sacre du printemps* a fundamental improvement over Monteverdi's *Orfeo?* No, because if art evolves and renews itself, the artist has long since broken his links with the objective description of nature and its reconstruction into an "ideal beauty." According to Matisse's terms, the artist "organizes his sensations," "releases his emotions" in order to solicit those of the viewer (or the listener) and touch his subjectivity.

The artist thus seems "freer" than the scientist to define the rules of his creation, and the rules in fact do vary from one artist to another. These rules actually characterize an artist's style. For example, for Matisse, "what I dream of is an art of *balance,* of *purity,* of *tranquility,* without any worrisome or troublesome subject, an art that would be, for any cerebral worker . . . something that calms and soothes the brain, like a comfortable armchair that relaxes and cures one from physical tiredness." Conversely, Marcel Duchamp announces the "death of art" by invoking humor and derision. For Ben (Vautier), a painter based in Nice, France, one of the functions of art is to distract, to capture the eye. The French painter François Morellet, with his "Geome-trees," attempts "a freak marriage between Pythagoras and Buffoon" by evoking, through strictly abstract shapes, trees, curly locks of hair, and copulations. In the musical domain, Pierre Boulez searches for "slippages over overlays" ("les glissements effectués sur leurs superpositions"), the contrast of tones, disturbances, and accidents in "a universe where consonance and dissonance are abolished." Among many contemporary artists, a return to the origins of creation, to its brain-based mechanisms, gives rise to a pictorial fiction, to some extent moving against the grain of time, leaving the spectator free to complete the creative process by the greatest number of possible routes. The random generator of the diversity of mental representations is in a sense re-created with the automatic writing of the surrealists, the "dionysian dance" of Pollock's "dripping," the "conscious awkwardness" of Cy Twombly's scribbles, Dubuffet's *"psychosites,"* Carcassonne's *"neurographies,"* the production of Frank Stella's "images [that] lead into each other while always continuing to distort themselves," and that are like as many "neuromotor pantomimes" (Jean Clair) of internal experience.

In the course of history, creators have thus invented "rules" that characterize their styles. But these rules are not set in stone, and they evolve. The perspective in painting, like the temperament in music, tries to seem "right" or to "ring true," but in fact deceives the eye and ear. The internalization of these rules implies a long and rather irreversible apprenticeship, similar to the learning of a language. The study of babies' listening strategies by Trehub and Trainor (1994) shows that they treat relations of pitch and the passage of time in the same way as adults. Babies spontaneously prefer "salient" musical forms with perfect fifth and keynote intervals. However, at the age of six months, Western and Javanese infants can detect wrong notes in melodies based in the Western major scale *and* the Javanese *pelog* scale, while adults are able only to recognize wrong notes from the musical scale of the culture in which they were raised. This drop in performance, which can be thought of as a "perceptual calibration" by selection of innate patterns (Changeux, 1983; Changeux and Danchin, 1976), severely limits the widespread notion of our perceptual system's virtually limitless plasticity. This process, in accordance with the theory of epigenesis by selective stabilization, finds itself in opposition to the hypothesis of composers such as Boulez or Schoenberg, according to whom adult listeners may acquire all imaginable musical structures with the same ease with which they were able to perceive or acquire conventional musical structure as children. In this study, Trehub and Trainor emphasize the double constraint of innate dispositions, of "neural forms" proper to the species, and of epigenetic selection based in individual and cultural history.

In wanting to return to the very origins of creation, wouldn't art be returning to that "natural chaos," those "confused shapes" that it is, to the contrary, supposed to organize? No, because, in my opinion, art possesses an essential function at the societal level. It plays a part in the production of *relevant* (Sperber and Wilson, 1989) forms that respond to the virtual (but nevertheless real) landscape of human societies' "subjective expectations" and because of this it contributes to the *religere,* "careful reflection," of individuals in the social group.

Louise Bourgeois (1995) writes that the sculpture *Silent Black Woman* (*Silencieuse femme noire*) represents the protest marches of the 1960s. And she continues: "There are many types of tensions, but the one I am trying to resolve, to soothe, is social tension." Here, we approach the "noble ideas" *(belles idées)* of the *exemplum* that Nicolas Poussin invites us to illustrate by our own actions. The work of art, through its capacity to awaken and make aware, thus allows one to pass on an ethical message. And in spite of this, one may wonder why dreaded human blindness, which caused the deaths of the Children of Bethel, as Laurent de la Hire has shown us, still prevails over our planet? Does not the irresponsibility of certain scientists who, with "professional conscience," reiterate in horror—even with good intentions—the tragedy of the Children of Bethel, deserve to be unmasked under any circumstances? Cannot art—news photography, for example—cry out loudly enough to prevent humanity from such straying off the right path of science?

I began this chapter with the image of a fortune-telling tortoise shell from the Shang Dynasty, emphasizing how humans, in the beginning of civilization, projected meaning onto that which had none. With the assets of universal scientific knowledge, human beings should make a commitment to use the creative faculties they possess in their brains to give meaning to that which calls out for it the most: humanity itself. It is our responsibility to urgently invent an "ethical model," which breaks with the violence, the intolerance, the crimes of our cultural past, and ensures more efficiently survival and well-being for all human lives.

References

Alberti, L. B. 1970 [1435]. *On painting (Della pittura)*. Translated with introduction and notes by John R. Spencer. New Haven: Yale University Press.

Boulez, P. 1971. *Boulez on music today (Penser la musique aujourd'hui)*. London: Faber.

Bourgeois, L. 1995. *Catalogue d'exposition*. Paris: Musée d'art moderne de la ville de Paris.

Changeux, J.-P. 1983. *L'homme neuronal*. Paris: Fayard.

——— 1994. *Raison et plaisir*. Paris: Odile Jacob.

Changeux, J.-P., and Connes, A. 1989. *Matière a pensée*. Paris: Odile Jacob.

Changeux, J.-P., and Danchin, A. 1976. The selective stabilization of developing synapses: A plausible mechanism for the specification of neuronal networks. *Nature, 264,* 705–712.

Changeux, J.-P., and Dehaene, S. 1989. Neuronal models of cognitive functions. *Cognition, 33,* 63–109.

Changeux, J.-P., and Chavaillon, J., eds. 1995. *Origins of the human brain*. Oxford: Clarendon.

Creager, A. N. H., and Gaudillière, J.-P. 1996. Meanings in search of experiments and vice-versa: The invention of "allosteric regulation" in Paris and Berkeley (1959–1967). *Historical Studies in the Physical and Biological Sciences, 27 (1),* 1–89.

Damasio, A. 1995. *L'erreur de Descartes*. Paris: Odile Jacob.

Debru, C. 1983. *L'esprit des proteines*. Paris: Hermann.

Dretske, F. 1995. *Naturalizing the mind*. Cambridge: MIT Press.

Droulez, J., and Berthoz, A. 1988. Servo-controlled conservative versus topological (projective) modes of sensory motor control. In *Disorders of posture and gait,* ed. W. Bles and T. Brandt, 83–97. Amsterdam: Elsevier.

Edelman, G. 1992. *Biologie de la conscience*. Paris: Odile Jacob.

Fellemann, D., and Van Essen, D. 1991. Distributed hierarchical processing in primate visual cortex. *Cerebral Cortex, 1,* 1–47.

Franck, M. 1995. *Collège de France: Figures et travaux*. Paris: Imprimerie nationale.

Furster, J. 1980. *The prefrontal cortex*. New York: Raven Press.

Georgopoulos, A., Taira, M., and Lukashin, A. 1993. Cognitive neurophysiology of the motor cortex. *Science, 260, 47–51*.

Grésillon, A. 1992. Ralentir travaux. *Genesis, 1, 9–31*.

Hebb, D. 1949. *The organization of behavior*. New York: Wiley.

Lawrence, P. 1992. *The making of a fly*. Oxford: Blackwell.

Le Bihan, D., Turner, R., Zeffiro, T., Cuénod, C., Jezzard, P., and Bonnerot, V. 1993. Activation of human primary visual cortex during visual recall: A magnetic resonance imaging study. *Proc. Natl. Acad. Sci. (USA), 90,* 11802–11805.

MacAdams, S., and Bigand, E., eds. 1994. *Penser les sons*. Paris: PUF.

Mazoyer, B. M., Tzourio, N., Frak, V., Syrota, A., Murayama, N., Levrier, O., Salomon, G., Dehaene, S., Cohen, L., and Mehler, J. 1993. The cortical representations of speech. *J. Cognitive Neurosci., 5,* 467–469.

Miyashita, Y., and Chang, H. 1988. Neuronal correlate of pictorial short-term memory in the primate temporal cortex. *Nature, 331,* 68–70.

Moller, A. P. 1992. Female swallow preference for symmetrical male sexual ornaments. *Nature, 357,* 238–240.

Monod, J. 1970. *Le hasard et le nécessité.* Paris: Editions due Seuil.

Movshon, J. A., and Blakemore, C. 1974. Functional reinnervation in kitten visual cortex. *Nature, 251,* 504–505.

Perrett, D., May, K., and Yoshikawa, S. 1994. Facial shape and judgements of female attractiveness. *Nature, 368,* 239–242.

Perrett, D., and Oram, M. W. 1993. Neurophysiology of shape processing. *Image and Vision Computing, 11,* 317–330.

Perrett, D., Rolls, E. T., and Caan, N. 1982. Neurons responsive to faces in the monkey temporal cortex. *Experimental Brain Res., 47,* 329–342.

Peterhans, E., and Von der Heydt, R. 1989. Subjective contours: Bridging the gap between psychophysics and physiology. *Trends in Neuroscience, 14,* 112–118.

Posner, M., and Raichle, M. 1994. *Images of mind.* New York: Scientific American Library.

Pusher, M. 1993. Seeing the mind. *Science, 262,* 673–674.

Schwartz, A. 1994. Direct cortical representations of drawing. *Science, 265,* 540–542.

Seckel, H. 1988. *Les demoiselles d'Avignon.* Catalogue d'exposition. Paris: Réunion des musées nationaux.

Sereno, M., Dale, A., Peppas, T., Kwong, K., Belliveau, J., Brady, T., Rosen, B., and Tootel, R. 1995. Borders of multiple visual areas in humans revealed by functional magnetic resonance imaging. *Science, 268,* 889–893.

Sperber, D., and Wilson, D. 1989. *La pertinence.* Paris: Editions de Minuit.

Trehub, S., and Trainor, L. 1994. Les stratégies d'écoute chez le bébé: Origines du développement de la musique et de la parole. In *Penser les sons,* ed. S. MacAdams and E. Bigand. Paris: PUF.

Wiesel, T. N., and Hubel, O. H. 1965. Comparison of the effects of unilateral and bilateral eye closure on cortical unit responses in kittens. *J. Neurophysiol., 28,* 1029–1040.

Zeki, S. 1993. *A vision of the brain.* Oxford: Blackwell.

Discussion: Section 6

STANISLAS DEHAENE: I would like to make a comment about [Nigel] Holmes's paper. I enjoyed it because it reminds us of how much our brains fill in when we see a picture. A lot of what we see is actually provided by the brain, not by the stimulus. In the earlier sections there was very much a dichotomy between either picture processing, which was bottom-up, or imagery which was pure top-down in the absence, in most cases, of any external stimulus. I think the real challenge for us in the brain sciences is to understand as we see a picture, the interplay of both bottom-up and top-down, which must be going on as you are showing, very nicely.

NIGEL HOLMES: I'm always reminded of the sculptor Henry Moore's comment that he would never read any critique of his work, because he might find out what he was doing. And I'm not quite like that, and I'm not Henry Moore. But that's nice, thank you.

STEPHEN KOSSLYN: In your very first demonstration with the scissors, you cannot see where your hand is. Do we know where our hands are when we're not looking at them? If not, then your findings are not as surprising as they at first seem. Do we, Marc?

MARC JEANNEROD: In fact, we performed a small experiment where we asked people to draw lines. We used a device that allowed them to see themselves drawing a line in one direction, but in fact, they were drawing it in another direction. And then we asked them, on each trial, to tell us, by using a chart, in which orientation they saw their hand move. And they always said what they saw, and not what they properly felt. So apparently we are very much bound to what we see and not to what we do.

HOLMES: And that is borne out by people of my generation who grew up drawing and now use a computer to draw—where we are drawing down here and what appears is up there. And we're not thinking about the marks we make here, we are looking at the marks that are made, that are left on the screen. And I thought that this would be a very difficult thing to do, but it wasn't.

MARK WEXLER: I have some data that show that there is systematic distortion of your imagined position of your hand when you can't see it. In fact, you always tend to anticipate a little bit the position of your hand.

FROM THE FLOOR: Zaltman, I may be the only one in the room who needs it, but could I just ask for some clarification? Is this enterprise an exploration of mind? Is it some form of therapy? Or what?

GERALD ZALTMAN: In this case, a pharmaceutical company was considering one of its products that related to cholesterol, and they wanted to have a better understanding of how people thought about the management of their cholesterol. Thus we used a variety of "therapeutic techniques" to elicit a rich set of feelings about that process that are commonly shared by a large number of people. This information in turn leads to some very practical guidelines, since mental models influence how we respond to the treatment and how we think about the illness as well as what we do about it.

ANNE HARRINGTON: Jerry, I wanted to pick up on the idea of tacit knowledge that you started with and ask you whether you think, and it's sort of an attractive idea, that in some ways metaphors are a particularly effective means whereby we translate what used to be unconscious or tacit knowledge into some kind of consciously accessible form? So in that sense, we almost have a sense of discovery when we hear, see what metaphors emerge in the course of talking. And this resonates with psychoanalytical thinking and things like that.

ZALTMAN: Yes, I think metaphors are very powerful for bringing tacit knowledge to a level of explicit awareness. And part of the power of metaphor and other figurative speech is not simply what they reveal but what they also hide. And so by pursuing a particular metaphor and trying to find out what it may also be hiding, you're able to get at yet other kinds of knowledge we're not aware of having. And I think that's quite important.

KOSSLYN: Jean-Pierre [Changeux], I found your evolutionary ideas very stimulating, and wondered if you could expand a bit on them. In particular, you sometimes talk about evolution in Lamarckian terms, which is rather out of favor in the United States.

JEAN-PIERRE CHANGEUX: Very distinguished scientists have said that evolution is following a Lamarckist kind of trend, which means that in fact that there would be direct imprinting by cultural objects into the human brain. In fact, there are two levels of selection. The first one is of course for the long-term memory, and the second is in the utilization of memory, I would say the retrieval mechanism. First of all in the storage of memory, there is drastic selection that may involve the system of emotion, for instance. And we know from very old studies on retrieval, that there is a recombination or reconstruction of memories. This simply means that we do not store things passively. And we don't reproduce memories passively, either. This view also was developed by Richard Dawkins in his concept of memes, "idea units," which he compared to viruses that infect a population of brains.

STEPHEN JAY GOULD: The only obvious thing to say is that, from a strictly Darwinian point of view, there is no objection whatsoever to invoking Lamarckian metaphors with respect to what happens in the lifetime of an individual, where I assume that things that get encoded and not just read out randomly, as in a pure Darwinian system, I don't like Dawkins's concept of memes for another reason, but there's no objection to it in the sense that human cultural change of course is Lamarckian, because whatever we achieve in our lifetime culturally we can pass on to future generations. The only objection a Darwinian has, and I don't think Jean-Pierre is making such a suggestion, would be to argue that in some way that material during someone's lifetime can get into the hereditary system and be passed in a directional or adaptive way to offspring. That's the only sense in which a Darwinian objects to Lamarckian exploits, but that's not being suggested here. That cultural evolution is Lamarckian is indeed fine. That's why it's rapid and directional compared with biological change; there are directional aspects of an individual psyche through the lifetime, which are analogous to Lamarckian processes.

CHANGEUX: They are not Lamarckian in the sense that it's not a direct imprint of things that are taking place. But that there are combinatorial-plus-selection mechanisms, of course, has nothing to do with your genes; all this is epigenetic. I also want to say that it's difficult to imagine a pure constructivist scheme not only for learning, but also for cultural evolution, of the sort that is now becoming popular and based mostly on a kind of Lamarckian view. I think that this kind of scheme is really too soft, because there are clearly constraints, developmental constraints first of all, that apply to learning processes in the child and also constraints for communication. And also for having some kind of signal entering the brain and being stored. In fact, you cannot have a child at any age store any kind of information. Every developmental scientist knows that there is a sensitive period where a given sort of information can get into the brain.

GOULD: A pure Lamarckian scheme couldn't possibly work; it would give you directionality without constraint. What you're saying is that you have two checks upon it in an individual's lifetime. One is the constraint of how the brain works and what you can't read out or in. And second, there probably is a genuinely metaphorically Darwinian component of purely selected-out random inputs.

CHANGEUX: And I think there is also one other aspect, which is that the whole thing is top-down. You may have a pre-organization of representations, and then depending on the fitness, I shouldn't use the word, of the combination with the goal, a given representation is then selected. So that's also another way of looking at it.

BARBARA GROSZ: I would like to take a step back. It strikes me that there were three themes that might tie back to verbal language. So let me say briefly what they are, especially in the first two papers. The first talk was entitled "The Gap between Seeing and Drawing," but there was also mention of how people perceived what you saw. And then in the second talk, I heard several mentions of the underlying purpose of communication to the viewer of the drawing. It wasn't just a natural scene out there, but rather the artist produced something—which I think is reminiscent of producing language for people. So I sensed that intention was a theme running through these tasks—and by contrast was explicitly not a major influence on the approach taken in the third, at least not conscious intention. Finally, in the last talk, it is clear that the artist's intentions have a major role in what he or she paints. So I wondered what the artists thought about intention and how that might play a role?

The second theme came to mind as Rhonda [Shearer] showed the pictures of fractals; I wondered whether you would say that there was some visual correlate of rhythm or tune, which we heard about yesterday as something special in language, when Jacques Mehler talked about rhythm distinguishing between languages. And I wondered if there were visual analogues to such auditory phenomena?

And the third theme that struck me was the role of context, particularly social context, which Catherine Snow brought up yesterday and I thought Marc Jeannerod brought up with respect to motion.

RHONDA SHEARER: Let me begin by addressing your point about rhythm. I do feel that when it gets down to it, you're talking about pattern and noise and proportions. And I think as we do more and more brain-imaging research we'll see that these relationships between modalities are operating in the same kind of part-whole hierarchical relationship. When I'm doing my own art, in one sense you could say that my work has some aspects of theater or books, because there is text—but it is nonlinear text, in terms of the sequencing. But I think that from the point of view of drawing, there is something like rhythm.

HOLMES: I'm not sure about the rhythm aspect, but I'm certainly trying to communicate when I make drawings. One of the problems, as you know, as a presenter when you only have a short time, is that you can only focus on a very tiny thing. The ultimate point of what I'm doing is indeed to communicate with somebody else, but in a simple way. And if you look at things and break them down into little bits and pieces you can come up with a drawing that communicates what the thing is or what the idea is. And in fact at lunch I confessed to Jerry that I feel like I'm the person in Tiananmen Square with this huge tank coming toward me, and you, the members of the audience, are the tank. And he confessed that he had almost the same feeling. In order to remind me of his remark, I drew a little picture of that. But I didn't draw the picture that everybody knows, which is a three-dimensional picture coming toward you. I drew a profile of the tank and a little person in front of it. Because that communicates that idea to me more.

GOULD: I thought it might be worth exploring the idea that just because we come to a geometric view rather late—it's not [truly] late (because who knows what the future is), but late in our known history so far—[this] probably bears very little relationship to some hard-to-define almost Platonic concept of importance in the actual world. Here we are, the end result of one paltry little evolutionary lineage with our modalities as we find them. I suspect the universe is just full of so many ways to know that we have no access to. And that's what is so fascinating about this brain research, that if we ever figure out this poor little contingently built brain of ours, with its limited modes of seeing the world, we might have an idea of where we get some sense. I suspect that most of the reason why we have no knowledge or sense of how to formulate interesting questions about eternity and the age of the universe and related things, is that we're just not built to do it. And I think we mustn't fall into the habit of thinking that because it might be difficult to think about fractals, therefore they may be unimportant in the universe. Probably the only reason we came to them late is we're not very good at it. It just makes me think, I know this is unanswerable, what else might be out there that we can't access at all? My other two comments, to Holmes, is use a camera lucida. And to Zaltman, Oh my God, I hope that woman has no problem more serious than high cholesterol in her life. God forbid.

KOSSLYN: The papers in this section were all focused on external representations. And the theme of the meeting is languages of the brain, which focuses on things internal. I'm wondering about your thoughts about the role of the external world as supporting representations that are used internally. I am curious what the speakers have to say about what we can learn about languages of the brain from studying these modes of manipulating the external world to represent and communicate?

SHEARER: Since the nineteenth century, or even before, when art historians started writing about landscapes and still lifes, landscapes were considered unimportant or inferior—because it's nature and not allegorical. And there were actual hierarchies created. For example, flower paintings were something for women to paint, not for men. The men would do the heroic sculptures and allegorical paintings. We tend to believe our categories, because even when we set up a categorization scheme to describe reality, we're looking through that category scheme. It's not reality. And so when you shift that category scheme you have another reality; we must be conscious that our belief systems aren't objectively real. Our measurements are approximate and our belief systems are constructed. And if we're married to them in any kind of fixed way, then we're trapped. This reminds me of what poor Bruno, who was burned at the stake, said: that images or symbols are simultaneously vehicles and chains, they are both. And I think that that's, for me, the most important part of what I'm doing. I'm trying to be conscious of the difference. And be able to capitalize on that plastic aspect.

ZALTMAN: I am wondering whether there is a false dichotomy here, between the internal versus the external. I don't think that the mind is the possession of the individual. Although I think that the mental models we have are indicative of some kind of pattern of neural activity, for us to understand that pattern of activity, we need to have various cues, various devices to have someone articulate, in one way or the other, what those patterns are, what those mental models are. That often relies on external cues that have social meaning, that give context to what we have, hold privately, seemingly privately in our minds. So in fact, to talk about what's in here, languages in here versus languages out there, is an invention that may sometimes be helpful for us. But I think a bit misleading.

SHEARER: And I think our bias toward Euclidean geometry is a fantastic example. Because if you look in the world, where are straight lines? They're certainly the exception and not the rule. Our brains evolved in a fractal environment, and yet we prefer straight lines. By importing such a geometric category to our conceptual space, we end up using simple dichotomies (parts of space divided by a straight line) to organize our beliefs and our realities. There may be something about the organization of our brains that leads us to adopt certain geometrical ideas when organizing the world and our thoughts. For example, I think of Richard Gregory's story of a man blind from birth, who later gains sight. And apparently after five years of being sighted, he ended up sitting in a dark room both day and night because the irregularities of the natural world were so appalling to him. Paint peeling would drive him crazy. He had a Platonic perfection in his head of what the world was like. And he was terribly disappointed. This tells us something about how his brain worked and how he would project on the world a more fixed state than other people.

HOLMES: I think I agree with you, but I would think of this in terms of some kind of common language that you have to tap into in order to communicate. So there is an external, the external language, you have to believe is in other people, otherwise you're not going to communicate it. I make my living from explaining things to people. If I don't explain it, I don't get hired again. So if I get it wrong, then that is bad. So, it stands or falls each time I deliver a job. You are ringing the bell of recognition in somebody else whenever you say something. Do you understand it or don't you understand it—and that's true of language and visuals.

CATHERINE SNOW: Nigel's comment brings up a dimension that has been notably missing in this section, namely that all of these images and utilizations of communication systems presuppose learning and development. I would like to note that one direct way to understand their organization is to observe them emerging over age, and also observe the conditions under which they don't emerge predictably. This is a perspective that shouldn't be ignored.

Contributors

Nathaniel M. Alpert, Ph.D., Division of Nuclear Medicine, Massachusetts General Hospital, Boston, Mass.

Nalini Ambady, Ph.D., Department of Psychology, Harvard University, Cambridge, Mass.

Alain Berthoz, Ph.D., Laboratoire de Physiologie de la Perception et de l'Action, Collège de France, Paris, France.

David Caplan, M.D., Ph.D., Department of Neurology, Massachusetts General Hospital, Boston, Mass.

Alfonso Caramazza, Ph.D., Department of Psychology, Harvard University, Cambridge, Mass.

Jean-Pierre Changeux, Ph.D., Institut Pasteur, Paris, France.

Yves Christen, Ph.D., IPSEN Foundation.

Stanislas Dehaene, Ph.D., Department of Research in Imaging, Pharmacology, and Physiology, Service Hospitalier Frédéric Joliot, Atomic Energy Commission, Institut National de la Santé et de la Recherche Médicale, Orsay, France

Jean-François Démonet, M.D., Ph.D., Institut National de la Santé et de la Recherche Médicale, Hopital Purpan, Toulouse, France.

Michel Denis, Ph.D., Groupe Cognition Humaine, Centre National de la Recherche Scientifique, Université de Paris-Sud, Orsay, France.

Michiko Dohi, M.D., Department of Radiology, Jikei University, Tokyo, Japan.

Albert M. Galaburda, M.D., Division of Behavioral Neurology, Beth Israel Deaconess Medical Center, Boston, Mass.

Barbara J. Grosz, Ph.D., Division of Applied Science, Harvard University, Cambridge, Mass.

Mark Hallahan, Ph.D., Psychology Department, College of the Holy Cross, Worcester, Mass.

Nigel Holmes, Westport, Conn.

Pierre Jacob, Ph.D., Institut Jean Nicod, Centre National de la Recherche Scientifique, Paris, France.

Marc Jeannerod, Ph.D., Institut des Sciences Cognitives, Centre National de la Recherche Scientifique, Bron, France.

Isabelle Klein, M.D., Ph.D., Department of Research in Imaging, Pharmacology, and Physiology, Service Hospitalier Frédéric Joliot, Atomic Energy Commission, Institut National de la Santé et de la Recherche Médicale, Orsay, France.

Stephen M. Kosslyn, Ph.D., Department of Psychology, Harvard University, Cambridge, Mass.

Simon Lambrey, Laboratoire de Physiologie de la Perception et de l'Action, Collège de France, Paris, France.

Denis Le Bihan, M.D., Ph.D., Department of Research in Imaging, Pharmacology, and Physiology, Service Hospitalier Frédéric Joliot, Atomic Energy Commission, Institut National de la Santé et de la Recherche Médicale, Orsay, France.

Bernard Mazoyer, M.D., Groupe d'Imagerie Neurofonctionnelle, GIP Cyceron, University of Caen, Caen, France.

Jacques Mehler, Ph.D., Laboratoire de Sciences Cognitives et Psycholinguistique, Centre National de la Recherche Scientifique, Paris, France.

Emmanuel Mellet, M.D., Groupe d'Imagerie Neurofonctionnelle, GIP Cyceron, University of Caen, Caen, France.

Franck Ramus, Ph.D., Institute of Cognitive Neuroscience, University College London, London, United Kingdom.

François Recanati, Ph.D., Institut Jean Nicod, Centre National de la Recherche Scientifique, Paris, France.

Rhonda Roland Shearer, Turbo, Inc., New York, N.Y.

Catherine E. Snow, Ph.D., Harvard Graduate School of Education, Cambridge, Mass.

Elizabeth S. Spelke, Ph.D., Department of Psychology, Harvard University, Cambridge, Mass.

Guillaume Thierry, Ph.D., Institut National de la Santé et de la Recherche Médicale, Hôpital Purpan, Toulouse, France.

Nathalie Tzourio, M.D., Groupe d'Imagerie Neurofonctionnelle, GIP Cyceron, University of Caen, Caen, France.

Isabelle Viaud-Delmon, Ph.D., Laboratoire de Physiologie de la Perception et de l'Action, Collège de France, Paris, France.

Gloria Waters, Ph.D., Massachusetts General Hospital, Boston, Mass.

Gerald Zaltman, Ph.D., Harvard Business School, Boston, Mass.

Edgar Zurif, Ph.D., Department of Psychology, Brandeis University, Waltham, Mass.

Index